Official Journal of the

EAU
European Association of Urology

EORTC
European Organization for Research and Treatment of Cancer – Genito-Urinary Group

ESUOE
European Society for Urological Oncology and Endocrinology

European Urology

KARGER

Printed in Switzerland on acid-free paper by Druckerei Schüler AG, Biel

Appears monthly: 2 volumes per year (12 issues)

Guidelines for Authors

European Urology

Submission

Only original papers written in English are considered and should be sent to:

Prof. C.C. Schulman
S. Karger AG
Editorial Office European Urology
P.O. Box
CH–4009 Basel (Switzerland)
Telephone +41 61 306 1358
Fax +41 61 306 1434
E-mail b.brogli@karger.ch

Mailing address for courier deliveries only:

Allschwilerstr. 10
CH–4055 Basel (Switzerland)

Manuscripts should be submitted in triplicate (with three sets of illustrations of which one is an original), typewritten double-spaced on one side of the paper, with a wide margin.

Conditions

All manuscripts are subject to editorial review. Manuscripts are received with the explicit understanding that they are not under simultaneous consideration by any other publication. Submission of an article for publication implies the transfer of the copyright from the author to the publisher upon acceptance. Accepted papers become the permanent property of 'European Urology' and may not be reproduced by any means, in whole or in part, without the written consent of the publisher. It is the author's responsibility to obtain permission to reproduce illustrations, tables, etc. from other publications.

Arrangement

Title page: The first page of each paper should indicate the title (main title underlined), the authors' names, and the institute where the work was conducted. A short title for use as running head as well as the full address of the author to whom correspondence should be sent are also required.

Full address: The exact postal address complete with postal code must be given at the bottom of the title page. Please also supply phone and fax numbers, as well as your e-mail address.

Key words: For indexing purposes, a list of 3–10 key words in English is essential.

Abstract: Each paper needs an abstract of up to 16 lines structured with subheadings as follows: Objective(s), Methods, Results, Conclusion(s).

Small type: Paragraphs which can or must be set in smaller type (case histories, test methods, etc.) should be indicated with a 'p' (petit) in the margin on the left-hand side.

Footnotes: Avoid footnotes. When essential, they are numbered consecutively and typed at the foot of the appropriate page.

Tables and illustrations: Tables and illustrations (both numbered in Arabic numerals) should be prepared on separate sheets. Tables require a heading and figures a legend, also prepared on a separate sheet. For the reproduction of illustrations, only good drawings and original photographs can be accepted; negatives or photocopies cannot be used. Due to technical reasons, figures with a screen background should not be submitted. When possible, group several illustrations on one block for reproduction (max. size 181 × 223 mm) or provide crop marks. On the back of each illustration, indicate its number, the author's name, and 'top' with a soft pencil.

Color illustrations: Up to 6 color illustrations per page can be integrated with the text at the reduced price of CHF 660.– / USD 545.00 per page. Color illustrations are reproduced at the author's expense.

References: In the text identify references by Arabic numerals [in square brackets]. Material submitted for publication but not yet accepted should be noted as 'unpublished data' and not be included in the reference list. The list of references should include only those publications which are cited in the text. Do not alphabetize; number references in the order in which they are first mentioned in the text. The surnames of the authors followed by initials should be given. There should be no punctuation other than a comma to separate the authors. Cite all authors, 'et al' is not sufficient. Abbreviate journal names according to the Index Medicus system. (Also see International Committee of Medical Journal Editors: Uniform requirements for manuscripts submitted to biomedical journals. Br Med J 1988;296:401–405.)

Examples
(a) Papers published in periodicals: Sun J, Koto H, Chung KF: Interaction of ozone and allergen challenges on bronchial responsiveness and inflammation in sensitised guinea pigs. Int Arch Allergy Immunol 1997;112:191–195.
(b) Monographs: Matthews DE, Farewell VT: Using and Understanding Medical Statistics, ed 3, revised. Basel, Karger, 1996.
(c) Edited books: Parren PWHI, Burton DR: Antibodies against HIV-1 from phage display libraries: Mapping of an immune response and progress towards antiviral immunotherapy; in Capra JD (ed): Antibody Engineering. Chem Immunol. Basel, Karger, 1997, vol 65, pp 18–56.

Rapid Communication: Manuscripts intended for rapid communication must present new findings of sufficient importance to justify their accelerated acceptance. They should follow the general arrangement of research papers with the exception that no abstract or introduction are required. The first paragraph should include the reason for the study and the main findings. They should not exceed 8 double-spaced manuscript pages in length, including figures, tables and references. Proofs are checked by the Main Editor and not sent to the author. Review will be rapid, and once accepted, the paper will be included in the next planned issue.

Galley proofs

Unless indicated otherwise, galley proofs are sent to the first-named author and should be returned with the least possible delay. Alterations made in galley proofs, other than the correction of printer's errors, are charged to the author. No page proofs are supplied.

Reprints

Order forms and a price list are sent with the galley proofs. Orders submitted after the issue is printed are subject to considerably higher prices.

KARGER

Fax +41 61 306 12 34
E-Mail karger@karger.ch
www.karger.com

The Guidelines for Authors are available at:
www.karger.com/journals/eur/eur_gl.htm

European Urology

General Information

Publication data: 'European Urology' is published 12 times a year. Volumes 35–36 with 6 issues each appear in 1999.

Subscription rates: Subscriptions run for a full calendar year. Prices are given per volume.

Personal subscription:
Subscription + postage and handling
CHF 339.50 + CHF 23.50 Europe
CHF 339.50 + CHF 35.50 Overseas
USD 259.50 + USD 23.50
(Must be in the name of, billed to, and paid by an individual. Order must be marked 'personal subscription'.)

Institutional subscription:
Subscription + postage and handling
CHF 679.– + CHF 29.40 Europe
CHF 679.– + CHF 44.40 Overseas
USD 519.00 + USD 29.40

Airmail postage: CHF 36.–, USD 30.00.
(Extra per volume.)

Discount subscription prices:
European Association of Urology
European Organization for Research and Treatment of Cancer – Genito-Urinary Group
European Society for Urological Oncology and Endocrinology

Microforms: Please direct all enquiries and orders to: University Microfilms Inc.
300 North Zeeb Road, P.O. Box 1346
Ann Arbor, MI 48106-1346 (USA)

Subscription orders: Orders can be placed at agencies, bookstores, directly with the Publisher
S. Karger AG, P.O. Box,
CH–4009 Basel (Switzerland)
or with any of the following distributors:
Deutschland: S. Karger GmbH, Postfach
D–79095 Freiburg
France: Librairie Luginbühl
36, bd de Latour-Maubourg, F–75007 Paris
Great Britain, Ireland: S. Karger Publishers
58 Grove Hill Road
Tunbridge Wells, Kent TN1 1SP
USA: S. Karger Publishers, Inc.
26 West Avon Road, P.O. Box 529
Farmington, CT 06085
India, Bangladesh, Sri Lanka:
S. Karger India Subscription Agency
B–5/132 Safdarjung Enclave
New Delhi-110029
Japan: Katakura Libri, Inc.
2F, Marushima Bldg, 4-6-17, Yushima,
Bunkyo-ku, Tokyo 113-0034

Change of address: Both old and new address should be sent to the subscription source.

Single issues and back volumes: Information can be obtained through the Publisher.

Advertising: Correspondence and rate requests should be addressed to the Publisher.

Bibliographic indices: This journal is regularly listed in bibliographic services, including *Current Contents®*.

Copying: This journal has been registered with the Copyright Clearance Center (CCC), as indicated by the code appearing on the first page of each article.
For readers in the US, this code signals consent for copying of articles for personal or internal use, or for the personal or internal use of specific clients, provided that the stated fee is paid per copy directly to
Copyright Clearance Center Inc.
222 Rosewood Drive
Danvers, MA 01923 (USA)
A copy of the first page of the article must accompany payment. Consent does not extend to copying for general distribution, for promotion, for creating new works, or for resale. In these cases, specific written permission must be obtained from the copyright owner,
S. Karger AG,
P.O. Box, CH–4009 Basel (Switzerland).

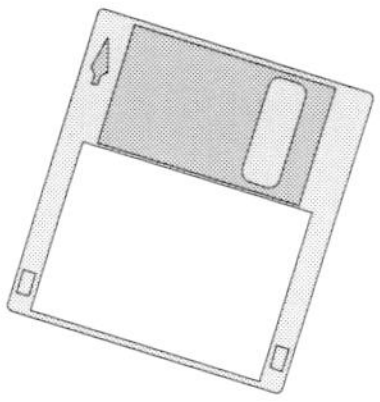

Disk Submission

A **comprehensive version** of these guidelines for the **submission of manuscripts and illustrations on disk** can be accessed online under **www.karger.com/journals/disksub.htm** or requested as a leaflet from the editorial department.

Please follow the general rules on style and arrangement in the **"Guidelines for Authors"** of the journal. Submit a **double-spaced printout** of your manuscript matching the file on disk exactly.

Technical Information

Store only data pertinent to this manuscript. Include your fonts (screen and printer fonts for Macintosh).
For a **text only** manuscript, use a 3.5 inch disk. For **text and illustrations,** use 3.5 or 5.25 Magneto Optical Disc; CD-ROM (DOS or hybrid); iomage Zip/DOS (100 MB), or 44 MB, 88 MB or 200 MB SyQuest. Compress extensive data using ZIP format.

Data Description

Label your disk with the **title of the journal or book** for which it is submitted; a **short version** of the paper's title; your **name,** postal and e-mail address, fax and phone number; **hard and software** used, including the version; and the **complete list of the file names.** File names consist of eight characters before the dot identifying the file and three characters after the dot identifying the application.

Text and Format

The **preferred word-processing package is MS-Word.** Other commonly used PC text programs and ASCII formats are accepted.
Update your data when you revise subsequent to the reviewer's or editor's decision and mark revisions clearly. Manuscripts accepted for publication are subject to **copy editing:** changes and/or questions will be marked in the manuscript, which will be returned to you with your disk and the galley proofs for checking.
Enter your text continuously flush left. Do not use any layout functions. Do not split words at the end of a line. **Do not use indentations.** Use a blank line before and a hard return at the end of paragraphs. **Arrange headings flush left.** Insert only **one space after punctuation marks.** Insert Greek letters, mathematical symbols etc. with your word-processing program. Use **boldface and italics** as well as sub- and superscript where appropriate.
Tables are part of the text and should be placed at the end of the text file. Separate the individual parts of a table by lines. Use the tabulator instead of spaces. Format operation data on one line in the same column. **Legends to illustrations are part of the text** and should also be listed at the end of the text file.

Illustrations

Store illustrations as separate files: do not embed them in your text. Export **line drawings/vector graphics** as TIF, EPS or WMF format. Use Photoshop for processing and retouching **scanned halftone images.** Save the original scan and the processed version. Export **black and white or color images** as TIF or EPS format in their anticipated size in print.
For detailed information on how to submit illustration data on disk please consult the leaflet or **www.karger.com/journals/disksub.htm.**

KARGER

Fax + 41 61 306 12 34
E-Mail karger@karger.ch
www.karger.com

The Journal Home Page is available at:
www.karger.com/journals/eur

KI 98 DISK

European
Urology

Strategies for the Chemoprevention of Prostate Cancer

Symposium, October 29–31, 1998, Brussels, Belgium

Editors
C.C. Schulman, Brussels, Belgium
G.J. Kelloff, Bethesda, Md., USA

61 figures, 21 in color and 61 tables, 1999

KARGER
Basel · Freiburg · Paris · London · New York ·
New Delhi · Bangkok · Singapore · Tokyo · Sydney

S. Karger
Medical and Scientific Publishers
Basel · Freiburg · Paris · London
New York · New Delhi · Bangkok
Singapore · Tokyo · Sydney

Drug Dosage
The authors and the publisher have exerted every effort to ensure that drug selection and dosage set forth in this text are in accord with current recommendations and practice at the time of publication. However, in view of ongoing research, changes in government regulations, and the constant flow of information relating to drug therapy and drug reactions, the reader is urged to check the package insert for each drug for any change in indications and dosage and for added warnings and precautions. This is particularly important when the recommended agent is a new and/or infrequently employed drug.

Printed in Switzerland on acid-free paper by
Druckerei Schüler AG, Biel

KARGER

Fax+ 41 61 306 12 34
E-Mail karger@karger.ch
www.karger.com

European Urology

Contents Vol. 35, No. 5–6, 1999

341 **Introduction**
Schulman, C.C. (Brussels); Kelloff, G.J. (Bethesda, Md.)

342 **Chemoprevention of Prostate Cancer: Concepts and Strategies**
Kelloff, G.J.; Lieberman, R.; Steele, V.E.; Boone, C.W.; Lubet, R.A.; Kopelovitch, L.; Malone, W.A.; Crowell, J.A. (Bethesda, Md.); Sigman, C.C. (Mountain View, Calif.)

Genetic and Environmental Factors in Prostate Cancer Genesis

351 **Molecular Biology of Progression of Prostate Cancer**
Nupponen, N.; Visakorpi, T. (Tampere)

355 **Androgen Metabolism and Prostate Cancer: Establishing a Model of Genetic Susceptibility**
Ross, R.K.; Coetzee, G.A.; Pearce, C.L.; Reichardt, J.K.V.; Bretsky, P. (Los Angeles, Calif.); Kolonel, L.N. (Honolulu, Hawaii); Henderson, B.E. (Los Angeles, Calif.); Lander, E.; Altshuler, D.; Daley, G. (Boston, Mass.)

362 **Genetic and Environmental Factors in Prostate Cancer Genesis: Identifying High-Risk Cohorts**
Ekman, P. (Stockholm)

370 **Epidemiology of Prostate Cancer Chemoprevention**
Boyle, P.; Severi, G. (Milan)

377 **Diet and Its Preventive Role in Prostatic Disease**
Denis, L. (Antwerp); Morton, M.S.; Griffiths, K. (Cardiff)

388 **Dietary Fat and Prostate Cancer Progression and Survival**
Fradet, Y.; Meyer, F.; Bairati, I.; Shadmani, R.; Moore, L. (Québec)

Molecular Targets for Chemoprevention of Prostate Cancer

392 **Vitamin D and Prostate Cancer Risk**
Peehl, D.M. (Stanford, Calif.)

395 **Lipoxygenase Inhibition in Prostate Cancer**
Myers, C.E.; Ghosh, J. (Charlottesville, Va.)

399 **Angiogenesis, p53, *bcl-2* and Ki-67 in the Progression of Prostate Cancer after Radical Prostatectomy**
Moul, J.W. (Washington, D.C./Bethesda, Md.)

408 **Changes in Gene Expression and Targets for Therapy**
Bussemakers, M.J.G. (Nijmegen)

413 **Mechanism of Androgen Receptor Activation and Possible Implications for Chemoprevention Trials**
Klocker, H.; Culig, Z.; Eder, I.E.; Nessler-Menardi, C.; Hobisch, A.; Putz, T.; Bartsch, G. (Innsbruck); Peterziel, H.; Cato, A.C.B. (Karlsruhe)

420 **New Agents for Chemoprevention of Prostate Cancer**
Sporn, M.B. (Hanover, N.H.)

424 **Retinoids in Chemoprevention**
Whelan, P. (Leeds)

429 **Evaluation of Biomarker Modulation by Fenretinide in Prostate Cancer Patients**
Urban, D.; Myers, R.; Manne, U.; Weiss, H. (Birmingham, Ala.); Mohler, J. (Chapel Hill, N.C.); Perkins, D.; Markiewicz, M. (Birmingham, Ala.); Lieberman, R.; Kelloff, G. (Bethesda, Md.); Marshall, M.; Grizzle, W. (Birmingham, Ala.)

439 **Factors Controlling the Expression of 5α-Reductase in Human Prostate: A Possible New Approach for the Treatment of Prostate Cancer**
Habib, F.K.; Ross, M.; Bayne, C.W. (Edinburgh)

443 **Certain Aspects of Molecular Endocrinology That Relate to the Influence of Dietary Factors on the Pathogenesis of Prostate Cancer**
Griffiths, K.; Morton, M.S. (Cardiff); Denis, L. (Antwerp)

Preclinical Models for Drug Discovery

456 **High-Grade Prostatic Intraepithelial Neoplasia in Dogs**
Waters, D.J. (West Lafayette, Ind.)

KARGER

Fax+41 61 306 12 34
E-Mail karger@karger.ch
www.karger.com

Access to full text and tables of contents, including tentative ones for forthcoming issues:
www.karger.com/journals/eur/eur_bk.htm

459 **Use of Animal Models in Defining Efficacy of Chemoprevention Agents against Prostate Cancer**
Bosland, M.C. (New York, N.Y.)

464 **Chemoprevention of Hormone-Dependent Prostate Cancer in the Wistar-Unilever Rat**
McCormick, D.L.; Rao, K.V.N. (Chicago, Ill.)

Surrogate Endpoint Biomarkers for Clinical Trials of Prostate Cancer Chemoprevention

468 **Subtle Morphological and Molecular Changes in Normal-Looking Epithelium in Prostates with Prostatic Intraepithelial Neoplasia or Cancer**
Montironi, R. (Ancona); Hamilton, P.W. (Belfast); Scarpelli, M. (Ancona); Thompson, D.; Bartels, P.H. (Tucson, Ariz.)

474 **Prostatic Intraepithelial Neoplasia: A Marker for High-Risk Groups and a Potential Target for Chemoprevention**
Sakr, W.A. (Detroit, Mich.)

479 **Genetic and Chromosomal Alterations in Prostatic Intraepithelial Neoplasia and Carcinoma Detected by Fluorescence in situ Hybridization**
Qian, J.; Jenkins, R.B.; Bostwick, D.G. (Rochester, Minn.)

484 **Tissue Architecture Analysis in Prostate Cancer and Its Precursors: An Innovative Approach to Computerized Histometry**
Bartels, P.H. (Tucson, Ariz.); Montironi, R. (Ancona); Duval da Silva, V. (Brasília/Porto Alegre); Hamilton, P.W. (Belfast); Thompson, D.; Vaught, L.; Bartels, H.G. (Tucson, Ariz.)

492 **Reversibility of Prostatic Intraepithelial Neoplasia: Implications for Chemoprevention**
Bostwick, D.G.; Neumann, R.; Qian, J.; Cheng, L. (Rochester, Minn.)

496 **Evolution of Isolated High-Grade Prostate Intraepithelial Neoplasia in a Mediterranean Patient Population**
Algaba, F. (Barcelona)

498 **Clinical Evolution of Prostatic Intraepithelial Neoplasia**
Zlotta, A.R.; Schulman, C.C. (Brussels)

504 **PIN I–III: When Should We Interfere?**
Newling, D. (Amsterdam)

508 **Prostatic Intraepithelial Neoplasia and Endocrine Manipulation**
van der Kwast, Th.H.; Labrie, F.; Têtu, B. (Rotterdam/Québec)

511 **The Utility of Prostate-Specific Antigen as a Surrogate Marker for Identification of High-Risk Cohorts and Assessing Response in Chemoprevention Trials**
Crawford, E.D. (Denver, Colo.)

Clinical Trial Designs for Chemoprevention of Prostate Cancer

515 **Practical Aspects of Clinical Trials on Chemoprevention of Prostate Cancer**
van der Meijden, A.P.M. ('s-Hertogenbosch)

519 **Statistical Considerations of Chemoprevention Clinical Trials in Prostate Cancer**
Sylvester, R.; Collette, L. (Brussels)

523 **Prostate Cancer Screening in Tyrol, Austria: Experience and Results**
Horninger, W.; Reissigl, A.; Rogatsch, H.; Volgger, H.; Studen, M.; Klocker, H.; Bartsch, G. (Innsbruck)

539 **The European Randomized Study of Screening for Prostate Cancer (ERSPC): An Update**
Schröder, F.H.; Kranse, R.; Rietbergen, J.; Hoedemaeker, R.; Kirkels, W. (Rotterdam); and members of the ERSPC

544 **Prostate Cancer Prevention Trial (PCPT) Update**
Coltman, C.A., Jr.; Thompson, I.M., Jr. (San Antonio, Tex.); Feigl, P. (Seattle, Wash.)

354, 423 **Congress Calendar**
548 **Author Index Vol. 35, No. 5–6, 1999**
549 **Subject Index Vol. 35, No. 5–6, 1999**
550 **Forthcoming Papers**
551 **Acknowledgement to the Reviewers**

552 **Author Index Vol. 35, 1999**
554 **Subject Index Vol. 35, 1999**
after 556 **Contents Vol. 35, 1999**

Curriculum in Urology 2.4

Infections and Stones
Prostatitis and Urethritis
Ludwig, M.; Weidner, W. (Giessen)

European
Urology

Introduction

Chemoprevention is the administration of drugs or other agents to prevent, inhibit or delay progression of cancer. Because of its long latency and high incidence, prostate cancer is an important target for chemoprevention. As with other cancers, development of rational chemopreventive strategies requires knowledge of major mechanisms of carcinogenesis in the prostate and identification of agents that interfere with these mechanism. Also, to identify suitable populations for evaluation of potential chemopreventive agents and for future chemopreventive intervention, risk factors such as the presence of early premalignant lesions and genetic predisposition should be well characterized. Because of the long time period for carcinogenesis and large cohort required for an evaluable study, cancer incidence is not usually a feasible endpoint for chemoprevention clinical trials. Thus, identification and characterization or intermediate biomarkers and their validation as surrogate endpoints for cancer incidence in clinical chemoprevention trials are significant components in the development of chemoprevention agents. Prostate cancer represents a prime target for chemoprevention studies because known risk factors, hormonal dependency and precursor lesions are well documented.

Promising chemopreventive drugs of the prostate include retinoids, antiandrogens, antioestrogens, steroid aromatase inhibitors, 5α-reductase inhibitors, vitamins D and E, selenium, lycopene and 2-difluoromethylornithine.

Several biomarkers can be used to monitor carcinogenesis in the prostate such as prostate-specific antigen (PSA), prostatic intraepithelial neoplasia (PIN), and nuclear and nucleolar morphometry. Epidemiological and clinical studies allow risk factors for prostate cancer incidence and progression (e.g. genetic polymorphisms in steroid 5α-reductase, increasing PSA levels following surgery to be seen. These studies are important for identifying cohorts suitable for chemoprevention intervention. Clinical trials range from evaluation of the effects of promising agents on intermediate biomarkers in men scheduled for prostatectomy, to phase II and phase III studies on reduction of PIN, and large phase III trials on inhibition of prostate carcinoma.

The concept of chemoprevention in prostate cancer is new and should in future have a significant impact on the incidence and mortality of this leading cancer threat in men.

Claude C. Schulman
Gary J. Kelloff

KARGER
Fax +41 61 306 12 34
E-Mail karger@karger.ch
www.karger.com

Accessible online at:
http://BioMedNet.com/karger

European
Urology

Eur Urol 1999;35:342–350

Chemoprevention of Prostate Cancer: Concepts and Strategies

Gary J. Kelloff[a] Ronald Lieberman[a] Vernon E. Steele[a] Charles W. Boone[a]
Ronald A. Lubet[a] Levy Kopelovitch[a] Winfred A. Malone[a]
James A. Crowell[a] Caroline C. Sigman[b]

[a]National Cancer Institute, Division of Cancer Prevention, Chemoprevention Branch, Bethesda, Md., and
[b]CCS Associates, Mountain View, Calif., USA

Key Words
Prostate · Chemoprevention · Drug development

Abstract
Chemoprevention is the administration of agents to prevent induction and inhibit or delay progression of cancers. For prostate, as for other cancer targets, successful chemopreventive strategies require well-characterized agents, suitable cohorts, and reliable intermediate biomarkers of cancer for evaluating chemopreventive efficacy. Agent requirements are experimental or epidemiological data showing chemopreventive efficacy, safety on chronic administration, and a mechanistic rationale for the observed chemopreventive activity. On this basis, promising chemopreventive drugs in prostate include retinoids, antiandrogens, antiestrogens, steroid aromatase inhibitors, 5α-reductase inhibitors, vitamins D and E, selenium, lycopene, and 2-difluoromethylornithine. Phase II trials are critical for evaluating chemopreventive efficacy. Cohorts in these trials should be suitable for measuring the chemopreventive activity of the agent and the intermediate biomarkers chosen as endpoints. Many cohorts proposed for phase II trials are patients with previous cancers or premalignant lesions. For such patients, trials should be conducted within the context of standard treatment. Two cohorts currently used in phase II prostate cancer chemoprevention trials are patients with PIN and patients scheduled for prostate cancer surgery. Biomarkers should fit expected biological mechanisms, be assayed reliably and quantitatively, measured easily, and correlate to decreased cancer incidence. Protocols for adequately sampling tissue are essential. Changes in PIN provide prostate biomarkers with the ability to be quantified and a high correlation to cancer. PIN measurements include nuclear polymorphism, nucleolar size and number of nucleoli/nuclei, and DNA ploidy. Other potentially useful biomarkers are associated with cellular proliferation kinetics (e.g. PCNA and apoptosis), differentiation (e.g. blood group antigens, vimentin), genetic damage (e.g. LOH on chromosome 8), signal transduction (e.g. TGFα, TGFβ, IGF-I, c-*erb*B-2 expression), angiogenesis, and biochemical changes (e.g. PSA levels).

Chemoprevention is the use of agents to slow the progression, reverse, or inhibit carcinogenesis – that is, to lower the risk of developing invasive or clinically significant disease. The features of prostate cancer – prevalence, long latency, deficient screening, significant mortality and morbidity – provide the need and opportunity for chemoprevention. Among US males, it is the most common can-

KARGER

Fax + 41 61 306 12 34
E-Mail karger@karger.ch
www.karger.com

0302–2838/99/0356–0342$17.50/0

Accessible online at:
http://BioMedNet.com/karger

Dr. Gary Kelloff, Chief, Chemoprevention Branch
Department of Health & Human Services
National Institutes of Health, National Cancer Institute
Bethesda, MD 20892 (USA)
Tel. +1 301 496 8563, Fax +1 301 402 0553

cer, accounting for 184,000 (29%) of all new cancers and 39,200 (13%) of cancer deaths in males [1]. Etiological and risk factors for prostate cancer include age >50 years, family history, high serum testosterone, high fat diet, prostatitis, and geographical background (prevalence being highest in US, Canada, and northwest Europe). Besides clinically evident disease, microscopic foci of adenocarcinoma have been found at autopsy in prostates of men who died from other causes. The frequency of such 'latent' tumors has been shown to increase with each decade of life from the 50s (5.3–14% incidence) to the 90s (40–80%) [2].

In most epithelial tissues, including the prostate, genetic progression [measured both as specific genetic lesions and more generally, as increased loss of heterozygosity (LOH) or gene amplification] and loss of cellular control functions are observed as the cell and tissue phenotype changes from normal histology to early dysplasia [prostatic intraepithelial neoplasia (PIN), then to increasingly severe dysplasia (high-grade PIN (HGPIN))], superficial cancers and finally invasive disease. These changes generally occur over a long time period. Particularly, in prostate, PIN develops over approximately 20 years [3]. From PIN to HGPIN and early latent cancer may take 10 or more years, and clinically significant carcinoma may not occur until 3–15 years later [3].

Chemoprevention versus Chemotherapy – Chemoprevention's Advantage

The scope of chemoprevention is throughout carcinogenesis, but before invasive disease is detected. Its advantage, particularly in slowly advancing prostate carcinogenesis, is that intervention occurs while cellular control mechanisms are intact, providing more defined targets than in invasive cancer, where many control mechanisms have been destroyed. Those controls that remain also may be inconsistent from cell to cell in the cancerous tissue. On the other hand, chemotherapeutics are given for short periods of time or in discrete cycles to cancer patients under continual physician's care, and so their side effects can be detected early and managed. Also, the potential net clinical benefit to the cancer patient allows a higher risk (more toxic) treatment. Chemopreventive agents are intended for relatively healthy subjects, many without detectable histological lesions (i.e., without detectable PIN), and so without clearly evident clinical benefit from intervention. Chemopreventive intervention is long term, even as long as lifetime. For these reasons, chemopreventive agents need to have minimal toxicity. However, since carcinogenesis is progressive, potential clinical benefits of chemopreventive intervention increase with the stage of progression. More toxicity is likely to be tolerable in chemopreventive agents targeted to regressing or inhibiting HGPIN than to those for lower risk subjects carrying a genetic polymorphism predisposing them to biosynthesizing high levels of activated testosterone (e.g., a polymorphism in the steroid 5α-reductase type II gene [4]; see table 1).

In clinical trials, treatment endpoints for cancer chemopreventives and chemotherapeutics are also quite different. Relatively few precancerous lesions, perhaps with the exception of severe dysplasia, progress to cancers. This low incidence and long latency make cancer incidence and mortality impractical endpoints for most chemoprevention trials. It is unlikely that adequate resources (time and numbers of eligible subjects) will be available to study cancer incidence reduction for more than a few agents. Effects on precancerous endpoints, providing they can be validated as surrogate measures of cancer incidence, are more feasible. Because of these factors, the development paths for chemotherapeutics [5] and chemopreventives [6] are very different. Nonetheless, there is some overlap both conceptually and practically between chemoprevention and chemotherapy. For instance, chemopreventive agents may be beneficial as adjuvant treatment to prevent recurrences or new primary tumors in patients already treated for cancer [e.g. 7]. Also, some mechanisms of chemopreventive and chemotherapeutic action are similar. Cytotoxicity was the primary mechanism of early generations of chemotherapeutic agents. Newer chemotherapeutics have mechanisms similar to those of some chemopreventive agents. For example, cytostatic agents are being explored as chemotherapeutics. Like some chemopreventive agents, the cytostatic chemotherapeutic agents slow the growth and progression of dysplastic cells (e.g., by inducing terminal differentiation). Similarly, angiogenesis inhibition may be effective for halting the spread of invasive cancer, as well as preventing progression of precancerous lesions.

Requirements for Successful Chemoprevention Strategies

In prostate, as in other major cancer target sites, three critical aspects govern the design and conduct of these trials – well-characterized agents, reliable biomarkers for measuring efficacy, and suitable cohorts. Developing ra-

Table 1. Prostate cancer: considerations and factors for chemoprevention

The Problem
In USA most common cancer in men
29% (184,500) of total new cancer cases (of top 10 cancer sites) in men (estimated 1998)
13% (39,200) of cancer deaths in men (estimated 1998)
Risk factors/risk markers
Age > 50 years
Familial history of prostate cancer
Germline mutation (e.g., PC-1)
High serum testosterone
High fat diet/high red meat consumption
Population/geographical background (highest incidences in Canada and northwest Europe)
Prostatitis
Genetic polymorphisms (e.g., in SRD5A2, gene for steroid 5α-reductase)
Low micronutrient levels (e.g., selenium, carotenoids, vitamin D)
Proposed chemopreventive mechanisms/chemical classes
Steroid 5α-reductase inhibitors (e.g., finasteride)
Retinoids (e.g., 9-*cis*-retinoic acid)
RAMBA (retinoic acid metabolism-blocking agent)
Antiproliferatives (e.g., DFMO, DHEA analogs)
Apoptosis inducers (e.g., perillyl alcohol and congeners)
Differentiating agents (e.g., vitamin D analogs)
Antioxidants (e.g., vitamin E, selenium, lycopene)
GSH-enhancing agents (e.g., oltipraz)
Antiestrogens (e.g., toremifene, tamoxifen, raloxifene, SERM-3)
Aromatase inhibitors (e.g., vorozole)
Antiandrogens (e.g., leuprolide, flutamide)
Angiogenesis inhibitors (e.g., linomide)
Signal transduction regulators (e.g., genistein)
Preclinical models of prostate cancer
Lobund-Wistar rats treated with MNU
Wistar rats treated with MNU then chronic testosterone
Noble rats treated with testosterone and estradiol (develop PIN)
Transgenic mouse with C3(1) and SV40 T-antigen
Rodents with human prostate xenografts (e.g., LNCaP)
Intermediate endpoint biomarkers
Histological: PIN (nuclear morphometry, nucleolar morphometry, nuclear texture, DNA ploidy)
Proliferation: PCNA, Ki-67 antigen expression
Differentiation: loss of high-molecular-weight cytokeratins (50–64 kD), altered blood group antigens (e.g., Lewis Y antigen), vimentin
Genetic/regulatory: c-*erb*B-2, TGFα, p53, *bcl*-2/bax, pc-1, chromosomal loss or gain (e.g., 8p, 9p and 16q), TGFβ, IGF-1
Biochemical: PSA levels, PAP levels
Angiogenesis: Microvessel density, vWF, VEGF
Clinical cohorts phase II
Patients scheduled for radical prostatectomy
Patients with PIN
Patients with cancer on biopsy, treated by watchful waiting
Patients at high risk for biochemical failure or rising PSA postradical prostatectomy
Subjects with positive family history
Clinical cohorts phase III
Patients with PIN
Men at high risk (e.g., PSA > 4 ng/ml and negative biopsy)
Men from general population, age ≥ 55 years, normal PSA and DRE

tional chemopreventive strategies for prostate requires knowledge of major mechanisms of carcinogenesis in the tissue and identification of agents that interfere with these mechanisms [8–11]. Also, to identify suitable populations for evaluation of potential chemopreventive agents and for future chemopreventive intervention, risk factors such as the presence of early premalignant lesions and genetic predisposition should be well characterized. The impracticality of cancer incidence as an endpoint for most chemoprevention trials was stated above. Thus, chemopreventive agent development depends on identifying and characterizing early intermediate endpoints and validating them as surrogate endpoints for cancer incidence in clinical chemoprevention trials [8–11]. The following sections of this paper cover issues on agents, biomarkers and chemoprevention trial design, both generally and as they pertain specifically to prostate.

Identifying Promising Chemopreventive Agents – Molecular Targets and Cellular or Tissue Effects

Basic research carcinogenesis has identified numerous molecular targets associated with the initiation and progression of precancers to invasive disease. Possible chemoprevention strategies use agents that interfere with the expression and/or activity of these molecules; examples of the mechanisms, their possible molecular targets in prostate, and agents that act at these targets are listed in table 2 [11].

Many potential chemopreventive agents have multiple chemoprevention-associated molecular activities. Examples using agents promising for prostate are shown in table 3 for the retinoid fenretinide, soy isoflavones, and selenium [11]. It is evident that many of these activities are interrelated, e.g., soy isoflavone inhibition of growth factor receptor tyrosine kinases may also cause other effects occurring along signal transduction pathways, such as inhibition of angiogenesis. Also, a single activity, even if it is the agent's predominant pharmacological activity, may not be the most important or the only one effecting chemoprevention. For example, besides being potent inhibitors of growth factor tyrosine kinases, the soy isoflavones are also weak estrogens and antiestrogens, and they potentially inhibit cytochrome P_{450}-catalyzed carcinogen activation, which could also contribute to their chemopreventive potential [reviewed in 12]. Such observations imply that molecular targeting should not be the only approach to identifying potential chemopreventive drugs,

Table 2. Mechanisms for chemoprevention in prostate with possible molecular targets

Mechanism	Possible molecular targets	Representative agents
Antimutagenesis		
Inhibit formation/activation of carcinogen	PG synthase hydroperoxidase, 5-lipoxygenase (inhibit)	NSAIDs, lipoxygenase inhibitors, COX-2 inhibitors
Deactivate/detoxify carcinogen	GSH/GST (enhance)	Oltipraz
Antiproliferation/antiprogression		
Modulate hormone/growth factor activity	Estrogen receptor (antagonize)	SERMS, isoflavones
	Androgen receptor (antagonize)	Bicalutamide, flutamide
	Steroid aromatase (inhibit)	Exemestane, vorozole, arimidex
	Steroid 5α-reductase (inhibit)	Finasteride, RAMBAs, retinoids
Inhibit oncogene activity	Farnesyl protein transferase (inhibit)	Perillyl alcohol
Inhibit polyamine metabolism	ODC activity (inhibit)	DFMO
	ODC induction (inhibit)	Retinoids
Induce terminal differentiation	TGFβ (induce)	Retinoids, RAMBAs, vitamin D and analogs
	Langherans' cells (enhance)	Vitamin E
Induce apoptosis	TGFβ (induce)	Retinoids, SERMs
	RAS farnesylation (inhibit)	Perillyl alcohol
	Telomerase (inhibit)	Retinoic acid
Inhibit angiogenesis	FGF receptor (inhibit tyrosine kinase)	Isoflavones
	Thrombomodulin (inhibit)	Retinoids
Antioxidant (antimutagen and antiproliferative)	Activated oxygen (quenching)	Lipoxygenase inhibitors, selenium, vitamin E, lycopene

Table 3. Potential chemopreventive activities of selected agents

Fenretinide	Soy isoflavones	Selenium
Angiogenesis inhibitor	Angiogenesis inhibitors	Antioxidant
Antiproliferative	Antiestrogens	Apoptosis inducer
Apoptosis inducer	Antioxidants	AA metabolism inhibitor
AA metabolism inhibitor	Apoptosis inducers	Catalase enhancer
Cytochrome P_{450} modifier	Cytochrome P_{450} modifiers	Cytochrome P_{450} modifier
Differentiating agent	EGFR inhibitors	GST/GSH enhancer
IGF-I inhibitor	Oncogene expression inhibitors (e.g., *jun*)	GSH peroxidase enhancer
Immunostimulant	ODC synthesis inhibitors	Immunostimulant
ODC synthesis inhibitor	PDGF inhibitors	UDP-glucuronyl-transferase enhancer
Protein kinase C inhibitor	Tyrosine kinase inhibitors	
TGFβ inducer		

but should be complemented by empirical screening which looks at chemopreventive effects at the cellular and tissue levels.

In fact, experimental and epidemiological carcinogenesis studies show that >90% of cancers are associated with mutation and cellular proliferation [13–15]. Normal functioning cells have three possible fates, which can be disrupted during carcinogenesis by mutation and are evidenced in carcinogenesis as uncontrolled proliferation. These are: (1) programmed cell death (from senescence, or in response to damage or environmental conditions such as overpopulation or hormone withdrawal); (2) maturation or differentiation, and (3) normal growth and proliferation. Mutagenesis can damage the cell and destroy normal growth controls, resulting in loss of programmed cell death and maturation pathways and increased (hyper)proliferation. And so, agents which inhibit mutagenesis and hyperproliferation, and which induce apoptosis or differentiation, have potential as chemopreventives regardless of their specific molecular targets [11].

Promising Agents for Prostate Cancer Chemoprevention

Candidate chemopreventive agents for prostate cancer have been identified using molecular targeting and screening in animal models, as well as observations from epidemiological studies and from clinical intervention studies where prostate cancer incidence reduction was not a primary endpoint. Currently promising agents include antiandrogens and antiestrogens (e.g., flutamide, toremifene, raloxifene, SERM-3 and steroid aromatase inhibitors), retinoids (e.g., fenretinide and 9-*cis*-retinoic acid), RAMBAs (retinoic acid metabolic blocking agents), vitamin E, organoselenium, lycopene, soy isoflavones (e.g., genistein), 2-difluoromethylornithine (DFMO), steroid 5α-reductase inhibitors (e.g., finasteride, dual type 1 and type 2 inhibitors), apoptosis inducers (e.g., perillyl alcohol), and differentiation agents (e.g., vitamin D analogs). Recent data showing growth inhibition of prostate cancer cells also suggest that anti-inflammatories such as lipoxygenase inhibitors [16] and selective COX-2 inhibitors [17] have promise as prostate cancer chemopreventives, as does the combination of selenium with vitamin E. A large (18,000 subjects) phase III clinical trial of finasteride (Proscar®), which inhibits the enzyme testosterone 5α-reductase, is in progress [18]. Early experimental data suggested that retinoids such as fenretinide and 9-*cis*-retinoic acid will be chemopreventive in the prostate, provided sufficient tissue levels are achieved [e.g., 19]. Ornithine decarboxylase (ODC) is found at high levels in the prostate and prostate neoplasms [20], so that DFMO appears to be a promising chemopreventive agent. In a study of subjects with previous skin cancers (melanoma and nonmelanoma), selenium in the form of selenized brewer's yeast (200 µg Se/day) was associated with a 63% reduction in prostate cancer in a cohort with prior nonmelanoma skin cancer compared with placebo-treated controls [21, 22]. In a study of Finnish smokers, a significant reduction in prostate cancer incidence of 32% (95% CI = 12–47%) was seen in those taking vitamin E (50 mg/day) compared with placebo or β-carotene [23]. Because testosterone and estrogen are believed to be involved in prostate carcinogenesis, antiestrogens and antiandrogens [24] may have potent chemopreventive activity individually, and in combination they may reduce such undesirable side effects of antiandrogens as gynecomastia. Epidemiologic studies suggest that increased serum levels of lycopene, the most abundant serum carotenoid, are associated with a decreased relative risk of prostate cancer [25]. The presence of vitamin D receptors in prostate cancers and low levels of vitamin D in the sera of prostate cancer patients [26] suggest vitamin D analogs as potential chemopreventive agents in men at risk.

Criteria for Intermediate Biomarkers Used as Surrogate Endpoints in Chemoprevention Studies

It is important to evaluate intermediate biomarkers as surrogates for cancer in the context of carcinogenesis at the target site, to insure that the biomarker is a precursor to cancer and not just indirectly associated. The assurance that chemopreventive agents can modulate the biomarker(s) chosen as the surrogate endpoint is clearly critical. Intraepithelial neoplasia has been shown to be modulatable, i.e., all-*trans*-retinoic acid caused CIN to regress [27] and sulindac caused regression if colorectal adenomas [28]. On this basis, PIN is regarded as a surrogate endpoint for prostate cancer.

The promise of PIN as a premalignant lesion and hence potential surrogate endpoint for prostate cancer, and the characteristics of PIN progression, have been described by Bostwick and Brawer [3, 29–33]. The evidence that PIN is a precancer includes morphology; the atypia observed in HGPIN is virtually indistinguishable from invasive cancer, except that in HGPIN the basal membrane is still intact. As PIN progresses, the likelihood of damage to the basal cell layer increases. PIN and prostate cancer share other phenotypic parameters. For example, certain cytoskeletal proteins, secreted proteins, and degree of glycosylation are shared by PIN and cancer, but not by benign prostatic hyperplasia or normal prostate epithelium. Also, PIN is associated spatially and temporally with prostate cancer, both being found primarily in the peripheral zone, and with far less prevalence in the transition zone. Based on several studies in which whole prostates were obtained, HGPIN was seen in 32% (of 876) of specimens without cancer and in 73% (of 731) of specimens with concomitant cancer. Increasing rates of aneuploidy and angiogenesis from low-grade PIN to HGPIN to cancer also are evidence that PIN is a precancer.

Hyperproliferation is another example of a biomarker that can be modulated. Lipkin [34] has described reduction of proliferation by calcium as measured by ^{3}H-thymidine uptake in patients at high risk for colon cancer. While they will more often be risk biomarkers, genetic lesions or their encoded products can in certain circumstances provide modulatable biomarkers. Although acquired genetic lesions would not be excised by a given agent, one can assume that some agents will confer a selective advantage to cells not carrying the lesion over those that do. The biomarker in this instance would be the quantitative reduction at the tissue level of genetically altered cells.

Also Westra and Sidransky [35] and Mao et al. [36] have cautioned against relying solely on a phenotypic biomarker such as dysplasia to evaluate chemopreventive effects and have underscored the need to evaluate genotypic changes in normal-appearing epithelia surrounding dysplastic lesions, since the phenotype of the whole tissue does not always reflect underlying genotypic changes that contribute to carcinogenesis.

The surrogate endpoint should have short latency compared with cancer incidence – ideally, months or a few years compared with the many years and decades required for cancers to develop. To ensure the design of efficient trials, a balance may be struck between short latency to occurrence of the biomarker and its temporal closeness to cancer. Some cohorts may be available for too short a period of time to allow modulation of the lesions most closely related to cancer. For example, treatment of presurgical cohorts in prostate (see below) primarily may explore changes in proliferation indices rather than actual progression of histological lesions. Despite the brevity of the associated trials, studies in these cohorts may be expected to provide valuable information on modulation of selected biomarkers that are proven to be associated with cancer risk. For all the biomarkers, it is highly desirable to measure modulation quantitatively as the difference (Δ) between the biomarker value at the end of treatment and baseline. Thus, baseline biopsies or other baseline tissue measurements are important.

Quantitative Measurement of Chemopreventive Efficacy Using Intermediate Biomarkers

The quantitative evaluation of chemoprevention endpoints is important, since it is very likely that qualitative measures will be too crude and lack the reproducibility to detect carcinogenesis-associated changes in small samples. Biomarkers measured by computer-assisted image analysis (CAIA), including both nuclear and nucleolar morphometry and cytophotometry, are valuable in this regard. Adequate performance ensures that a small trial with limited tissue availability will produce meaningful results. We expect that quantitative nuclear and nucleolar morphometric changes (i.e., changes in size, shape and texture of nuclear material) may be used to describe the histopathology that characterizes progression of PIN. In fact, these biomarkers are being evaluated in several ongoing phase II chemoprevention trials in prostate. Their promise is based on gradient changes associated with increasing PIN severity. Several computer-assisted imaging systems are commercially available and examples of their application in following carcinogenesis and chemopreventive effects in rat esophagus and mouse skin have been recently published [37]. These systems essentially consist of a light microscope, light sensor, digitizer to convert the light to computer-readable form, and a computer with appropriate software to analyze the tissue measurements. Examples of these measurements are nuclear size, shape, texture and pleiomorphism, and nucleolar number, size, shape, position and pleiomorphism. CAIA is also useful for cytometry, including measurements of cellular proliferation and DNA ploidy that typify IEN histopathology.

Sampling Issues in PIN as a Surrogate Endpoint for Cancer Incidence

Detection of PIN underscores sampling issues that must be addressed in chemoprevention studies using surrogate endpoints. As noted above, in men aged ≥ 50 years, HGPIN incidence exceeds 50%. However, of all sextant prostate biopsies taken in this subpopulation for any reason, when no cancer is present, only 5% HGPIN incidence is detected. In the general population, $<1\%$ HGPIN incidence is detected in sextant prostate biopsies. These discrepancies are most probably due to inability to ensure adequate tissue sampling in the prostate, and call for standardization of measurement methods. The number and location of samples from invasive cancer, HGPIN, and adjacent normal-appearing tissue, as well as the thickness/number of histologic sections processed and scored, are important parameters that affect variability, accuracy and reproducibility. Current approaches for refining the measurement of effects on the prevalence and extent of PIN involve calculating the percent of patients with PIN, mapping area and volume of PIN, and digital imaging of the prostate whole mount.

Table 4. NCI chemoprevention branch-sponsored or funded phase II/III clinical chemoprevention trials: prostate cancer

Agent	Cohort (treatment period)	Endpoint(s)
Phase II		
DFMO	Scheduled for prostate cancer surgery (48 weeks)	Histopathology (PIN grade, nuclear polymorphism, nucleolar polymorphism, ploidy), proliferation biomarkers (PCNA, Ki-67)
	Scheduled for prostatectomy (stage A or B prostatic carcinoma or bladder cancer without prostatic carcinoma and scheduled for cystoprostatectomy) (14 days)	Drug effect measurements: ODC activity (skin and prostate), polyamine levels (prostate); histopathology (TRUS-guided biopsies); biochemical biomarkers: PSA, PAP, testosterone
	Serum PSA 3–10 ng/ml (includes patients with prostatic carcinoma and PIN) (14 days to 1 year)	Drug effect measurements: ODC activity (skin and prostate), polyamine levels (prostate); histopathology (TRUS-guided biopsies); biochemical biomarkers: PSA, PAP, testosterone
Soy isoflavones	Scheduled for prostate cancer surgery (28 days)	Histopathology (PIN grade, nuclear polymorphism, nucleolar polymorphism, ploidy); proliferation biomarkers (PCNA, Ki-67), genetic/regulatory biomarkers (p53, *bcl*-2, pc-1, chromosome 8p loss)
Flutamide	Patients with HGPIN (12 months)	PIN grade and incidence, cancer incidence, nuclear polymorphism, nucleolar size, ploidy; other endpoints: PCNA, angiogenesis, apoptosis, LOH chromosome 8, growth factors, PSA
Flutamide/ leuprolide	Scheduled for radical prostatectomy (12 weeks)	PIN grade and incidence, nuclear polymorphism, nucleolar size, ploidy; other endpoints: PCNA, angiogenesis, apoptosis, LOH chromosome 8, growth factors, PSA
Flutamide/ finasteride, toremifene	Scheduled for radical prostatectomy (4–8 weeks)	PIN grade and incidence, nuclear polymorphism, nuclear size, ploidy
Fenretinide	Biopsy-proven nonmetastatic prostate adenocarcinoma, scheduled for radical prostatectomy (4 weeks)	Genetic/regulatory biomarkers: TGFβ, c-*myc*, p53, plasminogen activators (tPA, uPA), apoptosis
Fenretinide	Scheduled for prostate cancer surgery (48 weeks)	Histopathology: PIN grade, nuclear polymorphism, nucleolar polymorphism, ploidy; proliferation biomarkers: PCNA, Ki-67; differentiation biomarkers: Lewis Y antigen, genetic/ regulatory biomarkers: p53, EGFR, TGFα
Soy protein	Patients at high risk for biochemical failure postsurgery	Rising PSA, circulating prostate cancer cells (PSM-RT/PCR)
Phase III		
Finasteride	Men ≥ 55 years of age with normal DRE and PSA <3.0 ng/ml (7 years)	Prostate cancer incidence (grade and stage), BPH incidence and severity, overall and prostate-specific mortality, TURP, PSA levels
Selenized yeast	Skin cancer (melanoma, nonmelanoma) patients, low Se areas in USA (≈ 1 year)	PSA levels
l-Seleno-methionine	HGPIN (3 years)	Prostate cancer incidence (grade and stage), PIN grade, other histopathology and proliferation biomarkers

Cohorts for Chemoprevention Trials

Phase II trials are critical for evaluating chemopreventive efficacy, particularly for establishing intermediate endpoints as surrogate cancer endpoints [8–11]. Cohorts in these trials should be suitable for measuring chemopreventive activity of the agent and intermediate biomarkers chosen as endpoints. Also, many cohorts proposed for phase II trials are composed of patients with previous cancers or premalignant lesions. For such patients, the trials are conducted within the context of standard treatment. For example, a cohort currently used in phase II prostate cancer chemoprevention trials are patients scheduled for prostate cancer surgery. These patients are treated with the chemopreventive drug during the 2- to 8-week period between diagnostic biopsy and prostatectomy. As shown in table 4, changes in various biomarkers between the diagnostic biopsy tissue and biopsy tissue taken after prostatectomy are evaluated. Trials following this protocol are currently in progress with DFMO, fenretinide, flutamide, finasteride, flutamide + finasteride, toremifene and soy isoflavones. A study comparing 11 weeks of treatment with flutamide + leuprolide to no treatment is also in progress in the presurgical cohort. Another cohort for phase II and early phase III trials is patients with HGPIN without prostatic carcinoma. In this cohort, the primary endpoint is PIN regression and cancer incidence reduction, and the treatment period is up to 3 years. A trial of antiandrogen monotherapy (flutamide) is now in progress in this PIN cohort. A phase III trial of finasteride was cited above [18]. The cohort for this trial is essentially normal (PSA ≤ 3 ng/ml, no evidence of cancer on DRE), but high-risk (age ≥ 55 years) men. Bostwick [3] has described these and other potential cohorts for phase II and phase III chemoprevention trials. The other cohorts are men with prostate cancer for whom 'watchful waiting' rather than surgery is prescribed and men at high risk because of elevated PSA (>4 ng/ml).

Opportunities for Chemopreventive Intervention in Prostate Carcinogenesis

As suggested by the discussion above, there are many opportunities for inhibiting, delaying or modulating the natural history of prostate carcinogenesis. Examples of possible cohorts for chemopreventive intervention in phase II and phase III trials are defined by risk factors and include (by increasing risk): age >50 years; genetic polymorphism in 5α-steroid reductase 2 (SRD5A2); germline mutations (e.g., PC-1); elevated PSA with no other indication, and HGPIN. Potential surrogate endpoint biomarkers are also defined by these risk factors. The expected benefits of using such biomarkers in chemoprevention trials include enhanced identification of high-risk groups, more rapid assessment of efficacy based on modulation of the biomarker, and smaller sample size (important for pivotal phase II/III studies). A significant challenge for the next few years will be developing and improving the methodologies for sampling prostatic tissue and for quantitatively estimating the effects of intervention.

References

1 Landis SH, Murray T, Bolden S, Wingo PA: Cancer statistics, 1998. CA Cancer J Clin 1998; 48:6–29.
2 Kelloff GJ, Boone CW, Malone WF, Steele VE, Doody LA: Introductory remarks: Development of chemopreventive agents for prostate cancer. J Cell Biochem 1992;16(suppl H):1–8.
3 Bostwick D: Prostatic intraepithelial neoplasia: Current concepts. J Cell Biochem 1992; 16(suppl H):10–19.
4 Ross RK, Pike MC, Coetzee GA, Reichardt JK, Yu MC, Feigelson H, Stanczyk FZ, Kolonel LN, Henderson BE: Androgen metabolism and prostate cancer: Establishing a model of genetic susceptibility. Cancer Res 1998;58: 4497–4504.
5 O'Shaughnessy JA, Wittes RE, Burke G: Commentary concerning demonstration of safety and efficacy of investigational anticancer agents in clinical trials. J Clin Oncol 1991;9: 2225–2232.
6 Kelloff GJ, Johnson JJ, Crowell JA, Boone CW, DeGeorge JJ, Steele VE, Mehta MU, Temeck JW, Schmidt WJ, Burke G, Greenwald P, Temple RJ: Approaches to the development and marketing approval of drugs that prevent cancer. Cancer Epidemiol Biomarkers Prev 1995;4:1–10.
7 Hong WK, Lippman SM, Itri LM, Karp DD, Lee JS, Byers RM, Schantz SP, Kramer AM, Lotan R, Peters LJ, Dimery IW, Brown BW, Goepfert H: Prevention of second primary tumors with isotretinoin in squamous cell carcinoma of the head and neck. N Engl J Med 1990;323:795–801.
8 Kelloff GJ, Boone CW, Crowell JA, Steele VE, Lubet R, Doody LA: Surrogate endpoint biomarkers for phase II cancer chemoprevention trials. J Cell Biochem 1994;19:1–9.
9 Lippman SM, Benner SE, Hong WK: Cancer chemoprevention. J Clin Oncol 1994;12:851–883.
10 Kelloff GJ, Hawk ET, Crowell JA, Boone CW, Nayfield SG, Perloff M, Steele VE, Lubet RA, Sigman CC: Strategies for identification and clinical evaluation of promising chemopreventive agents. Oncology (Huntington) 1996;10: 1471–1480, 1484.
11 Kelloff GJ, Hawk ET, Karp JE, Crowell JA, Boone CW, Steele VE, Lubet RA, Sigman CC: Progress in clinical chemoprevention. Semin Oncol 1997;24:1–13.
12 Kelloff GJ, Crowell JA, Hawk ET, Steele VE, Lubet RA, Boone CW, Covey JM, Doody LA, Omenn GS, Greenwald P, Hong WK, Parkinson DR, Bagheri D, Baxter GT, Blunden M, Doeltz MK, Eisenhauer KM, Johnson K, Longfellow DG, Knapp GG, Malone WF, Nayfield SG, Seifried HE, Swall LM, Sigman CC: Clinical development plan: Genistein. J Cell Biochem 1996;(suppl 26):114–126.
13 Henderson BE, Ross RK, Shibata A, Paganin-Hill A, Yu MC: Environmental carcinogens and anticarcinogens; in Wattenberg L, Lipkin M, Boone CW, Kellof GJ (eds): Cancer Chemoprevention. Boca Raton, CRC Press, 1992, pp 1–317.
14 Kelloff GJ, Boone CW, Steele VE, Fay JR, Sigman CC: Inhibition of chemical carcinogenesis; in Arcos J, Argus M, Woo Y (eds): Chemical Induction of Cancer: Modulation and Combination Effects. Boston, Birkhäuser, 1995, pp 73–122.
15 Ruddon RW: The epidemiology of human cancers; in Ruddon RW (ed): Cancer Biology, ed 3. New York, Oxford University Press, 1995, chap 2, pp 19–60.

16 Ghosh J, Myers CE: Arachidonic acid stimulates prostate cancer cell growth: Critical role of 5-lipoxygenase. Biochem Biophys Res Commun 1997;235:418–423.

17 Liu XH, Yao S, Kirschenbaum A, Levine AC: NS398, a selective cyclooxygenase-2 inhibitor, induces apoptosis and down-regulates bcl-2 expression in LNCaP cells. Cancer Res 1998;58:4245–4249.

18 Feigl P, Blumenstein B, Thompson I, Crowley J, Wolf M, Kramer BS, Coltman CA Jr, Brawley OW, Ford LG: Design of the prostate cancer prevention trial (PCPT). Control Clin Trials 1995;16:150–163.

19 Pollard M, Luckert PH, Sporn MB: Prevention of primary prostate cancer in Lobund-Wistar rats by *N*-(4-hydroxyphenyl)retinamide. Cancer Res 1991;51:3610–3611.

20 Kadmon D: Chemoprevention in prostate cancer: The role of difluoromethylornithine (DFMO). Cell Biochem 1992;16(suppl H):122–127.

21 Clark LC, Combs GF Jr, Turnbull BW, Slate EH, Chalker DK, Chow J, Davis LS, Glover RA, Graham GF, Gross EG, Krongrad A, Lesher JL Jr, Park HK, Sanders BB Jr, Smith CL, Taylor JR: Effects of selenium supplementation for cancer prevention in patients with carcinoma of the skin. A randomized controlled trial. JAMA 1996;276:1957–1963.

22 Clark LC, Dalkin B, Krongrad A, Combs GF Jr, Turnbull BW, Slate EH, Witherington R, Herlong JH, Janosko E, Carpenter D, Borosso C, Falk S, Rounder J: Decreased incidence of prostate cancer with selenium supplementation: Results of a double-blind cancer prevention trial. Br J Urol 1998;81:730–734.

23 Heinonen OP, Albanes D, Virtamo J, Taylor PR, Huttunen JK, Hartman AM, Haapakoski J, Malila N, Rautalahti M, Ripatti S, Maenpaa H, Teerenhovi L, Koss L, Virolainen M, Edwards BK: Prostate cancer and supplementation wit α-tocopherol and β-carotene: Incidence and mortality in a controlled trial. J Natl Cancer Inst 1998;90:440–446.

24 Aquilina JW, Lipsky JJ, Bostwick DG: Androgen deprivation as a strategy for prostate cancer chemoprevention. J Natl Cancer Inst 1997;89:689–696.

25 Giovannucci EG, Ascherio A, Rimm EB, Stampfer MJ, Colditz G, Wallett WC: Intake of carotinoids and retinol in relation to risk of prostate cancer. J Natl Cancer Inst 1995;87:1767–1776.

26 Corder EH, Guess HA, Hulka BS, Friedman GD, Sadler M, Vollmer RT, Lobaugh B, Drezner MK, Vogelman JH, Orentreich N: Vitamin D and prostate cancer: A prediagnostic study with stored sera. Cancer Epidemiol Biomarkers Prev 1993;2:467–472.

27 Meyskens FL Jr, Graham V, Chvapil M, Dorr RT, Alberts DS, Surwit E: A phase I trial of β-all-*trans*-retinoic acid delivered via a collagen sponge and a cervical cap for mild or moderate intraepithelial cervical neoplasia. J Natl Cancer Inst 1983;71:921–925.

28 Giardiello FM, Hamilton SR, Krush AJ, Piantadosi S, Hylind LM, Celano P, Booker SV, Robinson CR, Offerhaus GJA: Treatment of colonic and rectal adenomas with sulindac in familial adenomatous polyposis. N Engl J Med 1993;328:1313–1316.

29 McNeal JE, Bostwick DG: Intraductal dysplasia: A premalignant lesion of the prostate. Hum Pathol 1986;17:64–71.

30 Bostwick DG, Brawer MK: Prostatic intraepithelial neoplasia and early invasion in prostate cancer. Cancer 1987;59:788–794.

31 Brawer MK: Prostatic intraepithelial neoplasia. Probl Urol 1990;4:392–407.

32 Brawer MK, Bigler SA, Sohlberg OE, Nagle RB, Lange PH: Significance of prostatic intraepithelial neoplasia on prostate needle biopsy. Urology 1991;38:103–107.

33 Brawer MK: Prostatic intraepithelial neoplasia. A premalignant lesion. Hum Pathol 1992;23:243–248.

34 Lipkin M: Prototypic applications of intermediate endpoints in chemoprevention. J Cell Biochem 1992;16(suppl G):1–13.

35 Westra WH, Sidransky D: Phenotypic and genotypic disparity in premalignant lesions: Of calm water and crocodiles. J Natl Cancer Inst 1998;90:1500–1501.

36 Mao L, El-Naggar AK, Papadimitrakopoulou V, Shin DM, Shin HC, Fan Y, Zhou X, Clayman G, Lee JJ, Lee JS, Hittelman WN, Lippman SM, Hong WK: Phenotype and genotype of advanced premalignant head and neck lesions after chemopreventive therapy. J Natl Cancer Inst 1998;90:1545–1551.

37 Boone CW, Bacus JW, Bacus JV, Steele VE, Kelloff GJ: Properties of intraepithelial neoplasia relevant to cancer chemoprevention and to the development of surrogate endpoints for clinical trials. Proc Soc Exp Med Biol 1997;216:151–166.

European Urology

Eur Urol 1999;35:351–354

Molecular Biology of Progression of Prostate Cancer

Nina Nupponen Tapio Visakorpi

Laboratory of Cancer Genetics, Institute of Medical Technology, University of Tampere, and Tampere University Hospital, Finland

Key Words
Hormone-refractory disease · Comparative genomic hybridization · Fluorescence in situ hybridization · Genetic alterations · Amplification · Deletion · Androgen receptor

Abstract
Despite the clinical importance of prostate cancer, the molecular mechanisms underlying the development and progression of prostate cancer are poorly understood. The lack of knowledge on the mechanisms has probably been one of the most important reasons why no new treatment modalities have been developed to cure the disease. Recent studies, especially those performed by comparative genomic hybridization, have revealed the frequent chromosomal alterations that most likely harbor the genes critical for the progression of prostate cancer. Such genetic aberrations include losses of 8p, 10q, 16q, and 13q as well as gains of 7p, 7q, 8q, and Xq. Unfortunately, the target genes for these alterations are, in most of the cases, not known. We have recently identified the androgen receptor (AR) gene as a target gene for the Xq12 amplification found in one-third of the hormone-refractory prostate cancer. The findings suggest that the AR gene amplification and overexpression is involved in the emergence of hormone-refractory prostate cancer.

Introduction

The incidence of prostate cancer has strongly increased during the past decades and it has now become the most common malignancy of men in many Western industrialized countries. Despite the clinical importance of the disease, the mechanisms underlying the development and progression of prostate cancer are incompletely understood [1]. About one-third of the patients are today diagnosed at a clinically advanced stage [2]. For these patients the androgen withdrawal therapy remains the only effective treatment. Most of the prostate cancer patients initially respond to hormonal therapy [1], but eventually the disease will progress. Unfortunately, no effective second-line treatment exists for such hormone-refractory tumors [1].

An accumulation of genetic changes affecting the expression of the critical genes is thought to underlie malignant transformation and cancer progression. Over the

KARGER

Fax +41 61 306 12 34
E-Mail karger@karger.ch
www.karger.com

0302–2838/99/0356–0351$17.50/0

Accessible online at:
http://BioMedNet.com/karger

Dr. Tapio Visakorpi, MD, PhD
Laboratory of Cancer Genetics
Institute of Medical Technology, University of Tampere, PO Box 607
FIN–33101 Tampere (Finland)
Tel. +358 3 2157725, Fax +358 3 2474168/2157710, E-Mail tapio.visakorpi@uta.fi

Table 1. The chromosomal alterations associated with the progression of prostate cancer during the hormonal therapy

Chromosome arm	Tumors showing alteration, %		Minimal region of alteration
	primary carcinoma	recurrent carcinoma	
Losses			
1p	7	54	1p36-pter
10q	10	46	10cen-q21, 10q26
19p and 19q	7	43	19pter-q13.1
20q	0	22	20cen-q22
Gains			
8q	6	73	8q21, 8q23-qter
18q	0	30	18q12
Xq	0	35	Xcen-q13

past 10 years, somatic chromosomal aberrations in prostate cancer have been studied with several techniques, such as classical cytogenetics, loss of heterozygosity (LOH), fluorescence in situ hybridization (FISH) and, most recently, by comparative genomic hybridization (CGH) analyses. These analyses have implicated several chromosomal regions in the development of prostate cancer. However, only very few genes have been directly implicated or suspected to be involved in the development of prostate cancer, and even less is known about the late progression and hormone resistance of prostate cancer. In this review, we try to describe what we have learnt about the genetic basis of the progression of prostate cancer and emergence of hormone-refractory disease.

Chromosomal Alterations

CGH is a fairly new molecular cytogenetic method which allows the detection of DNA sequence copy number changes throughout the genome in a single hybridization [3]. CGH is helpful in defining chromosomal regions that may harbor amplified oncogenes or deleted tumor suppressor genes as well as in investigating the clonal evolution of tumor progression. We have now analyzed both primary untreated and locally recurrent hormone-refractory prostate carcinomas using CGH [4, 5].

We have found that the recurrent tumors contain almost four times more alterations than the primary tumors by CGH. The most notable difference between these tumor types is that the gains and amplifications, which are almost completely missing in the hormone-dependent prostate carcinomas, are common in the hormone-refractory tumors. The results suggest that the early development of prostate cancer is attributable to the inactivation of tumor suppressor genes, whereas the late progression of the disease is also associated by activation of oncogenes. The most common genetic alterations in the locally recurrent hormone-refractory prostate carcinomas are losses of 8p, 13q, 1p, 22, 19, 10q, and 16q, and the gains of 8q, 7q, Xq, and 18q. The chromosome arms that are lost significantly more often in the hormone-refractory than the primary tumors are, e.g., 1p, 10q, 19p, 19q, 20p, and 20q. And, the chromosome arms that are gained more often seem to be 8q, 18q, and Xq (table 1).

In order to study the clonal evolution of prostate cancer during the hormonal therapy, we have also analyzed six primary and corresponding recurrent tumor pairs from the same patients [11]. Three of the cases showed a close genetic relationship as evidenced by high number of shared genetic alterations in the primary and the recurrent tumors, whereas in the rest of the cases, such a relationship was not that evident. The results emphasize that the androgen ablation therapy may act as a selection force, which may select a clone genetically very different than the primary tumor. The fact that recurrent tumors may share only few genetic alterations with the primary tumors suggest also that the biomarkers measured exclusively from primary tumors give only a restricted view on the hormone-refractory prostate cancer.

Genes Involved in the Progression of Prostate Cancer

The chromosomal alterations found by CGH and other methods pinpoint the regions where the genes, that are involved in the development and progression of malignancy, are located. Based on this information, it is possible to identify the target genes of the chromosomal alterations using positional cloning and related strategies. We have, so far, concentrated in two chromosomal regions, 8q and Xq, that are often gained in hormone-refractory prostate cancer.

By CGH, up to 30% of locally recurrent hormone-refractory prostate carcinomas contain an amplification at Xq11-q13, where a highly attractive positional candidate, the human androgen receptor (AR), gene is located. We have shown that the AR gene is amplified and overexpressed in 30% of hormone-refractory tumors [6, 7]. The amplified AR gene is almost always the wild-type gene suggesting that the overexpressed AR protein is functional [6, 7, Wallen et al., submitted 1998]. We have not found the AR gene amplification in any of the untreated prostate carcinomas indicating that the amplification is selected by the hormonal therapy. The results suggest that the amplified and overexpressed AR gene enables the cancer cells to utilize the remaining serum androgens after the castration. Or it may be that the overexpression of AR alters the function, for example the ligand specificity, of the receptor molecule. Altogether, it seems that hormone-refractory prostate cancers, of which growth was earlier considered to be androgen-independent, may as well be androgen-sensitive, or at least that the growth stimulation may be mediated through the AR.

The long arm of chromosome 8 (8q) is one of the most common regions of amplification in many cancer types, especially breast and prostate [4, 5, 8]. It was first described in prostate cancer by Bova et al. [9] using Southern analysis. In prostate cancer, up to 80% of hormone-refractory tumors, but only 5% of primary untreated tumors display 8q gains by CGH. The 8q gain seems to be associated with the aggressive phenotype in both breast and prostate cancer [10, 11]. The amplification of the 8q24 region has been shown to be associated with the presence of lymph-node metastases in prostate cancer [11]. In breast cancer, the 8q gain is associated with a poor prognosis [10]. Two independently amplified subregions, 8q21 and 8q23-q24 [5, 12], have been found by CGH, suggesting the presence of the several target genes for the amplification. A natural candidate target gene for the 8q24 amplification is the c-myc. We among others have shown that a subset of prostate cancer with the 8q gain shows a high-level amplification of c-myc [5, 13]. Nevertheless, it seems that there are other target genes for the 8q amplification as well. One of our major goals is to identify target genes for the 8q gain by using subtraction hybridization strategies.

Other frequently gained chromosomal regions in the hormone-refractory prostate carcinomas, we have found by CGH, are 7q, 7p, and 18q. Chromosome 7 contains several known genes, such as EGFR, CLK2, MDR1 and elongation factor-1-γ, of which altered function could theoretically be involved in the progression of prostate cancer. Recently, it was shown that the overexpression of the caveolin, located at 7q31, is often found in the metastatic lesions of prostate cancer [14]. In addition, the caveolin expression has been shown to be associated with androgen insensitivity in the mouse prostate cancer model [15]. We have applied FISH to study whether the caveolin gene is amplified in the tumors showing 7q gain by CGH. Although an increased copy number of the caveolin was found, no high-level amplifications of the gene were seen. Thus, it seems that the overexpression of the caveolin is not associated with the high-level amplification of the gene. The anti-apoptotic bcl-2 oncogene, which has commonly been found to be overexpressed in recurrent prostate carcinomas [1], is located in 18q21.3. Therefore, we have also analyzed the copy number of the bcl-2 in the recurrent prostate carcinomas showing the 18q gain by CGH. Once again, we have not found high-level amplifications of the gene suggesting that also the bcl-2 overexpression is not caused by the high-level amplification of the gene.

In conclusion, CGH analyses have revealed several chromosomal regions that are affected in prostate cancer. The amplification of 8q and Xq seems to be associated with the progression of the disease during the hormonal therapy. Thus, the identification of the target genes for these alterations would be of utmost importance.

References

1 Kallioniemi OP, Visakorpi T: Genetic basis and clonal evolution of human prostate cancer. Adv Cancer Res 1996;68:225–255.

2 Kosary C, Ries L, Miller B, Hankey B, Harras A, Edwards BE: SEER Cancer Statistics Review, 1973–1992, Tables and Graphs: National Institutes of Health Publication 96–2789. Bethesda, National Cancer Institute, 1995.

3 Kallioniemi A, Kallioniemi OP, Sudar D, Rutovitz D, Gray JW, Waldman F, Pinkel D: Comparative genomic hybridization for molecular cytogenetic analysis of solid tumors. Science 1992;258:818–821.

4 Visakorpi T, Kallioniemi AH, Syvanen AC, Hyytinen ER, Karhu R, Tammela T, Isola JJ, Kallioniemi OP: Genetic changes in primary and recurrent prostate cancer by comparative genomic hybridization. Cancer Res 1995;55: 342–347.

5 Nupponen NN, Kakkola L, Koivisto P, Visakorpi T: Genetic alterations in hormone-refractory recurrent prostate carcinomas. Am J Pathol 1998;153:141–148.

6 Visakorpi T, Hyytinen E, Koivisto P, Tanner M, Keinanen R, Palmberg C, Palotie A, Tammela T, Isola J, Kallioniemi OP: In vivo amplification of the androgen receptor gene and progression of human prostate cancer. Nat Genet 1995;9:401–406.

7 Koivisto P, Kononen J, Palmberg C, Tammela T, Hyytinen E, Isola J, Trapman J, Cleutjens K, Noordzij A, Visakorpi T, Kallioniemi OP: Androgen receptor gene amplification: A possible molecular mechanism for androgen deprivation therapy failure in prostate cancer. Cancer Res 1997;57:314–319.

8 Forozan F, Karhu R, Kononen J, Kallioniemi A, Kallioniemi OP: Genome screening by comparative genomic hybridization. Trends Genet 1997;13:405–409.
9 Bova GS, Carter BS, Bussemakers MJ, Emi M, Fujiwara Y, Kyprianou N, Jacobs SC, Robinson JC, Epstein JI, Walsh PC, et al: Homozygous deletion and frequent allelic loss of chromosome 8p22 loci in human prostate cancer. Cancer Res 1993;53:3869–3873.
10 Isola JJ, Kallioniemi OP, Chu LW, Fuqua SA, Hilsenbeck SG, Osborne CK, Waldman FM: Genetic aberrations detected by comparative genomic hybridization predict outcome in node-negative breast cancer. Am J Pathol 1995;147:905–911.
11 Van den Berg C, Guan XY, Von Hoff D, Jenkins R, Bittner M, Griffin C, Kallioniemi O, Visakorpi T, McGill J, Herath J, Epstein J, Saroscy M, Metzer P, Trent J: DNA sequence amplification in human prostate cancer identified by chromosome microdissection: Potential prognostic implications. Clin Cancer Res 1995; 1:11–18.
12 Cher ML, Bova GS, Moore DH, Small EJ, Carroll PR, Pin SS, Epstein JI, Isaacs WB, Jensen RH: Genetic alterations in untreated metastases and androgen independent prostate cancer detected by comparative genomic hybridization and allelotyping. Cancer Res 1996;56: 3091–3102.
13 Jenkins RB, Qian J, Lieber MM, Bostwick DG: Detection of c-myc oncogene amplification and chromosomal anomalies in metastatic prostatic carcinoma by fluorescence in situ hybridization. Cancer Res 1997;57:524–531.
14 Yang G, Truong LD, Timme TL, Ren C, Wheeler TM, Park SH, Nasu Y, Bangma CH, Kattan MW, Scardino PT, Thompson TC: Elevated expression of caveolin is associated with prostate and breast cancer. Clin Cancer Res 1998;4:1873–1880.
15 Nasu Y, Timme TL, Yang G, Bangma CH, Li L, Ren C, Park SH, DeLeon M, Wang J, Thompson TC: Suppression of caveolin expression induces androgen sensitivity in metastatic androgen-insensitive mouse prostate cancer cells. Nat Med 1998;4:1062–1064.

Congress Calendar

3.6.–5.6.1999 **İzmir** Turkey	11th World Video-Urology Congress Chairmen: Ziya Kırkalı, Arthur D. Smith	**Information:** Cem Güler, M. Uğur Mungan, Talatpasa Blv. 51/7, Alsancak – İzmir (Turkey 35220), Tel. +90 232 278 7477, ... 464 6766, ... 464 7372; Fax +90 232 278 7477, ... 464 7372, E-Mail: kirkali@likya.iyte.edu.tr or kirkaliz@cs.med.deu.edu.tr
18.6.–19.6.1999 **Warsaw** Poland	XXIX Scientific Congress of Polish Urological Association	**Information:** Department of Urology, Warsaw Medical School, 02-005 Lindleya 4, Warsaw (Poland), Tel./Fax +48 22 6281896, E-Mail: jj@pturol.org.p
27.6.–29.6.1999 **Paris** France	2nd International Consultation on Prostate Cancer	**Information:** Dr. Saad Khoury, Clinique urologique, Hôpital de la Pitié, 83, Bd de l'hôpital, F–75634 Paris Cedex 13 (France), Tel. +33 1 42 177120, Fax +33 1 42 177122, E-Mail: khoury@pratique.fr
1.7.–3.7.1999 **Paris** France	1st International Consultation on Erectile Dysfunction	**Information:** Dr. Saad Khoury, Clinique urologique, Hôpital de la Pitié, 83, Bd de l'hôpital, F–75634 Paris Cedex 13 (France), Tel. +33 1 42 177120, Fax +33 1 42 177122, E-Mail: khoury@pratique.fr
2.7.–3.7.1999 **Ancona** Italy	International Meeting on Radical Prostatectomy and Today's Alternative Options	**Information:** Prof. G. Muzzonigro, Cl. Urologica, Osp. 'Umberto I', University of Ancona, L.go Cappelli 1, I–60121 Ancona (Italy), Fax +39 071 2070501, E-Mail: clinuro@anvaxl.unian.it
17.7.1999	Die Knochenmetastase – ein interdisziplinäres Problem	**Information:** Mrs. U. Wagner Tel. +49 89 41 402507, Fax +49 89 41 402585, E-Mail: j.breul@lrz.tu-muenchen.de
31.8.–3.9.1999 **Herlev** Denmark	8th International Congress on Interventional Ultrasound	**Information:** Department of Ultrasound, Herlev Hospital, University of Copenhagen, DK–2730 Herlev (Denmark), Tel. +45 44 88 32 40, Fax +45 44 94 80 09, E-Mail: ultrasound@herlevhosp.dk

(Continued on page 423)

Genetic and Environmental Factors in Prostate Cancer Genesis

European Urology

Eur Urol 1999;35:355–361

Androgen Metabolism and Prostate Cancer: Establishing a Model of Genetic Susceptibility

R.K. Ross[a] G.A. Coetzee[b] C.L. Pearce[a] J.K.V. Reichardt[c] P. Bretsky[a] L.N. Kolonel[d] B.E. Henderson[a] E. Lander[e,f] D. Altshuler[e,g] G. Daley[e,g]

Departments of [a]Preventive Medicine, [b]Urology; [c]Institute for Genetic Medicine, USC School of Medicine, Los Angeles, Calif.; [d]Epidemiology Program, University of Hawaii at Manoa Cancer Research Center, Honolulu, Hawaii; [e]Whitehead Institute/MIT, Center for Genome Research, [f]Department of Biology, MIT, and [g]Department of Medicine, Massachusetts General Hospital, Boston, Mass., USA

Key Words

Prostatic neoplasms · Androgens · Genetics

Abstract

The prostate is an androgen-regulated organ, which has led to longstanding interest in the role of androgens in prostate carcinogenesis. Although evidence of a hormonal etiology for prostate cancer is strong, it is almost entirely circumstantial. Much of the problem in proving a causal relationship relates to the continued difficulties in reliably measuring human tissue-specific exposure to endogenous steroid hormones. The international and racial-ethnic variations in prostate cancer incidence, combined with the effects of migration on risk patterns, have suggested that genetic factors play a central role in determining prostate cancer risk. We are developing a polygenic model of prostate carcinogenesis, focused around a series of genes involved in androgen biosynthesis, transport and metabolism. We have begun to develop this model by utilizing sequence variants to study how polymorphic markers in two genes (SRD5A2 and AR) are related to prostate cancer risk within and between racial-ethnic groups. We are now collaborating with the Whitehead Institute/MIT, Center for Genome Research, to screen for single nucleotide polymorphisms in additional genes relevant to the androgen pathway and prostate cell growth. The model when fully developed can potentially provide a basis for targeting populations for screening interventions and for implementing primary preventive strategies.

The scientific community has been interested in the possible role of steroid hormones in cancer development for over 50 years [1, 2]. During that period, extraordinary amounts of indirect evidence has accumulated for a role of such hormones in the etiology of multiple human cancers [3]. Although there is some evidence that hormonal secretion and metabolism can be environmentally influenced, for example through dietary change, the control of hormonal patterns is also genetically regulated. Based on the extensive evidence of the hormone dependency of human prostate cancer, we are developing a polygenic model of prostate cancer susceptibility. We describe below the rationale on which this prostate cancer model is being built, the current model, and preliminary data that

KARGER

Fax + 41 61 306 12 34
E-Mail karger@karger.ch
www.karger.com

0302–2838/99/0356–0355$17.50/0

Accessible online at:
http://BioMedNet.com/karger

Brian E. Henderson, MD
USC/Norris Comprehensive Cancer Center
1441 Eastlake Ave., #4425
Los Angeles, CA 90033-0800 (USA)
Tel. +1 323 865 0419, Fax +1 323 865 0427, E-Mail behender@hsc.usc.edu

we and others have accumulated in support of this model. We also describe future research directions designed to expand the model to capture additional genes.

Prostate Cancer Epidemiology

By far the two most important risk factors for prostate cancer are age and race-ethnicity. Prostate cancer is extremely rare prior to age 40, but the rate of increase with aging is greater than for any other cancer; rates increase at approximately the 9–10th power of age [4]. For prostate cancer the rate of increase is steepest early in the age-specific curve and then gradually dissipates with age. This contrasts with some other epithelial cancers, such as colon and lung cancer, for which the relationship between age and incidence is strictly linear in log-log units.

African-American men have long been known to have the highest rates of prostate cancer in the world. Although rates vary somewhat among African-Americans across the US, rates average about 50–70% higher in African-Americans than whites [5]. The ratio of African-American to white incidence rates is highest early in the age-incidence cancers and then dissipates some with aging. Although historically there has been no totally adequate comparative data on prostate cancer rates among blacks in Africa, there is some recent data suggesting high rates of prostate cancer in some African populations [6]. Confirmation of these findings would support a strong genetic component to prostate cancer risk.

On the other end of the international and racial-ethnic spectrum of prostate cancer incidence, native Japanese and Chinese men (and probably other Asian populations such as Koreans) have the lowest prostate cancer rates in the world. Historically, it has been reported that the difference in incidence between African-Americans, on the one hand, and these native Asian populations, on the other, was approximately 50-fold [5]. We have, however, previously demonstrated that a major part of this difference is due to different detection strategies for prostate cancer between populations, and that the true difference in incidence is on the order of only 2- to 3-fold [7]. Nonetheless, Japanese- and Chinese-Americans have rates somewhat above those of men in their respective homelands, but their prostate cancer incidence rates never approach those of White Americans, much less African-Americans, even though Japanese, in particular, represent a highly acculturated immigrant population in the US [8].

Androgens and Prostate Cancer

Over the past two decades, we have published several detailed articles on the role of steroid hormones in carcinogenesis [3, 9]. Steroid hormones play a critical role in controlling cell proliferation in their primary target organs, and increased cell proliferation appears to be a common denominator in the pathogenesis of much human cancer [10], as this is a necessary event for the genetic changes required to activate proto-oncogenes or inactivate tumor suppressor genes. Genetic or environmental factors which alter the hormonal environment and, thus, the underlying rates of cell division in these target organs, would be expected to alter the underlying rate of malignant transformation in these target tissues as well [3].

The prostate is a hormonally regulated organ. Testosterone (T) diffuses freely into prostate cells where it is converted to its metabolically more active form, dihydrotestosterone (DHT), through the activity of the enzyme, steroid 5α-reductase type II. DHT (and with less binding affinity T) binds to the androgen receptor (AR); this complex binds to DNA resulting in transactivation of genes with androgen-responsive elements, including those that control cell division [11].

Among mammalian species, only men and dogs have a high naturally occurring incidence of prostate cancer [11], and prostate cancer has proven difficult to produce experimentally. This lack of both experimental and naturally occurring models of the disease has dampened progress in understanding the pathogenesis of prostate cancer. The first experimental model of prostate adenocarcinoma (the human histologic equivalent) was produced by Noble [12] in 1977, through administration of T subcutaneously, and all subsequent models have had at least some androgen requirement for tumor induction or progression.

Prostate cancer is androgen-dependent and androgen ablation or blockade have been a mainstay of treatment for early metastatic prostate cancer for decades [5]. It is widely believed that men with highly underdeveloped prostates, such as eunuchs or men with constitutional 5α-reductase deficiency, never develop prostate cancer [5].

While studies of hormone levels and prostate cancer risk are inherently complex due to inter- and intra-assay variability, cyclical and sporadic variations in the target hormone and the requirement for large prospective studies to name a few, one well-conducted prospective study recently found that prediagnostic circulating T levels were strongly predictive for prostate cancer development [13]. In that study, a strong trend of increasing prostate cancer risk with increasing levels of circulating free T was observed (risks by quartile were 1.0 (low), 1.4, 2.0 and 2.6 (high), p = 0.004 for trend).

As racial-ethnic variation in incidence is such a powerful feature of prostate cancer epidemiology, we have explored over the past decade whether there exist underlying differences in the androgen milieu of populations in the middle and at the extremes of prostate cancer incidence. We reported that T levels were higher in healthy young adult African-American than white men [14]. We later extended this study of hormone patterns in African-American and white men to include young Japanese men born and raised in rural Japan, a group of men with low expected lifetime risk of prostate cancer. These young Japanese men had T levels which did not differ significantly from either African-Americans or whites. However, in this extended study, we found that the Japanese men had circulating levels of 3α-androstanediol glucuronide, an index of in vivo 5α-reductase which was 25–35% lower than the African-American men and white men [15]. Chinese men in Hong Kong have been shown to have similarly low levels of this androgen metabolite [16].

These differences in prostate cancer incidence among African-Americans, US whites and Asians (Chinese, Japanese) might be explained by differences in T biosynthesis on the one hand, and T metabolism on the other. These T differences could be due to environmental influences, genetic control, or an interplay of genetic and environmental factors; we have initially focused on genetic control.

Genes and Cancer

There are two types of germline (constitutional DNA) genetic alterations which predispose to cancer [17]. Some germline genetic loci predispose directly to the disease. These single inherited genetic traits are uncommon in the population and, thus, carry with them low population attributable risks, even though individuals with these genetic traits may have a high absolute risk of developing the disease. One such candidate gene for prostate cancer has been located on 1q(24-25), although controversy exists as to its relevance [18].

Much more common are susceptibility genes with low absolute risk, but possibly high population attributable risk, as the higher risk genotype may be quite common in the population. These types of genes, such as those involved in androgen metabolism as discussed below, affect risk of cancer indirectly. Relevant sequence variants in several such genes in a common androgen pathway could give rise to a 'polygenic' etiology of cancer, thereby allowing the identification of individuals with high- or low-risk polygenic profiles [17].

Establishing a Genetic Model for Prostate Cancer

In developing a polygenic model of prostate carcinogenesis, genes involved in androgen biosynthesis, androgen activation and inactivation, and androgen transport as well as the 'downstream' genes transactivated through the AR, are all of interest (table 1). We have begun to explore a few such genes which: (1) encode products which potentially play an important role in inducing androgen stimulation of the prostate; (2) are polymorphic and (3) show substantial allelic variation among the racial-ethnic groups of greatest interest in terms of prostate cancer risk. There are two pathways through which androgens are metabolized in the testes. The 5δ pathway is more common in humans whereas the 4δ pathway is common in rodents [19]. The major metabolic androgen pathways pertaining to the prostate and the relevant sites of activity of the gene products of current interest as they pertain to the prostate are illustrated in figure 1.

We have initially focused on two genes in this pathway, the steroid 5α-reductase type II (SRD5A2) gene, which encodes the enzyme responsible for conversion of T to the metabolically more active (in terms of AR affinity) DHT, and the AR gene, which encodes the AR allowing for androgen binding and transport, DNA binding and transactivation of androgen-responsive genes.

Our primary initial goal was to demonstrate that the polymorphic markers of interest were related to prostate cancer risk, that the prevalence of high-risk genotypes correlates with the racial-ethnic variation in prostate cancer incidence and, when appropriate, that the genotypic variation correlates in the anticipated direction with biochemical variation in vivo. We have generally utilized the large Hawaii and Los Angeles multiethnic cohort for this series of studies [20]. This cohort of 215,251 individuals from five major ethnic groups was initiated in 1993.

Steroid 5α-Reductase Type II (SRD5A2) Gene

There are two distinct steroid 5α-reductase enzymes encoded by two different genes. There is only 50% homology in amino acid sequence between the two enzymes and

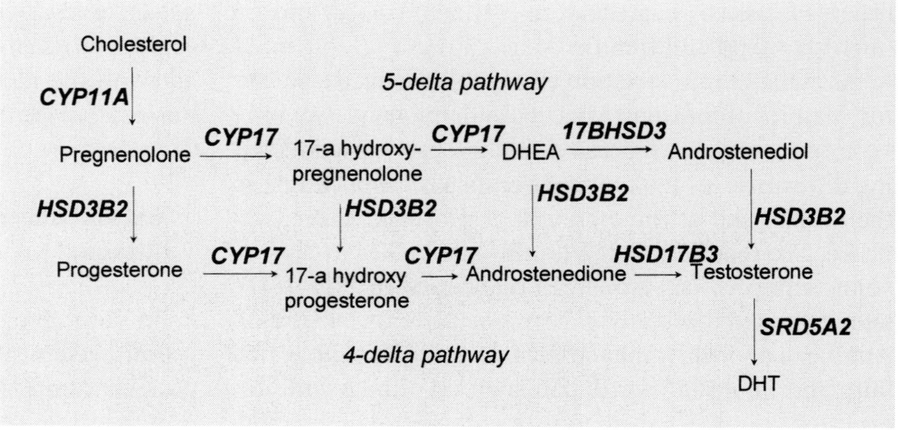

Fig. 1. The androgen metabolism pathway. The 5δ is more common in humans and rabbits and the 4δ pathway is more common in rodents [19].

Table 1. Genes potentially involved in prostate carcinogenesis by family

Family	Gene	Function
Cytochrome P_{450}	CYP11A	Androgen biosynthesis
	CYP17	Androgen biosynthesis
17β-Hydroxysteroid dehydrogenase	HSD17B3	Androgen biosynthesis
	HSD17B4	Androgen metabolism
3β-Hydroxysteroid (5δ) dehydrogenase	HSD3B1	Androgen metabolism
	HSD3B2	Androgen biosynthesis
Insulin-like growth factors	IGF1	Cell proliferation
	IGF2	Cell proliferation
Hormone receptors	AR	Androgen transport and transactivation
	LH/CG	Androgen biosynthesis
Other	LH	Androgen biosynthesis
	SHBG	Androgen transport
	SRD5A2	Androgen bioactivation
	PRL	Androgen receptor control
	GH1	Cell proliferation

a clear distinction in optimal pH. The type II enzyme encoded by the SRD5A2 gene on chromosome 2p contains five exons and is active primarily in the prostate and in genital skin [21]. Germline mutations of SRD5A2 have been identified in a highly inbred kindred in the Dominican Republic [22]. Boys with this mutated gene are phenotypically female and have a persistent vaginal pouch until puberty, at which time there is some phallic enlargement and development of some secondary sex characteristics, but the prostate remains highly underdeveloped.

We sequenced the SRD5A2 gene in a sample of men with either high or low circulating levels of 3α-androstanediol glucuronide (the biochemical serologic correlate of prostatic 5α-reductase activity in vivo) using single-strand conformation polymorphism (SSCP) followed by sequencing of any aberrant SSCP patterns identified. We identified seven missense mutations which resulted in an altered amino acid, and six nucleotide substitutions that were either silent (no amino acid change) or intronic. Only one of the seven missense mutations, the valine to leucine substitution at codon 89 (V89L substitution), was common among healthy men in the cohort [23]. We examined the distribution of this polymorphic marker in 286 control men from four racial-ethnic groups. The valine 89 homozygote genotype (VV) was the most common genotype in both African-Americans (59%) and whites (52%), but was much less common in Chinese and Japanese (30%). On the other hand, the leucine 89 homozygote genotype (LL) was most common in Chinese and Japanese (19%), but accounted for the genotype of only 10% of whites and 3% of African-Americans (the differences between Asians and the other two groups were highly statistically significant ($p < 0.001$)) [22]. After controlling for race-ethnicity, there was a strong correlation between the V89L genotype and circulating levels of androstanediol glucuronide.

A second missense mutation resulting in an alanine to threonine substitution at codon 49 (A49T) was uncommon in healthy men, so we did not at first evaluate it further in terms of prostate cancer risk. However, even though the allele frequency of this A49T mutation was only 0.5% in healthy high-risk African-American men and only 1.8% in healthy low-risk Latino men, it was considerably more common in men with prostate cancer, especially those presenting with advanced (i.e., clinically significant) disease [24]. Among African-Americans, the prevalence was 0.9% for men with early stage, low-grade prostate cancer and 6.1% for more advanced disease resulting in relative risk estimates of 1.9 and 10.6, respectively ($p = 0.001$ for presence of the T allele); for Latinos, the comparable figures were 4.6 and 7.0%, respectively, with resultant relative risks of 2.1 and 4.5 ($p = 0.04$ for presence of the T allele). We concluded that this single mutation, while very uncommon in healthy men, may actually be associated with nearly 10% of all advanced prostate cancers in these two populations [24].

The AR Gene

The AR gene, located on the long arm of the X-chromosome, codes for a transcription factor within the superfamily of steroid receptors. The large exon 1 encodes the transactivation domain that mediates target gene transcriptional activation. Exon 1 also encodes two polymorphic polyamino acid tracts, a poly-Q $(CAG)_n$ and a poly-G $(GGC)_n$ [25].

We have focused our attention on the $(CAG)_n$ sequence, since an expansion of this repeat is the cause of a rare, X-linked adult-onset motor neuron disease, spinal and bulbar muscular atrophy, or Kennedy's disease [26], associated with low virilization, reduced sperm production, testicular atrophy, and reduced fertility [26]. More than double the average number of CAG repeats are found in the AR of such patients. Among otherwise healthy men impaired sperm production and male infertility are associated with CAG repeat sizes in the long end of the 'normal' size distribution [27]. Thus AR activity appears to be negatively correlated with CAG size. Consistent with this notion, we hypothesized [28] and subsequently provided evidence [29] that shorter alleles of the $(CAG)_n$ could be associated with prostate cancer. Two independent epidemiological studies confirmed our original observations [30, 31], and a further two studies [32, 33] identified phenotypic subgroups among prostate cancer cases on the basis of CAG repeats.

We [34] and others [35] have observed an excess risk of prostate cancer in men with prostate cancer-affected brothers compared to those with prostate cancer-affected fathers. We have interpreted this to indicate either an X-linked or a recessive model of prostate cancer risk inheritance. Although the AR gene would be a strong candidate to explain such an inheritance pattern, a recent report found a strong linkage to the X chromosome far removed from the AR gene (Xq27-28), following a genome wide search in a large number of prostate cancer pedigrees [36]. Nonetheless, we have continued to pursue the issue of hereditary prostate cancer linked to the AR gene among African-American men. In this analysis, we analyzed a third polymorphic marker, a *Stu*I single nucleotidepolymorphism [37] (silent) at codon 211 (G1733A), roughly halfway between the two satellites. The S1 allele (uncut by the restriction enzyme) was associated with a statistically significant nearly 3-fold increased risk of prostate cancer among men under age 65 years. Moreover, an excess proportion of this allele (12 of 14, 86%) also was found among prostate cancer cases with an affected brother; the corresponding proportion among control men was 58% (118 of 204) [G. Coetzee, pers. commun.]. These preliminary data indicate that in African-American men non-$(CAG)_n$ genetic variation(s) in exon 1 might contribute to hereditary prostate cancer among brothers of men with this disease. Given the substantial distance between the AR and the putative linkage in the area of Xq27-28, it seems unlikely these two observations are directly related. However, both these early provocative results suggest multiple important research pathways for further understanding the contribution of the AR or some other major X chromosome gene to prostate cancer risk.

Expanding the Model

The early experience with SRD5A2 and AR suggests that the fundamental paradigm linking genetic polymorphisms to prostate cancer risk is plausible. In order to expand the number of potentially relevant genes and sequence variants, we have established a collaboration with Whitehead Institute/MIT, Center for Genome Research. A number of genes in the androgen pathway, as well as several others that affect cell growth through other pathways, have been selected for this project (table 1). We expect that additional candidate genes will be included. The transcribed regions of these genes are being sequenced by the Whitehead Institute/MIT, Center for Genome Research for single nucleotide polymorphisms (SNPs) [38]. We expect to identify novel SNPs and these will be incorporated, along with published SNPs, into large-scale genotyping of the prostate cancer cases and controls from the multiethnic cohort study.

The choice of genes in the androgen pathway and those associated with androgen biosynthesis and transport is biologically sound. The current epidemiologic literature suggests that these genes may play a role in prostate cancer etiology. If our findings continue to support a role for any or a combination of these genes it is possible that a prostate cancer 'risk profile' can be developed. The elucidation of such a risk profile for prostate cancer will allow for more careful screening and possibly less invasive treatment for this disease.

Acknowledgments

This work was supported by grants CA17054, CA54281, CA63464, CA72821, CA68581, and CA53890 from the National Cancer Institute, and 3IB-0082 from the State of California.

References

1 Bittner JJ: The causes and control of mammary cancer in mice. Harvey Lect 1947;42:221–246.
2 Huggins C, Hodges CV: Studies on prostatic cancer: Effect of castration, of estrogen, and of androgen injection on serum phosphatases in metastatic carcinoma of the prostate. Cancer Res 1941;1:293–297.
3 Henderson BE, Ross RK, Pike MC, Casagrande JT: Endogenous hormones as a major factor in human cancer. Cancer Res 1982;42: 3232–3239.
4 Cook PJ, Doll R, Fellingham SA: A mathematical model for the age distribution of cancer in man. Int J Cancer 1969;4:93–112.
5 Ross RK, Schottenfeld D: Prostate cancer; in Schottenfeld D, Fraumeni J (eds): Cancer Epidemiology and Prevention, ed 2. Oxford, Oxford University Press, 1996, pp 1180–1206.
6 Kehinde EO: The geography of prostate cancer and its treatment in Africa. Cancer Surv 1995; 23:281–286.
7 Shimizu H, Ross RK, Bernstein L: Underestimation of the incidence rate of prostate cancer in Japan. Jpn J Cancer Res 1991;82:483–485.
8 Bernstein L, Ross RK: Cancer in Los Angeles County. A Portrait of Incidence and Mortality, 1972–1987. Kenneth Norris Jr Comprehensive Cancer Center, University of Southern California, Los Angeles 1991.
9 Henderson BE, Ross RK, Bernstein L: Estrogens as a cause of human cancer: The Richard and Hinda Rosenthal Foundation Award Lecture. Cancer Res 1988;48:246–253.
10 Preston-Martin S, Pike MC, Ross RK, Henderson BE: Epidemiologic evidence for the increased cell proliferation model of carcinogenesis. Environ Health Perspect 1993;101(suppl 5):137–138.
11 Coffey DS: The molecular biology of the prostate; in Lepor H, Lawson RK (eds): Prostate Disease. Philadelphia, Saunders, 1993, pp 28–56.
12 Noble RL: The development of prostatic adenocarcinoma in Nb rats following prolonged sex hormone administration. Cancer Res 1977; 37:1929–1933.
13 Gann PH, Hennekens CH, Ma J, Longcope C, Stampfer MJ: Prospective study of sex hormone levels and risk of prostate cancer. J Natl Cancer Inst 1996;88:1118–1126.
14 Ross RK, Bernstein L, Judd H, Hanisch R, Pike MC, Henderson BE: Serum testosterone levels in healthy young black and white men. J Natl Cancer Inst 1986;76:45–48.
15 Ross RK, Bernstein L, Lobo RA, Shimizu H, Stanczyk FZ, Pike MC, Henderson BE: 5α-Reductase activity and risk of prostate cancer among Japanese and US White and Black males. Lancet 1992;339:887–889.
16 Lookingbill DP, Demers LM, Wang C, Leung A, Rittmaster RS, Santen RJ: Clinical and biochemical parameters of androgen action in normal healthy Caucasian versus Chinese subjects. J Clin Endocrinol Metab 1991;72:1242–1248.
17 Ross RK, Coetzee GA: The epidemiology and etiology of prostate cancer; in Petrovich Z, Baert L, Brady LW (eds): Diagnostic Imaging and Radiation Oncology. Berlin, Springer, 1996, pp 1–11.
18 Smith JR, Freije D, Carpten JD, Gronberg H, Xu J, Isaacs SD, Brownstein MJ, Bova GS, Guo H, Bujnovszky P, Nusskern DR, Damber JE, Bergh A, Emanuelsson M, Kallioniemi OP, Walker-Daniels J, Bailey-Wilson JE, Beaty TH, Meyers DA, Walsh PC, Collins FS, Trent JM, Isaacs WB: Major susceptibility locus for prostate cancer on chromosome 1 suggested by a genome-wide search. Science 1996;274:1371–1374.
19 Norman AW, Litwack G: Steroid hormones: Chemistry, biosynthesis, and metabolism; in Hormones, ed 2. New York, Academic Press, 1997, pp 1–71.
20 Kolonel LN, Henderson BE, Hankin JH, Nomura AMY, Wilkens LR, Pike MC, Stram DO, Monroe KR, Earle ME, Nagamine FS: A multiethnic cohort in Hawaii and Los Angeles: Baseline characteristics. Am J Epidemiol 1999, in press.
21 Wilson JD, Griffin JE, Russell DW: Steroid 5α-reductase 2 deficiency. Br J Cancer 1993;14: 577–593.
22 Thigpen AE, Davis DL, Gautier T, Imperato-McGinley J, Russell DW: The molecular basis of steroid 5-alpha reductase deficiency in a large Dominican kindred. N Engl J Med 1992; 327:1216–1219.
23 Makridakis N, Ross RK, Pike MC, Chang L, Stanczyk FZ, Kolonel LN, Shi C-Y, Yu MC, Henderson BE, Reichardt JKV: A prevalent missense substitution that modulates activity of prostatic steroid 5α-reductase. Cancer Res 1997;57:1020–1022.
24 Reichardt JKV, Makridakis NM, Ross RK, Pike MC, Kolonel LC, Henderson BE: A missense mutation in the SRD5A2 gene with a significant population-attributable risk for clinically apparent prostate cancer through increased dihydrotestosterone biosynthesis (in review).
25 Irvine RA, Yu MC, Ross RK, Coetzee GA: The CAG and GGC microsatellites of the androgen receptor gene are in linkage disequilibrium in men with prostate cancer. Cancer Res 1995;55: 1937–1940.

26 La Spada AR, Wilson EM, Lubahn DB, Harding AE, Fischbeck KH: Androgen receptor gene mutations in X-linked spinal and bulbar muscular atrophy. Nature 1991;352:77–79.
27 Tut TG, Ghadessey FJ, Trifiro MA, Pinsky L, Yong EL: Long polyglutamine tracts in the androgen receptor are associated with reduced trans-activation, impaired sperm production, and male infertility. J Clin Endocrinol Metab 1997;3777–3782.
28 Coetzee GA, Ross RK: Prostate cancer and the androgen receptor. J Natl Cancer Inst 1994;86: 872–873.
29 Ingles SA, Ross RK, Yu MC, Irvine RA, La Pera G, Haile RW, Coetzee GA: Association of prostate cancer risk with genetic polymorphisms in vitamin D receptor and androgen receptor. J Natl Cancer Inst 1997;89:166–170.
30 Hardy DO, Scher HI, Bogenreider T, Sabbatini P, Zhang ZF, Nanus DM, Catterall JF: Androgen receptor CAG repeat lengths in prostate cancer: Correlation with age of onset. J Clin Endocrinol Metab 1996;81:4400–4405.
31 Stanford JL, Just JJ, Gibbs M, Wicklund KG, Neal CL, Blumenstein BA, Ostrander EA. Polymorphic repeats in the androgen receptor gene: Molecular markers of prostate cancer risk. Cancer Res 1997;57:1194–1198.
32 Giovannucci E, Stampfer MJ, Krithivas K, Brown M, Brufsky A, Talcott J, Hennekens CH, Kantoff PW: The CAG repeat within the androgen receptor gene and its relationship to prostate cancer. Proc Natl Acad Sci USA 1997; 94:3320–3323.
33 Hakimi JM, Schoenberg MP, Rondinelli RH, Piantadosi S, Barrack ER: Androgen receptor variants with short glutamine or glycine repeats identify unique subpopulations of men with prostate cancer. Clin Cancer Res 1997;3:1599–1608.
34 Monroe KR, Yu MC, Kolonel LN, Coetzee GA, Wilkens LR, Ross RK, Henderson BE: Evidence of an X-linked genetic component to prostate cancer risk. Nat Med 1995;1:827–829.
35 Narod SA, Dupont A, Cusan L, Diamond P, Gomez JL, Suburu R, Labrie F: The impact of family history on early detection of prostate cancer. Nat Med 1995;1:99–101.
36 Xu J, Meyers D, Freije D, Isaacs S, Wiley K, Nusskern D, Ewing C, Wilkens E, Bujnovszky P, Bova GS, Walsh P, Isaacs W, Schleutker J, Matikainen M, Tammela T, Visakorpi T, Kallioniemi OP, Berry R, Schaid D, French A, McDonnell S, Schroeder J, Blute M, Thibodeau S, Trent J, Grönberg H, Emanuelsson M, Damber JE, Bergh A, Jonsson BA, Smith J, Bailey-Wilson J, Carpten J, Stephan D, Gillanders E, Amundson I, Kainu T, Freas-Lutz D, Baffoe-Bonnie A, Van Aucken A, Sood R, Collins F, Brownstein M, Trent J: Evidence for a prostate cancer susceptibility locus on the X chromosome. Nat Genet 1998;20:175–179.
37 Lu J, Danielsen D: Short report on DNA marker at candidate locus: A *Stu*I polymorphism in the human androgen receptor gene. Clin Genet 1996;49:323–324.
38 Wang DG, Fan JB, Siao CJ, Berno A, Young P, Sapolsky R, Ghandour G, Perkins N, Winchester E, Spencer J, Kruglyak L, Stein L, Hsie L, Topaloglou T, Hubbell E, Robinson E, Mittmann M, Morris MS, Shen N, Kilburn D, Rioux J, Nusbaum C, Rozen S, Hudson TJ, Lipshutz R, Chee M, Lander ES: Large-scale identification, mapping, and genotyping of single-nucleotide polymorphisms in the human genome. Science 1998;280:1077–1082.

European Urology

Eur Urol 1999;35:362–369

Genetic and Environmental Factors in Prostate Cancer Genesis: Identifying High-Risk Cohorts

Peter Ekman

Department of Urology, Karolinska Hospital, Stockholm, Sweden

Key Words
Prostate Cancer · Genetics · Environment · Diet · Receptors

Abstract
Prostate cancer is the most common malignancy found in males; however, little is as yet known regarding what initiates the disease. The incidence is highest among American Blacks and lowest in the East Asian population. Subtypes of the disease include familial clustering and a hereditary form (9%) supporting genetic events to be involved in prostate cancer pathogenesis. Chromosomal abberations so far identified as being frequently occurring in this disease seem to be related to later phases of disease progression. However, research finding the responsible promoting genetic alteration is rapidly progressing. To explain the varied geographical distribution of the disease, the environment also has to be taken into account. Risk factors identified so far include obesity, animal fat, red meat consumption and certain toxins containing cadmium, while vegetables, cereals and vitamin D seem to be protective. It is reasonable to believe that, in the near future, we will be able to identify persons at risk of acquiring the disease and then inform them how to adjust their lifestyle to avoid early progression of the malignancy.

Introduction

Prostate cancer is the most common malignancy of the male and one of the most common causes of cancer death. The continuously increasing mean survival of man leads to an increasing incidence of the disease and also an increasing number of men dying from the disease. Despite improved facilities for early detection and escalating attempts to cure the disease at an early stage, the death rate has so far not been influenced.

Major efforts are presently being made to try to identify genetic events responsible for the evolution and progression of prostate cancer aiming at explaining racial differences and variations in familial incidence of the cancer. Epidemiological studies try to explain the sometimes surprising geographic variation in prostate cancer incidence.

This report attempts to update risk factors known or thought to be involved in prostate cancer genesis.

Familial Cancer

Credit for the awareness of prostate cancer to be a familial disease has to be given to the Mormones in Salt Lake City [1]. Their meticulous geneology archives contain a most valuable source as an aid in the research on family aggregations of various diseases. Already in 1960 familial clustering of prostate cancer was reported by Woolf [1], indicating a 3 times higher risk of a relative to a

KARGER

Fax + 41 61 306 12 34
E-Mail karger@karger.ch
www.karger.com

0302–2838/99/0356–0362$17.50/0

Accessible online at:
http://BioMedNet.com/karger

Peter Ekman, MD, PhD
Professor and Chairman
Department of Urology
Karolinska Hospital
S–171 76 Stockholm (Sweden)

prostate cancer proband to acquire the disease himself. The modern era starts with 1982, when Cannon et al. [2] and Meikle and co-workers [3, 4] independently reported on the high risk of brothers to probands to acquire prostate cancer themselves (a 2- to 4-fold increase over the expected) as compared with their brothers-in-law, who supposedly lived under similar environmental conditions.

The interest in familial prostate cancer has, thereafter, grown substantially and today the literature contains numerous reports on this very topic. In 1990, Steinberg et al. [5] reported a 2.1 times increased risk in prostate cancer families; a later study by Isaacs et al. [6] from the same institution modified this figure to 1.8. These authors also failed to find any relation to other cancers, like breast cancer (see below). Other recent studies from Sweden and Canada set the relative risk to 1.7 [7, 8].

The figure also depends on the relationship in the family: A first-degree relative (father or brother) gives an odds ratio (OR) of 2, a second-degree relative (uncle) gives an OR of 1.7. If one has a first-degree as well as a second-degree relative, the risk increases to 8.8 [5]. The risk is also related to the number of affected family members: In cases with only 1 relative (father or brother with prostate cancer) the OR is 2.0. It increases to 5 with 2 relatives and to 11 with 3 first-degree relatives [7].

Twin Study

A further support that the disease may be hereditary and not only due to a similar lifestyle can be attained from the studies by Grönberg et al. [9] from 1995. These investigators used the well-established Swedish 'Twin Registry' and investigated the frequency of prostate cancer in twin brothers. The concordance rate among heterozygotic twins was 0.043 (comparable to familial cancer), whereas the concordance rate in monozygotic twins was 0.192, that is almost 5 times higher. This figure is markedly higher than for breast cancer (0.125). Lifestyle was not particularly studied in this report, which may have influenced the results, however probably only marginally. Lifestyle and diet were assumed to be similar in both twin groups. The same investigators also reported that the risk of acquiring prostate cancer was much higher when the prostate cancer in the fathers was diagnosed before age 70 than after 70. In sons to elderly men at diagnosis no difference could be seen over time regarding the risk of acquiring prostate cancer, but remained at 2.0 as expected in familial prostate cancer. In sons to younger men at diagnosis a markedly higher risk was seen for the sons at younger ages to develop the disease, a risk which gradually decreased by increasing age [7].

A lot of efforts are made today to find 'the gene' which induces the development of prostate cancer, the gene which makes a person a potential prostate cancer candidate. We and others have demonstrated a frequent occurrence of deletions at loci on chromosomes 8p, 10pq, and 16q (plus 18q) in prostate cancer [10–13]. In recent studies we have demonstrated a close relation between local tumor progression and loss of parts of chromosome 8p [14].

Loss of Heterozygosity

Patients, subjected to radical prostatectomy, whose tumors had retained their LPL locus on chromosome 8p had only a 20% risk of tumor progression at 3 years as compared with 75% when LPL was lost [15]. The difference as measured from Kaplan-Meier curves was highly significant ($p < 0.01$). The same relation was not seen at all for deletions on 16q (n.s.). Deletions of parts of 16q is anyway of great interest since it harbors the E-cadherin gene [16]. As described by Umbas et al. [17], loss of the function of E-cadherin is likely to promote tumor metastatic spread, since the E-cadherin protein is involved in cell-cell adhesiveness. Studies from our own laboratory by Pan et al. [15] demonstrated loss of parts of 16q in 70% of the metastatic cases as compared with 35% in localized cases, and, possibly these 35% were at risk of metastatic spread. As yet it has not been possible to link losses of chromosome 10q to any particular phenomenon, except that it usually occurs late in the process. The same thing is – in prostate cancer – true for the most widely studied tumor suppressor gene candidate: p53 on chromosome 17p. Losses of the Rb 1 gene on chromosome 13q is a rather common and probably early phenomenon in prostate cancer. However, studies in our own laboratory [18] indicate that losses on 13q usually occur distal to the Rb 1 gene. In summary, it is not very likely that we will find much of a promoter gene in any of these well-identified regions, all usually being later events, occurring once the cancer is already established. Linkage analysis of these regions have also been invariably disappointing.

Hereditary Cancer

Using segregation analyses studying familial prostate cancer, investigators at the Hopkins Hospital in Baltimore were able to make a further distinction, separating prostate cancer clusters in families into familial, and into true hereditary prostate cancer [19, 20]. This rare disorder (about 9% of all prostate cancers) was first described by Carter et al. [19] in 1992. The disease has a dominant mendelian inheritance with high penetrance. The criteria are: more than 3 affected family members, or that it is occurring in three generations, or that 2 family members have developed the disease before age 55.

HPC1 Gene

By means of linkage analyses on 95 American and Swedish hereditary prostate cancer families, the group at Hopkins finally succeeded in identifying a major susceptibility locus for prostate cancer on chromosome 1,24. This gene locus was called 'human prostate cancer gene 1' (HPC1) [21]. The gene was involved in 30% of the cases of hereditary prostate cancers studied. In practice, this means that 1 out of 500 men are affected with this genetic defect, a small number but the discovery marks a significant breakthrough. Studies in other series have failed to confirm the results [22]. These authors conclude that perhaps the HPC1 was involved only in families with at least 4 affected members. Yet another group has also failed to confirm the result but instead pointed out the locus at 1q42.2-43 as being mainly responsible [23]. The group at Johns Hopkins has continued their search for other genes and quite recently found a second locus on chromosome X, calling this gene HPCX [24]. The fact that the gene is localized on the X chromosome means that a son to a father with this genetic defect will not inherit the risk. In contrast, the daughters in the family will have a 100% risk of becoming carriers, and 50% of their sons in turn will inherit the risk factor. In the coming years we will probably witness a number of new candidate loci. It would also be of great interest to see if loci identified have any importance in identifying risk cohorts in a nonhereditary prostate cancer series.

Breast Cancer

Breast cancer has many features in common with prostate cancer when it comes to incidence, pathology, and hormone responsiveness. Breast cancer also occurs in a familial form, however, not as markedly as prostate cancer. In breast cancer, 2 TSG candidates have been identified supposedly linked to familial cancer, named BRCA1 (on chromosome 17q [25]) and BRCA2 (on chromosome 13q). Tulinius et al. [26] reported a relative risk of 1.5 for relatives in familial breast cancer. They also reported that prostate cancer was the most common second malignancy related to familial breast cancer plus that the prostate cancers were invariably highly progressive [27–30].

Link: Breast-Prostate Cancer

Gao et al. [31] later supported the theory of a link between breast and prostate cancer by finding a high frequency of losses of the BRCA1 gene in prostate cancer, however this was not based on linkage analyses. Recently several reports have favored a link between breast and prostate cancer, indicating an increased risk for sons to mothers with breast cancer to develop prostate cancer, as well as an increased risk for daughters of fathers with prostate cancer to develop breast cancer.

Murakami et al. [32] further confirmed the findings of frequent loss of heterozygosity of 17q in prostate cancer, and was also able to decrease the tumorigenicity of the prostate cancer cell line PPC-1 by transferring normal BRCA1 genes into it. Later, however, in the most recent report by Williams et al. [33] from the same group, it was notified that the loss was not exactly at the BRCA1 locus, but rather a bit distal from it. This is in complete agreement with data from our own laboratory in which, by using PCR-SSCP technique, no indications of losses at the BRCA1 locus could be demonstrated [18]. There also does not seem to be any link between the BRCA2 gene, located at the long arm of chromosome 13 (13q) and prostate cancer. As mentioned above, Isaacs et al. [6] also failed to find any relation between prostate and breast cancer. Moreover, the group in Umeå found a poor relation between familial breast and prostate cancer. These are so far unpublished data, in summary though, the true link between breast and prostate cancer is in doubt and needs further proof.

Environment

The wide difference in incidence of prostate cancer between Westerners and Asians has been well known and always looked upon as a genetic phenomenon. However, more intriguing has been to try to explain why the incidence of prostate cancer is getting so much higher in Japanese men living in the US, as described by Haenszel and Kurihara [34]. Apparently there must be some difference in lifestyle between East Asians and the Western culture, including dietary factors.

Incidence

In 1992, Carter et al. [35] reported that prostate cancer, indeed, was as common in Japan as in the US; however, the prostate cancer usually remained latent and seldom progressed to clinical cancer in Japan. Apparently some hitherto unknown factors might protect from tumor progression while others may induce this phenomenon. Attempts have been made to explain the difference also by using molecular genetic techniques. It has been reported by Watanabe et al. [36] and Konishi et al. [37] that p53 mutations are crucial for the evolution of clinical prostate cancer; this mutation is much more rare in Japanese men. Of interest is also the report by Takahashi et al. [38] demonstrating that androgen receptor mutations were more common in latent prostate cancer than in clinically manifest cancer. The hypothesis brought forward was that the mutation means a dead-end for the latent prostate cancer, effectively blocking further cellular expansion and progression.

CAG Repeats

The androgen receptor (AR) gene, located on the X-chromosome, is known to be polymorphic, having a highly variable trinucleotide microsatellite of CAG repeats in exon 1. The numbers of CAG repeats vary greatly in the population, with normal numbers ranging between 8 and 31, and average about 20 [39]. The longer AR variants have decreased transactivation activity and recently they were also shown to have decreased binding affinity for androgens [40]. This functional difference might be the factor associated with increased prostate cancer risk, since reduced androgen responsiveness of the long AR variants may be protective to the prostate, whereas the relative increased responsiveness of the short variants might predispose the prostate to chronic androgen overstimulation and a higher risk of developing cancer [41]. Several observations suggest indirectly that variation in the AR polyglutamine length, by modulating androgen activity, influences prostate carcinogenesis. African-Americans, who have generally shorter CAG repeat lengths in the AR, have a higher incidence and mortality rate from prostate cancer [42]. The AR is located on the X-chromosome, and evidence that prostate cancer has an X-linked genetic component is that a higher risk of prostate cancer occurs if a man's sibling rather than his father is affected with the disease [1, 5].

In a study by Ingles et al. [43] including 57 cases and 169 controls – men carrying an AR CAG allele with fewer than 20 repeats versus an allele with 20 or more repeats had an adjusted OR of 2.1 for prostate cancer. Results from the Harvard group provide strong evidence that the shorter AR CAG repeat lengths predict higher grade and more advanced stage of prostate cancer at diagnosis, and metastases and mortality from the disease.

IgF1 Levels

Recently, in a case-control study, a remarkable correlation was shown between the IgF levels in serum and the risk of developing prostate cancer. It has been shown that androgens can regulate the levels of growth-stimulating proteins and thereby modulate the IgF1 levels. On the other hand, IgF1 as well as IgF2 can upregulate the production of androgens from adrenals via the IgF1 receptor. This is possibly an important source of androgen stimulation in patients who fail following surgical or medical castration.

Epidemiology

Epidemiological data have to be intrepreted with caution. If one does not have large enough series, just by chance significant differences may occur. Several factors may coincide in the same group – the true underlying cause not being identified. Also the statistics when calculating relative risk (RR), OR and standard incidence ratio is tricky. A situation with an OR of 1.5 but with a range of 0.95–4.5 is not statistically significant because the lower figure has to be over 1.0. However, a much lower value like 1.2 may become significant if the range is 1.05–1.35.

Fat

Fat consumption is probably the most widely investigated parameter linked to risk of developing prostate cancer. Data by Key [44], reviewing the literature, found a mean RR of 1.25 in obese men in general. Meat, milk and total fat equaled at 1.3. In particular it seemed as if animal fat consumers suffered the greatest risk with a RR of 1.54. Vegetable fat in contrast seemed not to be linked at all to prostate cancer risk, and cereals even seemed to have a protective role; less prostate cancer was seen in cereals consumers [45, 46]. Grönberg et al. [47] found a clear relation between heavy eating in general and prostate cancer. As a consequence, body mass index was significantly related. Red meat was also a significant risk factor. Experimental data support the importance of fat in prostate carcinogenesis. Dunning tumors in rats fed a fat-free diet grew significantly slower [48, 49]. Hormone levels in South African Blacks increased significantly when they were given a Western diet [50].

Carrots

Other factors which have been discussed are the consumption of vegetables, in particular carrots. Men consuming large amounts of carrots had a RR value of only 0.66 [44]. A comparison was made with men treated with purified carotene, data accumulated from a carotene cancer prevention study [44]. Surprisingly, carotene as such had little influence on the disease (RR 0.99), so apparently there was something else in the carrots that protects from prostate cancer, or other factors in the lifestyle of carrot consumers. In 1988, Oishi et al. [51] reported a RR value of 2.13 in men with low carotene intake as compared with controls, however, these authors also based their calculations on food containing carotene. These authors also found a link to a low dietary intake of vitamin A – RR value 1.94. Somewhat confusing, however, also men with an extremely high intake of vitamin A suffered an increased risk of developing prostate cancer, possibly the 'therapeutic window' is small [52].

Phytoestrogens

The dramatic difference in incidence of clinical prostate cancer in Japanese men as compared to Caucasians may not be only explained by subjecting ourselves to various risk factors, but may, as well, be due to differences in protecting factors. There is a wide difference in consumption of various phytoestrogens (lignans and isoflavonoids) which are common in various legumes, grains, and, in particular, soyabeans. Another rich source of phytoestrogens, in particular isoflavonoids, is rye. A diet rich in rye products is popular in the north-eastern part of Finland, an area known to have the lowest prostate cancer incidence in the country [53]. A recent study using the Dunning R3327 prostate adenocarcinoma animal model showed that rats fed a rye bran or heat-treated rye bran diet or soy fluor grow much slower than tumors in control animals [54]. The experiments have also been carried out using the LNCaP human prostate cancer cell line inoculated into nude mice. Animals fed a diet rich in rye hardly noticed any tumor progression as compared with control animals. However, when fat was added to the rye diet, the protective role of rye vanished [55].

Sexual Activity

Being an important genital organ it has been tempting to link prostate cancer to a vigorous sexual life [56]. The literature indeed contains some reports indicating that sexually more active men do have a higher likelihood of getting prostate cancer. Early sexual debut, venereal diseases, and number of partners before marriage have been supposed to increase the risk of acquiring prostate cancer. Theoretically, viral diseases (HPV) should be the source of pathogenesis [57]. However, more interesting would have been to instead study sexual activity during the marriage. In studies by Jackson et al. [58], Zumoff et al. [59] and Drafta et al. [60], it was found that testosterone values were higher in males suffering from prostate cancer than controls, even though the literature varies on this point [61, 62]. It is possible that sexually active men do enjoy a different hormonal milieu, which unfortunately also may increase their risk of getting prostate cancer. Young Blacks have been reported to have higher testosterone values than their White comrades [63, 64]. After all it is tempting to believe that there is something in the hormonal milieu which stimulates prostate cancer development. It should be remembered that there is a long lag period between tumor induction and clinical cancer, hence, our data on serum hormone levels in elderly men may be misleading [65].

Nuclear Power

Radiation from nuclear power has been blamed to cause serious diseases including several malignant disorders. In a small study from England, 136 nuclear power plant employees were investigated [66]. It was found that the power plant workers had a 2.36 times higher risk of developing prostate cancer than expected from a control population. The main risk factors were supposedly tritiated chromium, iron, cobalt, and, perhaps most importantly, zinc.

Sun

UV radiation has also been linked to prostate cancer. Data from Schwartz and Hulka [67] and Hanchette and Schwartz [68] demonstrated an almost identical geographical variation of UV radiation and incidence of prostate cancer in the US, in an inverse relationship. The further south, the more sun, the less cancer of the prostate. The explanation should supposedly be via vitamin D. The surplus of vitamin D we get through various food suppliers etc. is a fraction compared with what the sun gives us [69]! Vitamin D_3 inhibits cell growth, both in vitro and in vivo [70, 71]. It has also been shown that vitamin D_3 causes rodent prostate cancer cells to differentiate to a less malignant phenotype and that the expression of the c-myc oncogene is inhibited [72, 73].

Vitamin D Receptor and Polymorphism

In recent years, it has become clear that the active form of vitamin D, $1,25(OH)^2D$, causes both antiproliferative and prodifferentiation responses in prostate cancer cell lines [74]. There is also evidence from epidemiologic studies that a high $1,25(OH)^2D$ level in blood decreases the risk of prostate cancer [75]. The human vitamin D receptor is known to have polymorphisms that result in individual variation in the circulating level of vitamin D receptor-regulating protein, osteocalcin [76]. The vitamin D receptor polymorphism, recently reported to be associated with increased risk of prostate cancer, is due to an increased number of adenosines in a poly-A tract. In a study by Ingles et al. [43], the long vitamin D receptor alleles (with poly-A >18) were associated with a 4.6-fold greater risk of prostate cancer.

A surprising phenomenon has been the low incidence of prostate cancer in Central Africa as compared with the world's highest incidence in the genetic matches of North America [77]. A speculation has been that men living in Central Africa do very little to protect themselves from the burning sun, whereas Blacks in the US do very little to get some extra tan in summertime. Black people have more melanin under the skin than Whites, which protects them from the sunshine and the production of vitamin D. The prostate cancer incidence, age-matched, is very low in Central Africa (4–10/100,000), increases in South Africa (23/100,000), to reach its maximum in North America (60–65/100,000). These data are from the 1970s; more recently it has been suggested that the true incidence of prostate cancer in Central Africa is heavily underestimated. However, M'Buyamba-Kabangu et al. [78] found that among Zairians moving to Belgium, the serum level of vitamin D was directly related to the time they had spent in the country, continuously getting lower.

Farming

Against the sun theory speaks the increased risk of prostate cancer reported among farmers despite prostate cancer being rarer in rural than in urban areas [79]. Farmers are likely to spend quite some time outdoors – and are exposed to the sun. However, farmers are indeed today exposed to several other risk factors in their work with herbicides, pesticides and fertilizers. It seems from a report by Wiklund and Dich [80, 81] including 20,025 farmers that it was mainly those employed as pesticide workers, who suffered the increased risk of getting prostate cancer, the younger ones having a 2.03 times increased risk. The increased risk has been supposed to be associated with the exposure to cadmium, a common ingredient in fertilizers. Cadmium has been reported to interfere with the vitamin D synthesis, hence, a plausible link to the UV radiation theory [82–84].

Conclusion

In conclusion, a substantial amount of promising research is going on at various centers. Using modern techniques like linkage analyses in familial and hereditary prostate cancer, an increasing number of responsible genes are likely to be found, and exploring other new techniques in the explosively developing world of molecular genetics, further important progress is to be expected. In studies of environmental factors, which are bound to be of great importance, epidemiologists seem to eventually be making progress and make the various pieces in this marvellous jigsaw puzzle fit. So, in the near future, identified high-risk carriers know how to adjust their lifestyle to delay the onset, and possibly retard the progress of the disease as long as possible.

References

1 Woolf CM: An investigation of familial aspects of carcinoma of the prostate. Cancer 1960;13: 739–744.

2 Cannon L, Bishop DT, Skolnick M, Hunt S, Lyon JL, Smart CR: Genetic epidemiology of prostate cancer in the Utah Mormon Genealogy. Cancer Surv 1982;1:47–69.

3 Meikle AW, Stanish WM: Familial prostatic cancer risk and low testosterone. J Clin Endocrinol Metab 1982;54:1104–1108.

4 Meikle AW, Smith JA, West DW: Familial factors affecting prostatic cancer risk and plasma sex-steroid levels. Prostate 1985;6:121–128.

5 Steinberg GD, Carter BS, Beaty TH, Childs B, Walsh PC: Family history and the risk of prostate cancer. Prostate 1990;17:337.

6 Isaacs SD, Kiemeney LALM, Baffoe-Bonnie A, Beaty TH, Walsh PC: Risk of cancer in relatives of prostate cancer probands. J Natl Cancer Inst 1995;87:13.

7 Grönberg H, Damber L, Damber JE: Familial prostate cancer Sweden. A nation-wide register cohort study. Cancer 1996;77:138–143.

8 Aprikian AG, Bazinet M, Plante M, Meshref A, Trudel C et al: Family history and the risk of prostatic carcinoma in a high risk group of urological patients. J Urol 1995;154:404–406.

9 Grönberg H, Damber L, Damber JE: Studies of genetic factors in prostate cancer in a twin population. J Urol 1994;152:1484–1489.

10 Carter HB, Piantadosi S, Isaacs JT: Clinical evidence for and implications of the multistep development of prostate cancer. J Urol 1990; 143:742–746.

11 Carter BS, Ewing CM, Ward SW et al: Allelic loss of chromosome 16q and 10q in human prostate cancer. Proc Natl Acad Sci USA 1990; 87:8751–8755.

12 Bergerheim USR, Kunimi K, Collins VP et al: Deletion mapping of chromosomes 8, 10 and 16 in human prostatic carcinoma. Genes Chrom Cancer 1991;3:215–220.

13 Kunimi K, Bergerheim USR, Larsson IL et al: Allelotyping of human prostatic adenocarcinoma. Genomics 1991;11:530–536.

14 Matsuyama H, Yi P, Yoshihiro S, Häggarth L, Chunde L, Tribukait B et al: Deletion of chromosome 8p22 for the development of disease progression in prostate cancer. Cancer Res, submitted.

15 Pan Y, Matsuyama H, Naining W, Yoshihiro S, Häggarth L et al: Chromosome 16q24 deletion and decreased E-cadherin expression: Possible association with metastatic potential in prostate cancer. Prostate 1998;36:31–38.

16 Cher ML, Ito T, Weidner N, Carroll PR et al: Mapping of regions of physical deletion on chromosome 16q in prostate cancer cells by fluorescence in situ hybridization (FISH). J Urol 1995;153:249–254.

17 Umbas R, Schalken JA, Aalders TW, Carter BS, Karthaus H et al: Expression of the cellular adhesion molecule E-cadherin is reduced or absent in high-grade prostate cancer. Cancer Res 1992;52:5104–5109.

18 Chunde L, Larsson C, Futreal A, Lancaster J et al: Identification of two distinct deleted regions on chromosome 13 in prostate cancer. Oncogenes 1998;16:481–487.

19 Carter BS, Beaty TH, Steinberg GD, Childs B, Walsh PC: Mendelian inheritance of familial prostate cancer. Proc Natl Acad Sci USA 1992; 89:3367.

20 Bastacky SI, Wojno KJ, Walsh PC, Carmichael MJ, Epstein JI: Pathological features of hereditary prostate cancer. J Urol 1995;153:987–992.

21 Smith JR, Freier D, Carpten J, Grönberg H et al: Major susceptibility locus for prostate cancer on chromosome 1 suggested by a genomic wide search. Science 1996;274:1371–1373.

22 Eels RA, Durocher F, Edwards S, Teare D et al: Linkage analysis of chromosome 1q markers in 136 prostate cancer families. Am J Hum Genet 1998;62:633–638.

23 Barriton P, Valerie A, Kenakenile A, Drellan E et al: Predisposing gene for early-onset prostate cancer, localized on chromosome 1q 42.2-43. Am J Hum Genet 1998;62:1416–1424.

24 Xu J, Schleutker J, Berry R, Grönberg H, Smith J et al: Evidence for a prostate cancer susceptibility locus on the X chromosome. Nat Genet 1998;20:175–179.

25 Hall JM, Lee MK, Newman B, Morow JE, Anderson LA: Linkage of early-onset familial breast cancer to chromosome 17q21. Science 1990;250:1684–1689.

26 Tulinius H, Eglsson V, Olafsdóttir GH, Sigvaldason H: Risk of prostate, ovarial and endometrial cancer among relatives of breast cancer patients. BMJ 1992;305:855–857.

27 Arason A, Barkardóttir RB, Egilsson V: Linkage analysis of chromosome 17q markers and breast-ovarian cancer in Icelandic families, and possible relationship to prostatic cancer. Am J Hum Genet 1993;52:711–717.

28 Xiang G, Zacharek A, Salkowski A, Grignon DJ, Sakr W et al: Loss of heterozygosity of the BRCA1 and other loci on chromosome 17q in human prostate cancer. Cancer Res 1995;55: 1002–1005.

29 Anderson DE, Badzioch MD: Familial effects of prostate and other cancers on lifetime breast cancer risk. Breast Cancer Res Treat 1993;28: 107–113.

30 Sellers TA, Potter JD, Rich SS, Drinkard CR, Bostick RM: Familial clustering of breast and prostate cancers and risk of postmenopausal breast cancer. J Natl Cancer Inst 1994;86:24.

31 Gao X, Zacharek A, Salkowski A, Grignon DJ, Wael S, Porter AT, Honn KV: Loss of heterozygosity of the BRCA1 and other loci on chromosome 17q in human prostate cancer. Cancer Res 1995;55:1002–1005.

32 Murakami YS, Brothman AR, Leach RJ, White RL: Suppression of malignant phenotype in a human prostate cancer cell line by fragments of normal chromosomal region 17q. Cancer Res 1995;55:3389–3394.

33 Williams BJ, Jones E, Xiao LZ, Steele MR, Stephenson RA et al: Evidence for a tumor suppressor gene distal to BRCA1 in prostate cancer. J Urol 1996;155:720–725.

34 Haenszel W, Kurihara M: Studies of Japanese migrants. I. Mortality from cancer and other diseases among Japanese in the United States. N Natl Cancer Inst 1968;40:43–68.

35 Carter HB, Piantadosi S, Isaacs JT: Clinical evidence for and implications of the multistep development of prostate cancer. J Urol 1990; 143:742–746.

36 Watanabe M, Ushijima T, Kaiuchi H, Shiraishi T, Yatani R et al: p53 gene mutations in human prostate cancers in Japan: Different mutations spectra between Japan and Western Countries. Jpn J Cancer Res 1994;85:904–910.

37 Konishi N, Hiasa Y, Hayashi I, Matsuda H, Tsuzuki T et al: p53 mutations occur in clinical, but not latent, human prostate carcinoma. Jpn J Cancer Res 1995;86:57–63.

38 Takahashi H, Furusato M, Allsbrook WC Jr, Niishii H, Wakui S et al: Prevalence of androgen receptor gene mutations in latent prostatic carcinomas from Japanese men. Cancer Res 1995;55:1621–1624.

39 Edwards A, Hammond HA, Lin J, Caskey CT, Chakraborty R: Genetic variation at five trimeric and tetrameric tandem repeat loci in four human population groups. Genomics 1992;12: 241–253.

40 McLean HE et al: Abnormal androgen receptor binding affinity in subjects with Kennedy's disease (spinal and bulbar muscular hypertrophy). J Clin Endocrinol Metab 1995;80:508–516.

41 Irvine RRA et al: The CAG and GGC microsatellites of the androgen receptor gene are in linkage disequilibrium in men with prostate cancer. Cancer Res 1995;55:1937–1940.

42 Coetzee GA, Ross RK: Re: Prostate cancer and the androgen receptor. J Natl Cancer Inst 1994; 86:872–882.

43 Ingles SA, Ross RK, Yu NC, Irvine RA et al: Association of prostate cancer risk with genetic polymorphism in vitamin D receptor and androgen receptor. J Natl Cancer Inst 1997;89: 166–170.

44 Key T: Risk factors for prostate cancer. Cancer Surv 1995;23:63.

45 Kolonel LN: Nutrition and prostate cancer. Cancer Causes Control 1996;7:83–94.

46 Morton MS, Griffiths K, Blacklock N: The preventive role of diet in prostatic disease. Br J Urol 1996;77:481–493.

47 Grönberg H, Damber L, Damber JE: Total food consumption and body mass index in relation to prostate cancer risk: A case-control study in Sweden with prospectively collected exposure data. J Urol 1996;155:969–974.

48 Clinton SK, Palmer SS, Spriggs CE et al: Growth and Dunning transplantable prostate adenocarcinomas in rats fed diets with various fat contents. J Nutr 1988;118:908.

49 Pollard M, Luckert PH: Promotional effects of testosterone and dietary fat on prostate carcinogenesis in genetically susceptible rats. Prostate 1985;6:1.
50 Hill P, Wynder EL, Garbaczewski L, Garnes H, Walker ARP: Diet and urinary steroids in black and white North American men and black South African men. Cancer Res 1979;39:5101.
51 Oishi K, Okada K, Yoshida O, Yamabe H, Ohno Y et al: A case-control study of prostatic cancer with reference to dietary habits. Prostate 1988;12:179–190.
52 Kolonel LN, Hankin JH, Yoshawa CN: Vitamin A and prostate cancer in elderly men: Enhancement of risk. Cancer Res 1987;47: 2982–2985.
53 Kleemola P, Virtanen M, Pietinen P: The 1992 diet survey of Finnish adults, vol B2/1994. Helsinki, Helsinki National Public Health Institute, Department of Nutrition, 1994.
54 Landström M, Zhang JX, Hallmans G, Åman P et al: Inhibitory effects of soy and rye diets on the development of Dunning R3327 prostate adenocarcinoma in rats. Prostate 1998;36: 151–161.
55 Bylund A, Zhang JX, Bergh A, Damber JE et al: Rye bran and soy protein delay growth and increase apoptosis of human LNCaP prostate adenocarcinoma in nude mice. Submitted.
56 Steele R, Lees REM, Kraus AS et al: Sexual factors in the epidemiology of cancer of the prostate. J Chron Dis 1971;24:29–37.
57 Sitas F: Geographical epidemiology of prostate cancer: Is there an association with infection? Cancer Surv 1995;23:79.
58 Jackson MA, Ahluwalia BS, Herson J et al: Characterization of prostatic carcinoma among blacks: A continuation report. Cancer Treat Rep 1977;61:167–172.
59 Zumoff B, Levin J, Strain GW et al: Abnormal levels of plasma hormones in men with prostate cancer: Evidence toward a 'two-disease' theory. Prostate 1982;3:579–588.
60 Drafta D, Proca E, Zamfir V et al: Plasma steroid levels in benign prostatic hypertrophy and carcinoma of the prostate. J Steroid Biochem 1982;17:689–693.
61 Harper ME, Peeling WB, Cowley T et al: Plasma steroid and protein hormone concentrations in patients with prostatic carcinoma, before and during oestrogen therapy. Acta Endocrinol 1976;81:409–426.
62 Habib FK, Lee IR, Stich SR et al: Androgen levels in the plasma and prostatic tissues of patients with benign hypertrophy and carcinoma of the prostate. J Endocrinol 1976;71:99–107.
63 Schuman LM, Mandel J, Blackard C et al: Epidemiologic study of prostatic cancer: Preliminary report. Cancer Treat Rep 1977;61:181–186.
64 Rotkin ID: Studies in the epidemiology of prostatic cancer: Expanded sampling. Cancer Treat Rep 1977;61:173–180.
65 Krain LS: Some epidemiologic variables in prostatic carcinoma in California. Prev Med 1974;3:154–159.
66 Rooney C, Beral V, Maconochie N, Fraser P, Davies G: Case-control study of prostatic cancer in employees of the United Kingdom Atomic Energy Authority. BMJ 1993;307: 1391–1397.
67 Schwartz GG, Hulka BS: Is vitamin D deficiency a risk factor for prostate cancer? Anticancer Res 1990;10:1307–1312.
68 Hanchette CL, Schwartz GG: Geographic patterns of prostate cancer mortality. Cancer 1992;70:2861–2869.
69 Preece MA, Tomlinson S, Ribot CA, Pietrek J, Korn HT et al: Studies of vitamin D deficiency in man. Q J Med 1975;176:575–589.
70 Eisman JA, Barkla DH, Tutton PJ: Suppression of in vivo growth of human solid tumor xenografts by 1α,25-dihydroxyvitamin D_3. Cancer Res 1987;47:21–25.
71 Abe M, Miyayra C, Sakagami H et al: Differentiation of mouse myeloid leukemia cells induced by 1α,25-dihydroxyvitamin D_3. Proc Natl Acad Sci USA 1981;78:4990–4994.
72 Chida K, Hashiba H, Fukushima M, Suda T, Kuroki T: Inhibition of tumor promotion in mouse skin by 1α,25-dihydroxyvitamin D_3. Cancer Res 1985;45:5426–5430.
73 Reitsma PH, Rothberg PG, Astrin SM et al: Regulation of myc gene expression in HL-60 leukaemia cells by a vitamin D metabolite. Nature 1983;306:4992–4994.
74 Peehl DM et al: Antiproliferative effects of 1,25-dihydroxyvitamin D_3 on primary cultures of human prostatic cells. Cancer Res 1994;54: 805–810.
75 Corder EH, Guess HA, Hulka BS, Friedman GD, Sadler M et al: Vitamin D and prostate cancr: A prediagnostic study with stored sera. Cancer Epidemiol Biomarkers Prev 1993;2: 467–472.
76 Morrison NA et al: Contribution of trans-acting factor alleles to normal physiological variability: Vitamin D receptor gene polymorphism. Proc Natl Acad Sci USA 1992;89:6665–6669.
77 Kovi J, Heshmat MY: Incidence of cancer in Negroes in Washington, DC, and selected African cities. Am J Epidemiol 1972;96:401–413.
78 M'Buyamba-Kabangu JRM, Fagard R, Lijnen P, Bouillon R, Lissens W, Amery A: Calcium, vitamin D-endocrine system, and parathyroid hormone in black and white males. Calcif Tissue Int 1987;41:70–74.
79 Morrison H, Savitz D, Semenciw R, Hulka B, Yang M et al: Farming and prostate cancer mortality. Am J Epidemiol 1993;137:270–280.
80 Wiklund K, Dich J: Cancer risks among male farmers in Sweden. Eur J Cancer Prev 1995;4: 81–90.
81 Dich J, Wiklund K: Prostate cancer in pesticide applicators in Swedish agriculture. Prostate 1998;34:100–112.
82 Piscator M: Role of cadmium in carcinogenesis with special reference to cancer of the prostate. Environ Health Perspect 1981;40:107–120.
83 Larsson SE, Lorentzon T: The effect of cadmium exposure on vitamin D metabolism; in Norman A (ed): Vitamin D and Problems Related to Uremic Bone Disease. Berlin, de Gruyter, 1975, pp 67–73.
84 Waalkes MP, Rehm S: Cadmium and prostate cancer. J Toxicol Environ Health 1994;43: 251–269.

Genetic and Environmental Factors in Prostate Cancer Genesis

European Urology

Eur Urol 1999;35:370–376

Epidemiology of Prostate Cancer Chemoprevention

Peter Boyle Gianluca Severi

Division of Epidemiology and Biostatistics, European Institute of Oncology, Milan, Italy

Key Words
Prostate cancer · Epidemiology · Chemoprevention · Ageing

Abstract
In absolute terms, prostate cancer is a public health problem of major and increasing importance particularly as the population ages. Prostate cancer control comprises a series of actions ranging from primary prevention, through screening to improvements in therapy for prostate cancer. An exciting approach lies in the possibility of chemoprevention to reverse the process of carcinogenicity and prevent prostate cancer by this route. Indeed, there are several very interesting ideas being tested at this moment. One major difficulty is the long length of time which can elapse between exposure and the time at which clinical cancer can be found and diagnosed. In cases where delays are long, then preventative treatment should be initiated at an early age. This, and many other issues, current in prostate cancer, are rendered problematic by the age distribution of prostate cancer in the population. Although it is decreasing now, around the early 1990s, the median age of diagnosis of prostate cancer was around 75 in some European countries although considerably lower in population groups in the United States. The median age at death is between 77 and 80 in most countries. These special circumstances must be taken into account when discussing clinical trials of chemoprevention of prostate cancer. The importance of developing reliable intermediate endpoints which can be used in such studies in highlighted.

Introduction

Prostate cancer is an important public health problem with over a quarter of a million new cases diagnosed world-wide in the single year 1985 [Parkin et al., 1993]. It was predicted that in the USA alone, 40,400 men would die of prostate cancer in 1995, while in the countries of the European Community it accounts for more than 35,000 deaths each year [Wingo et al., 1995; Jensen et al., 1990].

The incidence of the disease is increasing rapidly in most regions of the world [Alexander and Boyle, 1994] and will pass 500,000 cases annually by the end of this century if risk remains fixed at 1980 levels or will reach 700,000 if the observed trends in increase continue [Boyle, 1994]. Whereas there are large increases in the incidence of prostate cancer apparent throughout the world, the mortality rate has remained constant in generations of men born since the early years of this century [Boyle et al., 1995].

The evidence that prostate cancer risk has important environmental determinants is compelling. Briefly, different populations around the world experience different levels of prostate cancer and these levels change with time usually in an orderly and predictable manner: international variation in incidence is around two orders of magnitude [Boyle et al., 1995]. However, when migration takes place groups of migrants tend to acquire the prostate cancer pattern of their new home [Haenszel and Kurihara, 1968]. Furthermore, groups within a community whose lifestyle habits differentiate themselves from other members of the same community generally have notably

KARGER
Fax + 41 61 306 12 34
E-Mail karger@karger.ch
www.karger.com

0302–2838/99/0356–0370$17.50/0

Accessible online at:
http://BioMedNet.com/karger

Peter Boyle, PhD
Division of Epidemiology and Biostatistics
European Institute of Oncology, Via Ripamonti, 435
I–20141 Milan (Italy)
Tel. +39 02 57 48 98 15, Fax +39 02 57 48 98 13

different prostate cancer rates, e.g. Seventh Day Adventists and Mormons [Boyle and Zaridze, 1993]. For reasons such as these it is widely accepted that the risk of prostate cancer has environmental determinants, defining 'environment' in its broadest sense to include a wide range of lifestyle factors including dietary, social and cultural factors. Although these are theoretically avoidable, for prostate cancer no avoidable causes have been clearly identified although a large number of factors have been investigated.

The prostate gland is regarded as a primarily androgen-dependent gland controlled essentially by levels of plasma testosterone, of which 90–95% of the daily 6–7 mg production is synthesized and secreted by the testes [Lipsett, 1970]. In research directed to the search for endocrine or biochemical factors that could be implicated in prostatic carcinogenesis, determination of steroid and peptide hormone concentrations in plasma of patients with the disease has failed to consistently identify any endocrine disturbance, or any difference from the normal asymptomatic male which could lead to a greater understanding of prostate cancer aetiology [Griffiths and Khoury, 1994]. Although it is clear that the 'causes' of prostate cancer are hormonal in origin, at the present time there is no consistent evidence of any primary endocrine disturbance that is necessarily implicated in the aetiology of prostate cancer. Further, there is little known with certainty regarding the environmental determinants of prostate cancer risk. However, despite this situation there have been some clues of sufficient strength to consider interventions in otherwise healthy men to reduce their incidence of prostate cancer. These are described in some of the chapters in this volume and will not be dealt with here.

Public Health Importance of Prostate Cancer: 2000

In many countries of the world, prostate cancer is the second most common form of cancer in men [Boyle, 1994]. If the prevalence of the prostate cancer is defined to include cancer patients who are alive between up to 5 years after diagnosis, there are estimated 1,014,000 patients throughout the world with prostate cancer, who require medical care, which comprise approximately 16% of all 5-year prevalent cancer cases in males. Of these prostate cancer prevalent cases, 896,000 originated in developed and 118,000 in developing countries [Parkin et al., 1995]. In developed countries prostate cancer is the most prevalent malignancy in males primarily because of high incidence of the localized tumours and relatively good survival.

The incidence of prostate cancer is increasing steadily in many countries around the world. The highest increase in incidence rates is reported from the African-American population in the USA with an overall increase taking place in most western countries. Although the incidence of prostate cancer is remarkably lower in the developing world, the increase is also quite substantial [Boyle et al., 1995].

In the twelve Member States of the European Community in 1980, it was estimated that there were 85,000 new cases of prostate cancer, making this the second commonest form of cancer (after lung cancer) in men [Jensen et al., 1990]. In the USA, prostate cancer has overtaken lung cancer in terms of absolute incidence although it remains second to lung cancer as a cause of cancer death [Wingo et al., 1995]. Most importantly, given that in several countries the increased number of children born after World War II will be in their mid-50s in the early part of the 20th century (at an age when cancer risk is becoming an important consideration) and coupled with the trends in increasing life expectancy [see Brody, 1985] for example, the consequence will be an increase in absolute terms in the number of cases of prostate cancer diagnosed [Boyle, 1994]. In the absence of treatment improvements and with prospects for prevention by modification of lifestyle remote within current knowledge, there will also be an increase in the number of deaths from prostate cancer world-wide. The situation would be further augmented by the presence of a temporal trend in risk which is widely reported from many countries and unlikely to be entirely artefact [Boyle, 1994].

The number of cases of prostate cancer in the year 2000 and beyond are set to increase. For a disease which currently presents more than 15% lifetime risk in North Americans, knowledge of risk factors is extremely limited and, consequently, prospects for primary prevention are poor. The rise in the number of cases of prostate cancer requiring treatment will have important implications for the provision of treatment facilities including the training and supply of specialists competent to treat these patients. If it stopped here, it would merely reflect an economic challenge but, unfortunately, increased numbers of cases will bring with it increased numbers of deaths from the disease. The prospects for preventing the situation building up for the year 2000 are poor and work in hand today needs to progress to help limit the impact of the continuing expansion in absolute numbers of cases set to take place throughout the early decades of the next century.

For this reason, prostate cancer of great importance in public health, a major effort is required to reduce the impact of these unavoidable increases.

Impact of the Ageing of the Population on the Prostate Cancer

Life expectancy at birth has increased dramatically throughout this century. In many westernized countries, life expectancy of a boy or girl born today can be expected to approach 80 years. Over the coming years physicians are likely to see an increased number of patients reporting prostatic problems simply because the world population is ageing. By the year 2020, up to a 200% increase of the population over 65 years of age is expected [Kirby et al., 1994]. At the start of this century, only 25% of the US population lived to 65 years of age. Currently, 70% are living to this age, with 30% reaching their eighth decade. Before the end of this century, life expectancy is likely to exceed 80 years in several countries [Brody, 1985], and every other man can expect to reach an age when he has a 40% chance of developing clinical prostate cancer. Furthermore, the post-World War II baby boom is approaching the age of 50 and early next century will attain an age when both cancer and lower urinary tract symptoms (LUTS) becomes an important health concern. Sadly there has been little work undertaken to quantify the impact of this ageing process in years to come. However, the effect of the ageing which has already gone on is evident in the increasing burden of urological cancers around the world.

The ageing of the US population has been well described by Brody [1985]. In Europe, less work has been done although some data are available from United Nations publications in recent years. In qualitative terms it is clear where the major changes will take place in the elderly population in Europe:

(1) In *Northern Europe,* the all-ages population will increase between 1975 and 2000 by 3% in men and 2% in women. The population of Northern Europe for those over 60, will increase by 4% in men and 1% in women.

(2) In *Western Europe,* the overall changes will be 3% in men and 1% in women. However, in the over 60 years, there will be major changes with a 20% increase in men and an 11% increase in women.

(3) In *Eastern Europe,* the all-ages population will increase by 15% in men and 13% in women. Lower life expectancy will limit the increases in the over 60 years population to 12% in both sexes.

(4) In *Southern Europe,* the all-ages population will increase by 15% in men and 14% in women. The over 60 population will increase by 24% in men and 27% in women.

With a disease so strongly linked to age, such as is the case with prostate cancer, the greatest qualitative increase in the absolute numbers of cases of prostatic diseases will be experienced in Southern Europe with substantial increases taking place also in Eastern Europe and in men in Western Europe, the latter related to the loss of life in generations who experienced the two major wars which Europe experienced this century.

Prostate Cancer Control

The ultimate goal of all cancer research and cancer treatment is to prevent people dying from the disease in question. Knowledge has been accruing regarding actions and interventions which *could* lead to a reduction in death from prostate cancer either by reducing the risk of developing the disease, identifying the disease at a stage when it is more curable or by improving the outcome of therapy. Such a package of actions is aimed at prostate cancer control, where progress will eventually come through contributions from the various elements of a control and prevention strategy.

One potential contributory factor could be screening, particularly with prostate-specific antigen (PSA) testing, although it is difficult to imagine a more controversial issue in public health or oncology at present than whether widespread testing for PSA should be widely applied as a screening test for prostate cancer. In the absence of completed randomized trials, the medical community and the general public depend on the reasoned arguments of experts in the field for guidance. There is a very wide range of opinion, ranging from those who advocate widespread PSA testing in the population to those, equally informed, who believe that there are no circumstances in which PSA testing should be conducted.

The accepted criteria for screening [Wilson and Jungner, 1969] are still unfulfilled in certain respects for prostate cancer [Schröder and Boyle, 1993] although there has been a continual progress in our understanding of prostate cancer in recent years. There is a need for results from randomized trials and these are underway. There is also need for data regarding prostate cancer incidence and mortality from areas where a large proportion of the relevant male population has been screened (at least over half) and cancer registration and mortality data are fairly complete. The group of articles recently published in the *Annals of Oncology* present a series of opinions about key questions in prostate cancer screening at the present time [Barry, 1998; Svetec and Thompson, 1998; de Konig and Schröder; Neal and Donovan, 1998; Ciatto et al., 1998; Boyle, 1998b]. Each stops short of recommending general population screening based on the available evidence and outlines a series of supporting arguments. But the situation is not so straightforward that men can be told to hold-off having a PSA measured until findings from randomized studies become available early next century. There will certainly be men whom the urologist feels should be tested and there will be many men, increasingly informed by the Internet, who will request to be tested. Such men must make an informed decision in discussion with their physician.

The concept of chemoprevention is that by administering a compound to individuals without the disease in question, the probability that they will develop the disease is thereby reduced. There are several potential study designs for testing a potential chemotherapeutic agent. Observational studies are the most frequently used study design in epidemiology. This type of study is characterized by the lack of control which the investigator has over which treatment is assigned to each study subject. Undoubtedly, randomized clinical trials are the best method of providing evidence of the relative efficacy of cancer prevention strategies. One major consequence of this conclusion is that such evaluations will be of necessity long and expensive.

However, it is extremely important when designing a cancer prevention trial to pay close attention to the biological features of carcinogenesis. Although the precise mechanism and time course of carcinogenesis is not known for any form of cancer, there is strong evidence that the process may take a considerable time for some cancers. Thus, there can frequently be a long period between exposure and the appearance of the cancer: this will have consequences for prevention trials aimed at intervening on some risk factor. For example, age at menarche is a widely accepted risk factor for breast cancer, but breast cancer is uncommon before the age of 30; cigarette smoking is commonly initiated before the age of 20 but lung cancer may not appear for 20–40 years following the initiation of exposure, and asbestos exposure is held to cause mesothelioma if the individual was exposed to asbestos and at least 20–40 years have passed since exposure was initiated.

Events involved in the carcinogenic process are identified into early-stage and late-stage factors [Bertram et al., 1987]: historically this was referred to the periods of initiation and promotion (table 1). When considering cancer control, the focus is not the disease ('cancer') but rather it is the process ('carcinogenesis'): this has been well described by Sporn [1993]. The whole issue of design for prevention trials is summarized below but is well laid out elsewhere in considerable detail [Piantadosi and Byar, 1989].

Table 1. Conceptual outline of carcinogenesis indicating where preventive strategies could occur and where to target cancer prevention studies [from Bertram et al., 1987]

Primary prevention	Initiation	
Secondary prevention	Promotion	Prevention trials
Tertiary prevention	Pre-cancer	
Screening		
Treatment	Cancer	Treatment trials

Primary prevention trials are designed to prevent initiation and these trials would be expected to be the largest because the further to the beginning of the process we go, the lower the risk of developing cancer. Examples of primary prevention trials include smoking prevention among teenagers, avoidance of sunlight or use of sun blocks to prevent malignant melanoma or skin cancer, and possibly some dietary modifications. *Secondary prevention* attempts to remove or effect promoting factors. Examples may include smoking cessation, changes in diet or the use of a micronutrient or trace metal supplement. *Tertiary prevention* trials are those designed to test the effects of interventions on preneoplastic lesions such as leukoplakia of the mouth, cervical and oesophageal dysplasia or early skin cancers.

There have been five phases of research on cancer control established [Greenwald and Cullen, 1985]: Phase I, the phase of hypothesis development; Phase II, the phase of methods development; Phase III, the phase of intervention trials; Phase IV, the phase of defined-population studies, and Phase V, the implementation phase of results and conclusions as policy.

The initial trials of pharmacological agents in humans are usually referred to as Phase I studies; such studies are usually to obtain basic information on permissible doses and toxicity. This phase is relevant for cancer prevention trials using trace elements, drugs or other agents which could conceivably have toxicity. Such studies are not needed for trials involving modification of lifestyle such as smoking cessation or dietary changes.

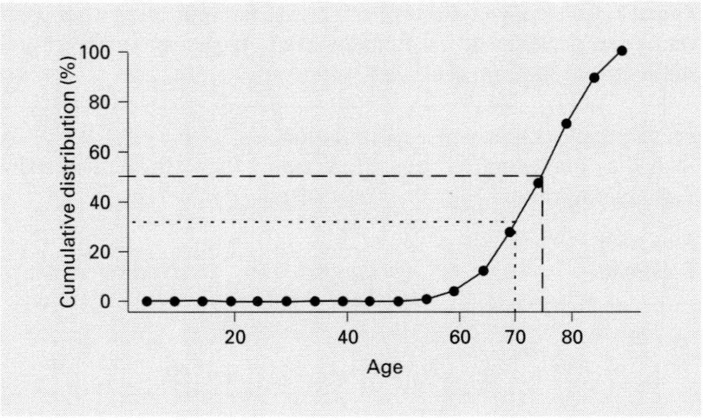

Fig. 1. Prostate cancer incidence in England and Wales, 1988–1990.

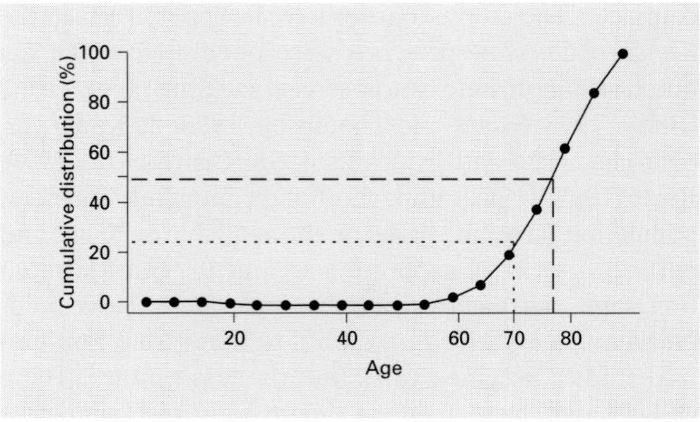

Fig. 2. Prostate cancer mortality in England and Wales, 1988–1990.

In the therapeutic model of pharmacological agents, Phase II studies attempt to estimate response rates when, for example, a chemotherapeutic agent is administered to subjects with different kinds of cancer. This phase of research generally only applies to tertiary cancer prevention studies when agents may be tried in small uncontrolled trials to determine whether or not they have any effect on preneoplastic lesions.

The role of Phase I and Phase II studies in the process of evaluating some preventive strategies in humans has been supplemented by epidemiological studies which have demonstrated convincingly several associations such as those between cigarette smoking and lung cancer or increased fat intake and colorectal cancer.

Phase III studies are generally designed to compare promising therapies to no treatment or placebo, to standard treatment or to each other. The methodology for designing and conducting Phase III studies of cancer treatments translates directly to the issues in many cancer prevention trials.

Phase IV studies are concerned primarily with long-term safety and efficacy. This idea is an important one to consider for cancer prevention studies. Although most preventive agents are believed to have low toxicity, their administration over a long period of time to a large population will almost certainly result in some unanticipated effect in a subgroup of subjects. In the language of cancer prevention studies, Phase IV studies are termed 'defined population studies'. Phase V studies apply interventions to a population at large and are intended to reduce cancer rates by a widespread application of proven methods.

There are several major consequences of the differences between prevention trials and treatment trials which are essential to consider before contemplating a chemoprevention trial. The ideas for treatment trials come from a variety of sources such as drug screening, basic research in surgery, radiation medicine, immunology and molecular genetics whereas many of the ideas for prevention trials come from findings from epidemiological studies or animal experiments. Treatment trials employ interventions such as chemotherapy, surgery, radiation, biologic response modifier, gene therapy and hormonal therapy whereas prevention trials employ methods such as lifestyle change or treatment with micronutrients, vitamins and hormones. Therefore, treatment trials require the substantive expertise of oncologists, surgeons, radiotherapists and immunotherapists whereas prevention trials are more likely to require substantive input from social psychologists and nutrition experts.

However, the most important difference between Phase III trials of treatment and prevention is likely to be in the sample size, where treatment trials are relatively small, involving between 100 and 1,000 subjects in each arm of the study followed for 3 months to 5 years and costing hundreds of thousands of dollars, whereas prevention trials require to be much larger involving thousands to millions of subjects per arm of the study and with a follow-up extending to 5–15 years (or more) and costing millions to tens of millions to over 100 million dollars.

Chemoprevention Trials of Prostate Cancer

Once there is a good hypothesis and a strong candidate intervention, the first concept to define is at what stage of the carcinogenesis process the intervention needs to be made. This has immediate consequences for the size and duration of the study because the earlier that intervention is required the larger the sample size requires to be and the longer the follow-up since it is farther from the stage of clinical cancer. The situation is further complicated by the age structure of prostate cancer in the community.

For example, consider prostate cancer incidence in England and Wales between 1988 and 1990 [Parkin et al., 1997]. For the 3 years covered by these data, the *effective* population is 74 million men, corresponding (approximately) to a country with a total population of 160 million. During this period, there were 38,317 incident cases of prostate cancer diagnosed in this population. Of these, there were 140 (0.37% of the total) incident cases before age 50 in this population and 1,690 (4.41%) incident cases before age 60 in this population. The median age of cases was 75.5 (fig. 1). Similarly with regard to mortality data for the same period of time, there were 23,417 deaths from prostate cancer in this population of which there were 59 (0.25% of all prostate cancer deaths) deaths before age 50 in this population and 648 (2.77%) deaths before age 60 in this population. The median age at death was 78 (fig. 2). This is similar in other populations around the same time period (table 2).

Consequently, the population selected for an intervention trial of prostate cancer needs to be older, since the disease occurs at a later age, and larger, since there are many more competing causes of death at older age groups than for any other form of cancer. These trials will, by definition, be among the most complicated of randomized clinical trials to conduct.

Table 2. Median age at death and median age at diagnosis for prostate cancer in the world

	Median age at death	Median age at diagnosis
Australia	77.15	73.90
Australia, Victoria		74.56
Canada	77.96	72.92
Italy	78.48	
Italy, Varese		75.05
France	80.41	
France, Calvados		72.99
Denmark	77.54	75.10
Norway	79.05	75.52
Sweden	78.64	74.95
Scotland	77.75	74.94
USA, San Francisco, Non-Hispanic White		72.40
USA, San Francisco, Black		71.54
USA, Detroit, White		71.91
USA, Detroit, Black		71.23
USA, SEER, White		72.36
USA, SEER, Black		70.79
USA	78.01	

The estimates are computed using data from WHO, from Cancer Incidence in Five Continents VII (IARC Lyon 1997). Mortality generally refers to 1992 and incidence to 1988–1992 data.

Conclusions

Within conventional study designs, it is obvious that prevention trials are more complicated (sample size, duration, costs) than treatment trials. Furthermore, the unusual age structure of prostate cancer introduces an extra layer of complexity and these trials will be notoriously difficult to mount and to run properly: the implications for costs are enormous.

We live in exciting times. It appears that there are applications for chemoprevention which could be of significance for cancer control. There is a great need at the present time for research to develop nontoxic compounds and to develop them in a systematic manner on a biological basis. For breast cancer we have not reached our goal yet, but appear to be on the right pathway. For prostate cancer we are at an earlier phase of developing this research.

Better measures, biological markers of intermediate endpoints, and improved statistical methodologies are required to make essential trials more feasible. It is neither practical, realistic nor, arguably, ethically appropriate, to have to commit to a number of large mega-trials, involving large numbers of subjects followed up for a very long period of time. The alternative must be to prioritize the identification of intermediate endpoints, frequently referred to as biological markers. This must be our current research priority in the area of chemoprevention, particularly in the context of prostate cancer.

Acknowledgements

It is a pleasure to acknowledge that this was conducted within the framework of support from the Associazione Italiana per la Ricerca sul Cancro (Italian Association for Research on Cancer).

References

Alexander FE, Boyle P: The rise in prostate cancer: Myth or reality? In Garraway MJ (ed): The Epidemiology of Prostate Diseases. Edinburgh, Churchill Livingstone, 1994.

Auvinen A, Tammela T, Stenman UH et al: Screening for prostate cancer using serum prostate-specific antigen: A randomised, population-based pilot study in Finland. Br J Cancer 1996; 74:568–572.

Barry MJ: PSA screening for prostate cancer: The current controversy. A viewpoint. Ann Oncol 1998;9:1279–1282.

Bertram JF, Kolonel LN, Meyskens FL: Strategies and rationale for chemoprevention of cancer in humans. Cancer Res 1987;47:3012–3031.

Boyle P: Prostate cancer 2000: Evolution of an epidemic of unknown origin; in Denis L (ed): Prostate Cancer 2000. Heidelberg, Springer, 1994, pp 5–11.

Boyle P: Invited discussant of Labrie et al (ref 8). Los Angeles, ASCO, 1998a.

Boyle P: PSA screening for prostate cancer: The current controversy. Ann Oncol 1998b;9: 1263–1264.

Boyle P, Maisonneuve P, Napalkov P: Geographical and temporal patterns of incidence and mortality from prostate cancer. Urology 1995; 46:47–55.

Boyle P, Napalkov P, Barry MJ, Bishop DT, Correa R, Gu FL, Guess H, Jacobsen S, Kiemeney LA, Nagy G, O'Leary M, Padley R, Pontes E, Richard F, Saitoh M, Vesey SG: Epidemiology and natural history of prostate cancer; in Murphy G, Denis L, Chatelain C, Griffiths K, Khoury S, Cockett AT (eds): First International Consultation on Prostate Cancer, Monaco, June 20–21 1996. Scientific Communication International Ltd, 1997, pp 1–29.

Boyle P, Zaridze DG: Risk factors for prostate and testicular cancer. Eur J Cancer 1993;29:1048–1055.

Brody J: Prospects for an aging population. Nature 1985;315:463–466.

De Konig HJ, Schröder FH: PSA screening for prostate cancer: The current controversy. Ann Oncol 1998;9:1293–1296.

Griffiths K, Khoury S (eds): Primer on Molecular Control of Prostate Growth. Whitehouse Station, NJ, Merck & Co. Inc., 1994.

Greenwald P, Cullen JW: The new emphasis in cancer control. J Natl Cancer Inst 1985;74: 543.

Haenszel W, Kurihara M: Studies of Japanese migrants. I. Mortality from cancer and other diseases among Japanese in the United States. J Natl Cancer Inst 1968;40:43–68.

Jensen OM, Esteve J, Moller H, Renard H: Cancer in the European Community and its member states. Eur J Cancer 1990;26:1167–1256.

Kirby R, Fitzpatrick J, Kirby M, Fitzpatrick A: A shared care for prostatic diseases. ISIS Medical Media, 1994.

Kramer BS, Brown ML, Prorok PC et al: Prostate cancer screening: What we know and what we need to know. Ann Intern Med 1993;119:914–923.

Labrie F, Dupont A, Candas B et al: Decrease of prostate cancer death by screening: First data from the Quebec prospective and randomised study. 1998 ASCO Proc, Los Angeles. Am Soc Clin Oncol 1998;17:2A.

Lancet News: PSA screening said to reduce prostate cancer deaths, or does it? Lancet 1998;351: 1563.

Neal DE, Donovan JL: Screening for prostate cancer. Ann Oncol 1998;9:1289–1292.

Parkin DM, Pisani P, Ferlay J: Estimates of the world-wide incidence of eighteen major cancers in 1985. Int J Cancer 1993;54:594–606.

Parkin DM, Pisani P, Ferlay J: Worldwide burden of cancer; in Biennial Report 1994–1995. Lyon, IARC, 1995, pp 14–15.

Parkin DM, Muir CS, Whelan S, Gao YT, Ferlay J, Powell J (eds): Cancer incidence in five continents, vol VI: IARC Sci Publ No 120. Lyon, IARC, 1992.

Piantadosi S, Byar DP: Design of prevention trials; in Moon TE, Micozzi MS (eds): Nutrition and Cancer Prevention: Investigating the Role of Micronutrients. New York, Dekker, 1989, pp 441–472.

Schröder F, Boyle P: Screening for prostate cancer: Necessity or nonsense? Eur J Cancer 1993;5: 656–661.

Sporn MB: Chemoprevention of cancer. Lancet 1993;342:1211–1213.

Svetec D, Thompson IM: PSA screening. Current controversy. Ann Oncol 1998;9:1283–1288.

Wilson JMG, Jungner G: Principles and Practice of Screening for Disease. Publ Health Paper No 34. Geneva, WHO, 1969.

Wingo PA, Tong T, Bolden S: Cancer statistics 1995. CA Cancer J Clin 1995;45:8–30.

Zappa M, Ciatto S, Bonardi R, Mzzotto A: Overdiagnosis of prostate carcinoma by screening: An estimate based on the results of the Florence Screening Pilot Study. Ann Oncol 1998;9: 1297–1300.

Genetic and Environmental Factors in Prostate Cancer Genesis

European Urology

Eur Urol 1999;35:377–387

Diet and Its Preventive Role in Prostatic Disease

L. Denis[a] M.S. Morton[b] K. Griffiths[b]

[a]Oncology Centre, Antwerp, Belgium, and [b] Tenovus Cancer Research Centre, University of Wales College of Medicine, Cardiff, UK

Key Words
Diet · Prostate cancer · Chemoprevention · Phyto-oestrogens

Abstract
Asian men have much lower incidences of prostate cancer and possibly of benign prostatic hyperplasia (BPH) than their Western counterparts. Vegetarian men also have a lower incidence of prostate cancer than omnivorous males. Both Asian and vegetarian men consume low-fat, high-fibre diets which provide a rich supply of weak dietary oestrogens. These plant or phyto-oestrogens have been proposed as chemopreventive agents, particularly for Asian men and to a lesser extent, for vegetarian men also. The three principal classes of phyto-oestrogens are the isoflavonoids, flavonoids and lignans. Many foods of plant origin contain varying amounts of these compounds and hundreds of plants manifest some degree of oestrogenic activity. Soya, a dietary staple in many parts of Asia, is a major source of the isoflavonoids, daidzein and genistein. Flavonoids are present in high concentration in many fruits, vegetables and crop species. In particular, apigenin and kaempferol are regarded as major flavonoids because of their common occurrence in plants, and their significant concentrations when present. Apples, onions and tea-leaves are excellent sources of flavonoids. Plant lignans are present in many cereals, grains, fruits and vegetables, and give rise to the mammalian lignans, enterodiol and enterolactone; however, the richest source is linseed (flaxseed) and other oilseeds. In addition to their oestrogenic activity, many of these plant compounds can interfere with steroid metabolism and bioavailability, and also inhibit enzymes, such as tyrosine kinase and topoisomerase, which are crucial to cellular proliferation.

Introduction

The marked differences in the incidence of certain types of cancer between various countries or regions of the world suggest that particular dietary factors can influence the biological processes related to carcinogenesis, either in a provocative or an inhibitory role. Estimates of the proportion of cancers attributable to dietary status habit vary from 10 to 70% [1–3], but data continues to accumulate supporting a role for such dietary factors [4, 5] and, although often contradictory, a pattern is recognizable which directs attention to the potential benefits for healthcare of preventative studies related to the intake of these factors. This relationship between dietary status and cancer has recently been reviewed [6].

KARGER

Fax + 41 61 306 12 34
E-Mail karger@karger.ch
www.karger.com

0302–2838/99/0356–0377$17.50/0

Accessible online at:
http://BioMedNet.com/karger

L. Denis, MD
Apartment 2, Block H
Lange Gasthuisstraat 35–37
B–2000 Antwerp (Belgium)
Tel. +32 3 202 7872, Fax +32 3 231 7477, E-Mail louis.denis@skynet.be

That geographical differences in cancer incidence are attributable to diet is supported by changes observed in the incidence rates in migrants who move from areas of low risk for particular cancers to countries where the risk is higher [7–9]. Such changes are illustrated by data from the migration of Japanese and Chinese men and women to Hawaii and to mainland USA, whose risk of developing prostate or breast cancer, previously low, increases to match that of the indigenous population within a few generations.

Miller et al. [5] considered that appropriate dietary changes could decrease the incidence of various cancers by reducing fat intake and increasing vegetable consumption in the case of breast and colorectal cancers, by reduction of obesity for endometrial cancer and diminishing intake of cured meats, salt-preserved foodstuffs and nitrite, whilst increasing fruit and vegetable consumption, in the case of stomach cancer. Such views are controversial [10, 11], particularly with regard to the relationship between dietary fat intake and cancer risk [10, 12].

Cancers of the prostate and breast, cardiovascular disease and osteoporosis feature prominently as 'Western diseases'. The Western diet is characterized by high animal fat content and protein and low in fibre, which contrasts with the diet of the Asian communities which is low in animal fat and rich in starches, legumes, fruit and vegetables – all of which have a high fibre content (fig. 1). Predictably, therefore, animal fat is readily seen as a *causative factor.* More recently, however, it has been the recognition [6,13] that *certain constituents of the Asian diet and that of the Mediterranean region protect against the development of these diseases,* and it is the lack of these constituents in the Western diet which is the important factor.

Some Geographical Differences in Prostate Cancer Incidence Rates

Carcinoma of the prostate belongs to the group of hormone-dependent cancers, those of breast, ovary and endometrium, the incidence and mortality rates of which are high in the Western world, relative to those in Asia and in Mediterranean countries (fig. 2).

Already prostatic cancer is recognized as a serious healthcare problem, one of the most commonly diagnosed cancers in the West [14, 15], with the lifetime risk in North American men being nearly 10%. A recent report [16] indicates that carcinoma of the prostate is now the second most common cancer after skin cancer in the male population of the USA and the second most common cause of death from cancer, after that of the lung. The highest mortality rates occur in the Black male population of the USA, twice that of the Whites [17–19]. The rate is 30 times less in Osaka, Japan and 120 times less in Shanghai, China, than that of Black males in North America [14, 20–22]. The low prevalence of prostate cancer in Japan is noteworthy, since their mean life expectancy and socio-economic standards are as high as their counterparts in the West. The incidence in Japan is, however, rising and Japanese migrants to the USA manifest an increased risk to approximately half that of the indigenous Americans[14, 23].

Since prostate cancer, as well as benign prostatic hyperplasia (BPH), clinically present over the age of 50, the prevalence of both later in life in relation to the increasing life expectancy in developed countries suggests that prostate disease will become an even more formidable health problem in the next millennium and emphasizes the importance of preventative measures.

Some Aspects of Dietary Status in Relation to Cancer Aetiology

The Western diet is deficient in fibre and evidence supports the concept that high fibre intake protects against colorectal cancer [24], possibly mammary cancer [25]. Vegetables are a source of fibre, but their protective role [26, 27] may now additionally be attributable to other *non-nutrient components* of plant products [28–30].

The belief that prostate cancer risk was related to a high animal fat intake merely originated from international rates of prostate cancer mortality [31, 32] with the positive correlation between occurrence and mortality, and per capita fat consumption. The United States Health Professionals Follow-Up Study of 47,855 men aged 40–75 [33] was one of the first studies to include an adjustment for total caloric intake. Total animal fat consumption was directly related to the risk of advanced cancer, although the linear trend fell just short of acceptable statistical significance. Other studies, however [34–36], failed to find this association. Moreover, dietary fat did not influence the incidence of experimental prostate cancer [37], although total caloric intake rather than percentage fat, was

Fig. 1. General characteristics of Western and Eastern diets.
Fig. 2. Highest and lowest incidence rates recorded world-wide for prostate cancer, breast cancer, endometrial cancer and ovarian cancer.

1

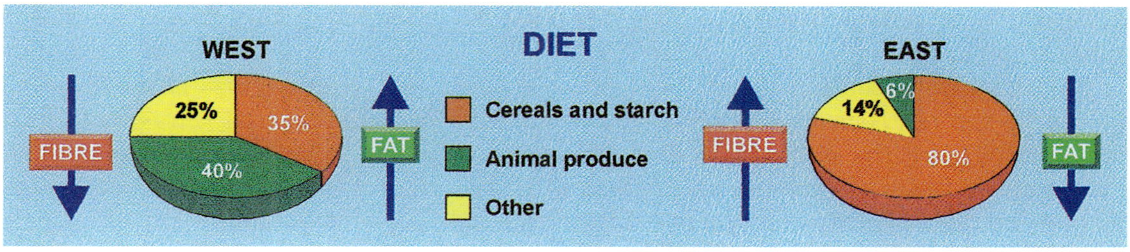

DIET
WEST
EAST
FIBRE
FAT
25%
35%
40%
Cereals and starch
Animal produce
Other
14%
6%
80%

2

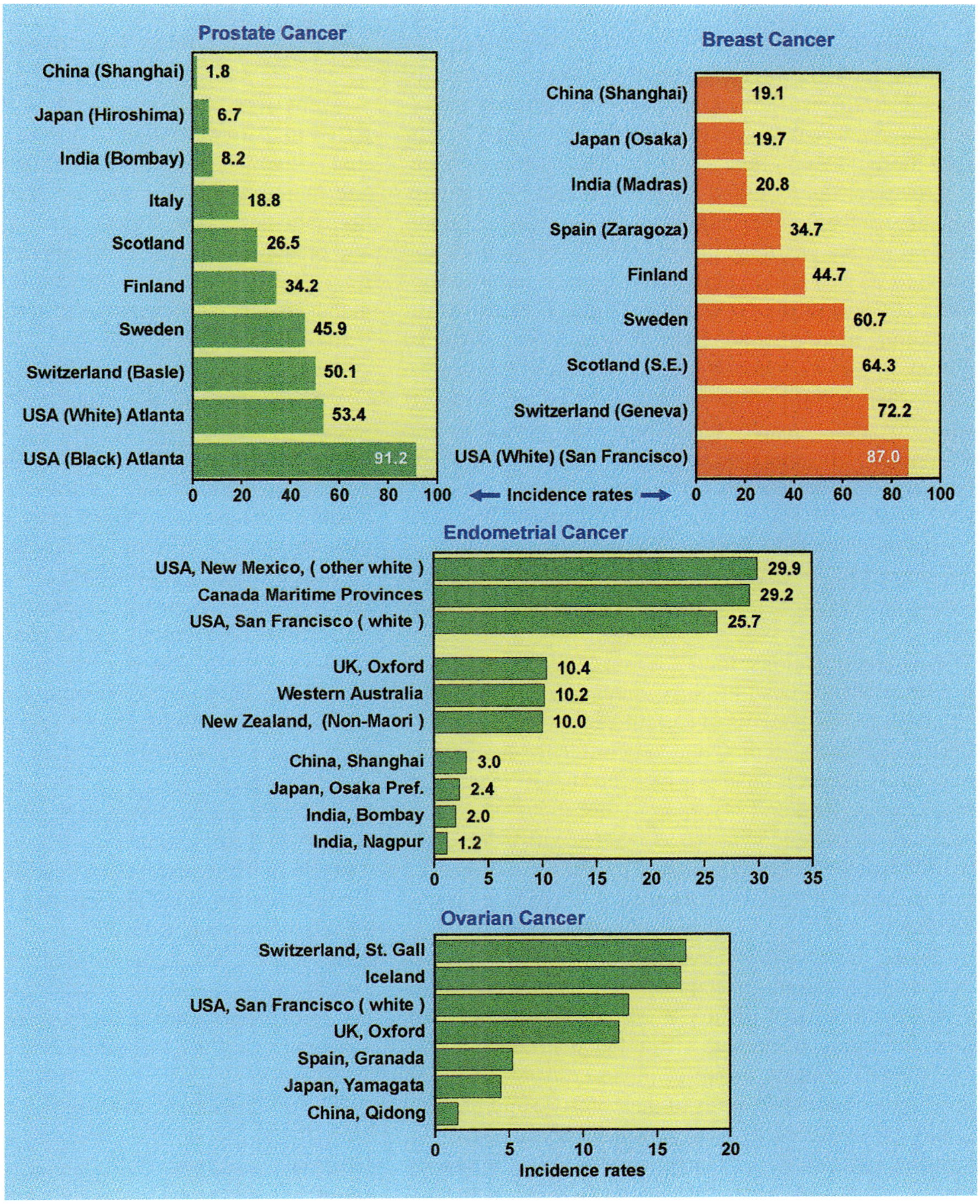

Prostate Cancer
China (Shanghai) 1.8
Japan (Hiroshima) 6.7
India (Bombay) 8.2
Italy 18.8
Scotland 26.5
Finland 34.2
Sweden 45.9
Switzerland (Basle) 50.1
USA (White) Atlanta 53.4
USA (Black) Atlanta 91.2
0 20 40 60 80 100
Incidence rates
Breast Cancer
China (Shanghai) 19.1
Japan (Osaka) 19.7
India (Madras) 20.8
Spain (Zaragoza) 34.7
Finland 44.7
Sweden 60.7
Scotland (S.E.) 64.3
Switzerland (Geneva) 72.2
USA (White) (San Francisco) 87.0
0 20 40 60 80 100
Endometrial Cancer
USA, New Mexico, (other white) 29.9
Canada Maritime Provinces 29.2
USA, San Francisco (white) 25.7
UK, Oxford 10.4
Western Australia 10.2
New Zealand, (Non-Maori) 10.0
China, Shanghai 3.0
Japan, Osaka Pref. 2.4
India, Bombay 2.0
India, Nagpur 1.2
0 5 10 15 20 25 30 35
Ovarian Cancer
Switzerland, St. Gall
Iceland
USA, San Francisco (white)
UK, Oxford
Spain, Granada
Japan, Yamagata
China, Qidong
0 5 10 15 20
Incidence rates

associated with tumorigenesis, a concept supported by Albanes [38] in man.

Epidemiologists tend to support the hypothesis that prostate cancer risk is increased by high levels of dietary fat. Unfortunately, few studies have used a satisfactory dietary methodology and putative associations are thereby weakened. Most failed to adjust for total caloric intake and made little reference to fruits, vegetables and cereals – rich sources of the non-nutrient components of the typical Asian diet [6, 13] and referred to as *phyto-oestrogens.*

Some have, however, reported a protective effect of vegetables against the risk of cancer, in particular, a 17-year Japanese cohort study [39–41] of 265,118 adults, aged more than 40 years, which investigated the relationship between lifestyle and disease risk. Daily consumption of green-yellow vegetables was found to be an important protective factor against cancers of the stomach and prostate, as well as ischaemic heart disease, atherosclerosis and liver cirrhosis. Green-yellow vegetables, defined as containing more than 600 μg of carotene/100 g, included pumpkin, carrots, spinach, green lettuce and green asparagus. The mortality from cancer of the breast was lower with increased consumption of soya bean paste soup and soya milk. Hirayama [39] speculated that β-carotene and possibly *other components of soya beans and vegetables* were implicated in the reduction of mortality. In a case-control study on the effects of diet on breast cancer risk in Singapore [42], noteworthy was the finding that soya protein was recognized as a protective component of the diet.

Both investigations, therefore, suggested the potential influence of soya bean products on cancer risk and drew attention to components of certain vegetables, present in the traditional Asian diet, that may influence carcinogenesis. In a study of Japanese men in Hawaii, Stemmermann and co-workers [34] reported that an increased consumption of rice and soya was associated with a decreased risk of prostate cancer. Soya-based foods such as tofu are a rich source of the phyto-oestrogens referred to as isoflavonoids [6, 13].

Several investigators have also demonstrated significant strong negative correlations between mortality from prostate cancer and dietary intake of cereals [43, 44]. Cereals contain precursors of the lignans found in men and women, another group of phyto-oestrogens [6, 45]. Furthermore, a cohort study of diet, lifestyle and prostate cancer in Seventh-Day Adventist men revealed that increasing consumption of beans, lentils, peas, tomatoes, raisins, dates and other dried foods were all associated with significantly decreased prostate cancer risk [46]. The Mediterranean-style diet, considered protective against endocrine cancer as well as cardiovascular disease [47, 48], features a high intake of fresh fruit, vegetables and pasta. Fresh fruit, citrus fruits and raw vegetables were found to be protective against many cancers, including that of the prostate, in several Italian studies [49–51].

The Phyto-Oestrogens: The Isoflavonoids, Flavonoids and Lignans

Many foods of plant origin contain constituents referred to as *isoflavonoids, flavonoids and lignans* (fig. 3), some of which possess weak oestrogenic activity (fig. 4) and therefore the potential for exerting an influence on hormone-dependent cancers such as those of the breast and prostate [6]. They can be equated with tamoxifen, the weakly oestrogenic agent universally used in breast cancer management. The presence of nonsteroidal substances with oestrogenic activity in certain foodstuffs of plant origin has been long recognized [52, 53]. Soya bean and red clover, members of the leguminosae family, are major sources of isoflavonoids [53]. Soya is consumed daily in large amounts in China and Japan and traditional diets of the Indian subcontinent, Africa, some Mediterranean countries and South America, have a high legume content including soya, lentils and chickpeas [53].

Soya beans contain the glycoside conjugates of the isoflavonoids, genistein and daidzein and their methylated derivatives, biochanin A and formononetin (fig. 5). These can be metabolized by the enzymes of the normal microflora of the gut to the aglycones, genistein and daidzein, which are then absorbed and appear in blood and ultimately in urine, primarily as glucuronide conjugates, and also sulphates [6].

The lignans also constitute a group of diphenolic compounds of plant origin [53, 54]. The plant precursors, matairesinol and secoisolariciresinol, are metabolized after ingestion by intestinal microflora to give rise to the weakly oestrogenic enterolactone and enterodiol respectively (fig. 6). The lignans are absorbed from the gut to appear in blood and other body fluids. The precursors of the lignans are found in many cereals, grains, fruits and vegetables but the richest source is linseed (flaxseed) [55].

The isoflavonoids and lignans are found in various body fluids [6], in urine, plasma, saliva and in semen. Expressed prostatic fluid contains enterolactone and equol [56], suggesting that dietary oestrogens can accumulate in the prostate and are components of prostatic secre-

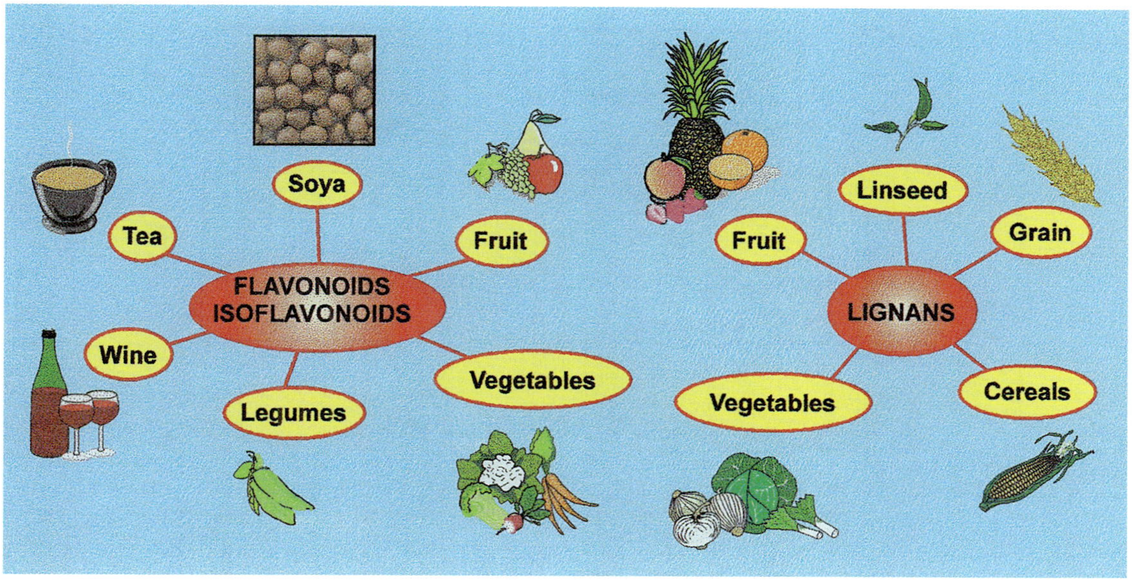

3

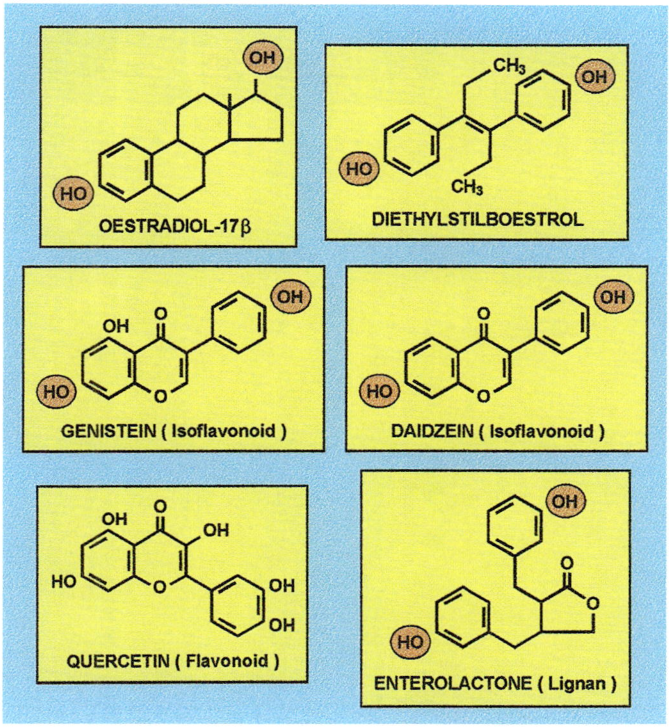

4

Fig. 3. Diagrammatic representation of certain sources of flavonoids, isoflavonoids and lignans.

Fig. 4. Relationship between the chemical structures of 17β-oestradiol, the synthetic oestrogen diethylstilboestrol and weak dietary oestrogens.

tion along with proteins such as prostate-specific antigen (PSA). The levels of isoflavonoids are high in the urine and plasma of the Japanese and Chinese men and women (fig. 7). Lignans and isoflavonoids are also excreted in large amounts in the urine of vegetarians [57] who consume large quantities of whole grain cereals, vegetables and fruits and who also have a lower incidence of prostate cancer than the general Western population.

Biological Effects of Phyto-Oestrogens: Relevance to the Prevention of Prostatic Disease

Oestrogenic Activity

Enterolactone, daidzein and genistein have a weak oestrogenic activity [58], although anti-oestrogenic properties have also been described. They compete with oestra-

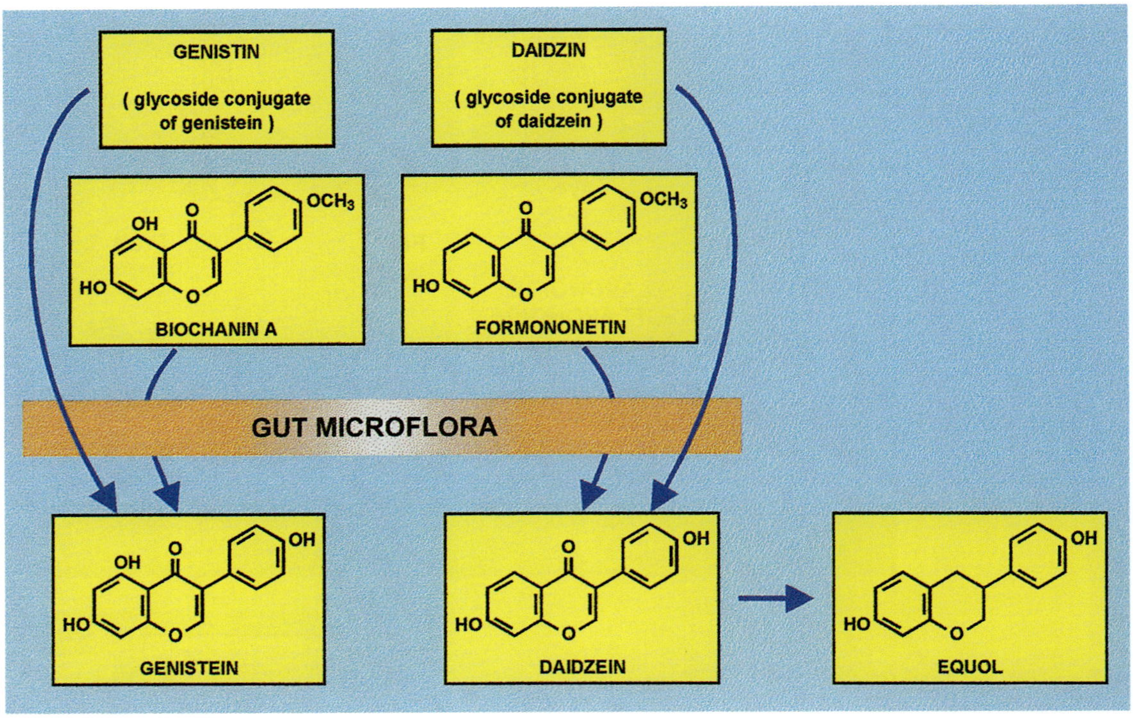

5

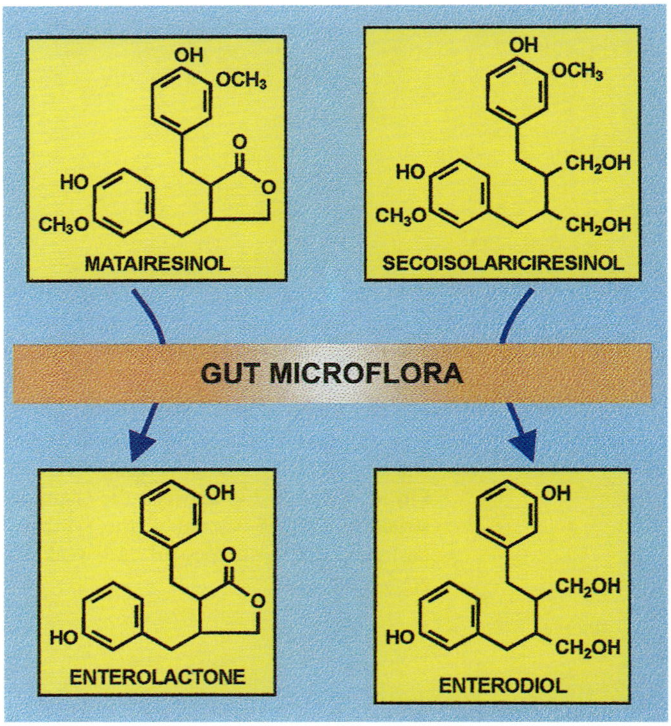

6

Fig. 5. Diagrammatic representation of metabolism by the normal gut microflora of dietary components into particular isoflavonoids and derivatives.

Fig. 6. Formation of lignans by gut microflora.

diol for binding to the nuclear oestrogen receptor [59] and stimulate the synthesis of sex hormone-binding globulin (SHBG) in the liver [60]. Of the total testosterone in plasma, only 2% is free and this biologically active fraction enters the prostate. Any increase in SHBG levels would decrease free plasma testosterone. Higher plasma SHBG and decreased free testosterone have been reported for vegetarian men [61] and Japanese and Chinese men [62].

Fig. 7. Comparison between the serum levels of isoflavonoids and lignans found in UK and Japanese males and females (age 40+).

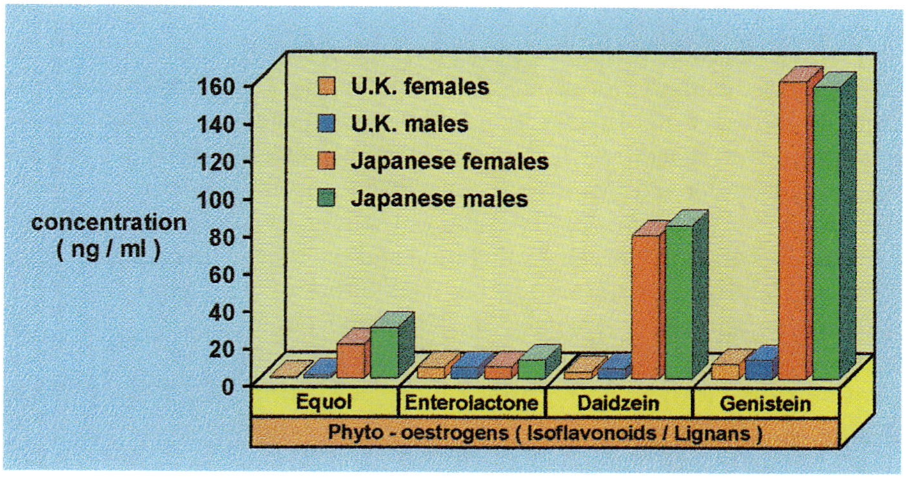

Fig. 8. Movement of blood vessels towards microfoci of cancer, under the influence of secreted angiogenic factors such as VEGF.

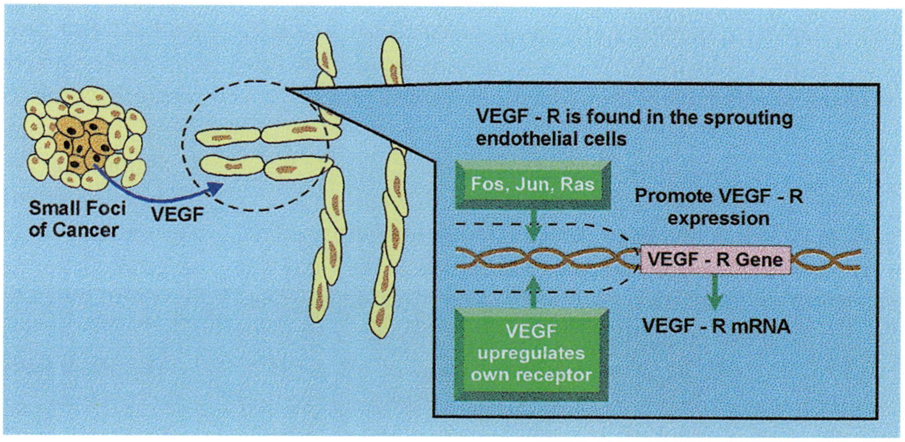

Inhibition of Steroid-Metabolizing Enzymes

Within the prostate, testosterone is metabolized to 5α-dihydrotestosterone (DHT) by the 5α-reductase (5α-R) enzyme [6]. DHT associates with the androgen receptor (AR) and is the DHT-AR complex which influences gene transcription [63].

Recent studies [64] confirm that phyto-oestrogens inhibit not only 5α-R, but also 17β-hydroxysteroid dehydrogenase, the latter regulating the reversible interconversion of testosterone and androstenedione, as well as oestrone and oestradiol.

There are substantial levels of plasma oestrogens in the human male, approximately 30% of the plasma oestrogen being synthesized and secreted by the testes and the remainder is derived from the peripheral aromatization of the adrenal C19 steroids such as dehydroepiandrosterone (DHA) and androstenedione. This oestrogen synthesis is regulated by the aromatase enzyme system in adipose and muscle tissue. Declining testicular activity and increasing aromatization after mid-life, around the age of 50, has been associated with an elevated SHBG level and a consequent rise in the plasma-free 17β-oestradiol concentration relative to the level of free testosterone [65, 66]. It would now be generally accepted [66] that this mid-life 'oestrogenic stimulus' is the predominant factor that induces stromal hyperplasia of the prostate, mediated through a synergistic action between oestradiol and DHT, that results in the stromal adenoma that causes bladder outflow obstruction. Studies [67–71] indicate that *certain phyto-oestrogens inhibit the human P450 aromatase enzyme system.*

A not unreasonable concept might be that the naturally ubiquitous phyto-oestrogens in the Asian and Mediterranean males influence the pathogenesis of clinical BPH by directly inhibiting the growth-promoting effect of DHT and oestradiol on the stromal tissue of their 'ageing' prostate glands.

Inhibition of Tyrosine-Specific Protein Kinases

Tyrosine-specific protein kinases are an integral part of the trans-cell membrane located receptor proteins that are required for the signal transduction pathways activated by various growth factors such as epidermal growth factor (EGF), platelet-derived growth factor, insulin and insulin-like growth factors [66, 72]. Tyrosine phosphorylation plays an important role in cell proliferation and cell transformation and tyrosine kinase-specific inhibitors offer potential as anticancer agents [73]. The isoflavonoid, genistein, has been shown to be a specific inhibitor of tyrosine kinase activity [74]. Furthermore, genistein induces apoptosis in human breast tumour cells [75], inhibits invasion of murine mammary carcinoma cells [76] and enhances adhesion of endothelial cells [77]. Genistein is also cytostatic, arresting cell cycle progression in G2M [78, 79] and induces apoptosis in immature human thymocytes by inhibiting DNA topoisomerase II [80].

Dietary Components, Angiogenesis and Prostate Cancer Progression

Attention has also been directed to the inhibitory effect of genistein on endothelial cell proliferation [81] and the process of angiogenesis or neovascularization. Angiogenesis involves the generation of new capillaries, a process invoking the proliferation and migration of endothelial cells. Normally the process is restricted to wound healing and to such processes as the formation of the corpus luteum, but angiogenesis is also enhanced in association with cancer growth. Folkman and co-workers [82–84] report that new capillary blood vessels are necessary for a cancer to expand beyond 2 mm in size.

Angiogenesis therefore exercises an important role in cancer progression and is essentially seen as the growth towards a focus of cancer of capillary sprouts and columns of endothelial cells from pre-existing capillaries (fig. 8). The process is probably promoted by the production of growth factors by the cancer cells and vascular endothelial growth factor (VEGF) and fibroblast growth factor-2 (FGF-2), or members of the FGF family, are recognized as potent angiogenic agents [73]. Blocking angiogenesis could inhibit cancer progression. Genistein inhibited the FGF-2 induced invasion of collagen by bovine microvascular endothelial cells, with a reported IC_{50} of approximately 150 μM. Endothelial cell proliferation in vivo was inhibited by lower concentrations of the isoflavonoid. Moreover, genistein significantly reduced the FGF-2-stimulated elevation of both the urokinase-type plasminogen activator (PA) and its physiological inhibitor (PAI-1) in vascular endothelial cells, factors associated with the proteolytic degradation of the extracellular matrix in angiogenesis. These effects may relate to the inhibition of the tyrosine kinase-associated FGF receptor [74].

There is therefore evidence for a protective role for genistein in restraining the progression and possible dissemination of foci of prostatic cancer by inhibiting neovascularization, the effects on angiogenesis and tumour suppression opening up encouraging concepts for an innovative cancer preventative measures.

Prostatitis and Dietary Factors

Coffey and co-workers [85] have observed that soya may play a protective role against the pathogenesis of nonbacterial prostatitis in rats. This is an inflammatory process localized primarily in the lateral lobe of the rat prostate, with which steroid hormones may be associated [86, 87]. Rats maintained on a soya-free diet for 11 weeks developed severe inflammation in the lateral prostate, whereas rats maintained on a diet with adequate soya, or commercial rat chow which contains soya, did not develop any signs of prostatitis.

The Way Forward

In proposing that dietary factors are responsible for the marked differences in the prostatic cancer incidence and mortality rates between East and West, there can rarely have been such convincing support than the identification of the large amounts relative to counterparts in the West, of isoflavonoids, flavonoids and lignans in the body fluids of Asian people as a consequence of a their high dietary intake. Moreover, this and a greater understanding of particular specific effects of the phyto-oestrogens on the biological processes associated with carcinogenesis thereby provide support for the belief that such compounds could restrain cancer development. Such information that is currently accumulating at a most impressive rate will be necessary to encourage those at the highest government level to strongly consider strategies for cancer, if not 'Western disease' prevention. The encouragement of individuals to recognize the probable healthcare benefits from such dietary change, or an increase in the intake of such phyto-oestrogens in food supplementation packages, through a lifetime, must also be seen as a major role for those now committed to such programmes for prevention.

Associated with this new emphasis on prevention must be the realization that the ultimate proof of real benefit will reside in statistical evidence available some years into the new millennium. It must be seen that the strategy for prevention must firstly be health education directed specifically to the incidence, morbidity and mortality associated with cancer, but particularly those of prostate and breast. The *'relative vulnerability', or degree of risk* to those people who enjoy a conventional Western diet, high in animal protein and low in cereals, legumes, fruit and vegetables, compared with the lesser risk of those with a soya-based Asian or Mediterranean vegetarian style of diet, must be emphasized.

Dietary advice could follow. Already there is government encouragement for people to increase their consumption of vegetables, especially legumes, fruit and cereals. More specifically, and with the intention of introducing soya and its isoflavonoid content into the diet, there would be mention of the availability of soya-based food supplements that taken daily enhance the levels of the phyto-oestrogens genistein and daidzein to those of the Chinese and Japanese people. Such soya preparations could be introduced into the regular diet such that there is minimal interference of the Western dietary style that most people would be loath to reject. The concept must be that the introduction of these dietary phyto-oestrogens offers the possibility that their potential restraining influence on those biological processes implicated in carcinogenesis can provide at best significant health benefit, but at worst, can do little damage.

With the often stated reluctance, even hostility to fundamental dietary change, the realization and acceptance that there is available, an 'easy fix' that provides a specific, dietary supplementation of isoflavonoids and lignans to be taken along with the individual food preferences must be seen as the way forward.

There have already been successful trials of a prototype supplement at the Tenovus Cancer Research Centre. Epidemiological studies have noted lesser incidence of prostate cancer in Eastern Europe and Finland and also in immigrant communities of these peoples in Canada and Australia, where the original dietary customs tend to be preserved. Their traditional bread contains rye and buckwheat flour, which is significantly richer in lignans than wheat flour and loaves which often have whole flaxseeds added. The resultant multigrain loaf is therefore a rich source of dietary lignans and, as bread, is consumed daily in quantity. This may have some relevance to the reduced occurrence of prostate cancer in these communities.

A necessary strategy of health education must also be envisaged in Asian countries to ensure knowledge of the existing health benefits of their traditional soya-based dietary habit. This is particularly necessary when population groups in Asia acquire any degree of affluence, since there already has been recognized, a willingness to encompass Western dietary habits that would be supported by the 'fast food' industry.

It remains to be determined whether the dietary constituents, the isoflavonoids, flavonoids and lignans exercise their biological effect as antioxidants, weak oestrogens, antioestrogens or, indeed, as inhibitors of those signalling pathways driven by the ubiquitous growth regulatory factors. Tamoxifen, which is recognized as acting as a weak oestrogen in its universal use in the clinical management of breast cancer as a weak oestrogen, is being investigated as to its efficacy in the prevention of the disease in women considered 'at risk'. Already recognized, however, is the beneficial influence it elicits with regard to cardiovascular disease and osteoporosis in women.

Hormone replacement therapy, which is essentially low-dose oestrogen therapy and controls menopausal problems such as hot flushes, also provides longer term benefits in restraining cardiovascular disease and osteoporosis. It is noteworthy that menopausal Japanese women have a lower frequency of hot flushes than their Western counterparts which presumably can be attributed to their soya-based diet and its associated weak oestrogen content.

Although probable, the benefits of dietary intervention can readily be promulgated, there might be concern amongst men a greater intake of weak oestrogens could produce certain undesirable side effects, such as feminization. Although understandable, reassurance would come from the absence of such effects in the vast male population of Asia, consuming a life-long traditional soya diet. The traditional Asian male assumes all aspects of a healthy male life and is abundantly fertile, whilst at the same time enjoying a significantly reduced risk of prostatic malignancy.

Appropriate chemopreventive trials of phyto-oestrogens may be difficult to establish and certainly may be seen as expensive. They must, however, be supported and although certain mild adverse side effects may emerge from current lack of knowledge of biological processes, this must be seen from our current understanding of the Asian people as being of minimal risk. Certainly, if the aim of such studies is to evaluate the influence of enhancing the concentrations of particular isoflavonoids or lignans in the study groups merely to the predetermined levels of the Asian people, it is reasonable to anticipate that any adverse effects would be negligible.

References

1 Wynder E, Gori G: Contribution of the environment to cancer incidence: An epidemiologic study. J Natl Cancer Inst 1977;58:825–832.
2 Higginson J, Muir C: Environmental carcinogenesis: Misconceptions and limitations to cancer control. J Natl Cancer Inst 1979;63:1291–1298.
3 Doll R, Peto R: The causes of cancer: Quantitative estimates of avoidable risks of cancer in the United States today. J Natl Cancer Inst 1981;66:1191–1308.
4 Hill MJ: Dietary fat and human cancer (review). Anticancer Res 1987;7:281–292.
5 Miller AB, Berrino F, Hill M, Pietinen P, Riboli E, Wahrendorf J: Diet in the aetiology of cancer: A review. Eur J Cancer 1994;30A:207–220.
6 Griffiths K, Adlercreutz H, Boyle P, Denis L, Nicholson RI, Morton MS: Nutrition and Cancer. Oxford, ISIS Medical Media, 1996.
7 Haenzel W, Kurihara M: Studies of Japanese migrants. Mortality from cancer and other diseases among Japanese in the United States. J Natl Cancer Inst 1968;40:43–68.
8 Buell P: Changing incidence of breast cancer in Japanese-American women. J Natl Cancer Inst 1973;51:1479–1483.
9 Shimizu H, Ropp RK, Bernstein L, Yatani R, Henderson BE, Mack TH: Cancers of the breast and prostate among Japanese and white immigrants in Los Angeles County. Br J Cancer 1991;63:963–966.
10 Skrabanek P: Invited viewpoints. Eur J Cancer 1994;30A:220–221.
11 McMichael AJ: Invited viewpoints. Eur J Cancer 1994;30A:221–223.
12 Anon: Diet and breast cancer. Nature 1992; 359:76.
13 Adlercreutz H: Western diet and Western diseases: Some hormonal and biochemical mechanisms and associations. Scand J Clin Lab Invest 1990;50(suppl 201):3–23.
14 Zaridze DG, Boyle P, Smans M: International trends in prostatic cancer. Int J Cancer 1984; 33:223–230.
15 Sondik E: Incidence, survival and mortality trends in prostate cancer in the United States; in Coffey DS, Resnick MI, Dorr FA, Karr JP (eds); A Multidisciplinary Analysis of Controversies in the Management of Prostate Cancer. New York, Plenum Press, 1981, p 9.
16 World Health Organisation: Trends in prostate cancer 1980–1988. WHO Weekly Epidemiol Rec 1992;67:281–288.
17 Dhom G: Epidemiology of hormone-dependent tumors; in Voigt KD, Knabbe C (eds); Endocrine Dependent Tumors. New York, Raven Press, 1991, pp 1–42.
18 Muir CS, Waterhouse JAH, Mack T, Powell J, Whelan S (eds); Cancer incidence in five continents, vol V: IARC Sci Publ No. 88. Lyon, IARC, 1987.
19 Zaridze DG, Boyle P: Cancer of the prostate: Epidemiology and aetiology. Br J Urol 1987; 59:493–503.
20 Skeet RG: Epidemiology of urological tumours; in Williams DI, Chisholm GD (eds); Scientific Foundations of Urology, vol II. London, Heineman Medical, 1976, pp 199–211.
21 Miller GJ: Diagnosis of stage A prostatic cancer in the People's Republic of China; in Coffey DS, Resnick MI, Dorr FA, Karr JP (eds); A Multidisciplinary Analysis of Controversies in the Management of Prostate Cancer. New York, Plenum Press, 1988, pp 17–24.
22 Parkin DM, Muir CS, Whelan S, Gao YT, Ferlay J, Powell J (eds); Cancer incidence in five continents, vol VI; IARC Sci Publ No 120. Lyon, IARC, 1992.
23 Boyle P, Levi F, Lucchini F, La Vecchia C: Trends in diet-related cancers in Japan: A conundrum. Lancet 1993;342:752.
24 Burkitt DP: Epidemiology of cancer of the colon and rectum. Cancer 1971;28:3–13.
25 Rose DP: Dietary fibre, phytoestrogens, and breast cancer. Nutrition 1990;8:47–51.
26 Trock B, Lanza E, Greenwald P: Dietary fibre, vegetables, and colon cancer: Critical review and meta-analysis of the epidemiologic evidence. J Natl Cancer Inst 1990;82:650–661.
27 Macquart-Moulin G, Riboli E, Cornee J, Charnay B, Berthezene P, Day N: Case-control study on colorectal cancer and diet in Marseilles. Int J Cancer 1986;38:183–191.
28 Steinmetz K, Potter J: Vegetables, fruit and cancer. I. Epidemiology. Cancer Causes Control 1991;2:325–357.
29 Steinmetz K, Potter J: Vegetables, fruit and cancer. II. Mechanisms. Cancer Causes Control 1991;2:427–442.
30 Ingram DM, Nottage E, Roberts T: The role of diet in the development of breast cancer: A case-control study of patients with breast cancer, benign epithelial hyperplasia and fibrocystic disease of the breast. Br J Cancer 1991;64: 187–191.
31 Wynder EL, Mabuchi K, Whitmore WF: Epidemiology of cancer of the prostate. Cancer 1971;28:344–360.
32 Boyle P, Zaridze DG: Risk factors for prostate and testicular cancer. Eur J Cancer 1993;29A: 1048–1055.
33 Giovannuucci E, Rimm EB, Colditz GA et al: A prospective study of dietary fat and risk of prostate cancer. J Natl Cancer Inst 1993;85: 1571–1579.
34 Severson RK, Nomura AM, Grove AS, Stemmerman GN: A prospective study of demographics, diet and prostate cancer among men of Japanese ancestry in Hawaii. Cancer Res 1989;49:1857–1860.
35 Stemmerman GN, Nomura AM, Heilbrun LK: Cancer risk in relation to fat and energy intake among Hawaii Japanese: A prospective study. International Symposium of the Princess Takamatsu Cancer Research Fund 1985;16:265–274.
36 Kolonel LN, Hankin JH, Nomura AM, Chu SY: Dietary fat intake and cancer incidence among five ethnic groups in Hawaii. Cancer Res 1981;41:3727–3728.
37 Simopoulos AP: Nutritional cancer risks derived from energy and fat. Med Oncol Tumor Pharmacother 1987;4:227–239.
38 Albanes D: Caloric intake, body weight and cancer: A review. Nutr Cancer 1987;9:199–217.
39 Hirayama T: A large-scale cohort study on cancer risks by diet – with special reference to the risk-reducing effects of green-yellow vegetable consumption; in Hayash Y et al (eds); Diet, Nutrition and Cancer. Utrecht, VNU Sci Press/Tokyo, Jpn Sci Soc Press, 1986, pp 41–53.
40 Hirayama T: Epidemiology of prostate cancer with special reference to the role of diet. Monogr Natl Cancer Inst 1979;53:149–155.
41 Hirayama T: Life-style and cancer: From epidemiological evidence to public behaviour change to mortality reduction of target cancers. Monogr Natl Cancer Inst 1992;12:65–74.
42 Lee HP, Gourley L, Duffy SW, Esteve J, Lee J, Day NE: Dietary effects on breast cancer risk in Singapore. Lancet 1991;337:1197–1200.
43 Kodama M, Kodama T: Interrelation between Western-type cancers and non-Western type cancers as regards their risk variations in time and space. II. Nutrition and cancer risk. Anticancer Res 1990;10:1043–1049.
44 Rose DP, Boyar AP, Wynder EL: International comparisons of mortality rates for cancer of the breast, ovary, prostate and colon and per capita food consumption. Cancer 1986;58:2363–2371.
45 Setchell KDR, Adlercreutz H: Mammalian lignans and phytooestrogens. Recent studies on their formation, metabolism and biological role in health and disease; in Roland IR (ed); Role of Gut Flora in Toxicity and Cancer. London, Academic Press, 1988, pp 315–345.
46 Mills PK, Beeson WL, Phillips RL, Frazer GE: Cohort study of diet, lifestyle and prostate cancer in Adventist men. Cancer 1989;64:598–604.
47 Block G, Patterson B, Subar A: Fruit, vegetables and cancer prevention: A review of the epidemiological evidence. Nutr Cancer 1992;18: 1–29.
48 Negri E, La Vecchia C, Franceschi S, D'Avanzo B, Parazzini F: The role of vegetables and fruit in cancer risk; in Hill MJ, Giacosa A, Caygill CPJ (eds): Epidemiology of Diet and Cancer. Chichester, Horwood, 1994, pp 327–334.
49 Buiatti E, Palli D, De Carli A et al: A case-control study of gastric cancer and diet in Italy. Int J Cancer 1989;44:611–616.
50 Buatti E, Palli D, De Carli A et al: A case-control study of gastric cancer and diet in Italy. II. Association with nutrients. Int J Cancer 1990; 45:896–901.
51 La Vecchia C, De Carli A, Negri E, Parazzini F: Epidemiological aspects of diet and cancer: A summary review of case-control studies from Northern Italy. Oncology 1988;45:364–370.
52 Bradbury RB, White DC: Oestrogens and related substances in plants. Vitam Horm 1954;12: 207–233.

53 Price KR, Fenwick GR: Naturally occurring oestrogens in food – A review. Food Addit Contam 1985;2:73–106.
54 Rao CBS (ed): The Chemistry of Lignans. Waltair/India, Andra University Press, 1978, pp 1–377.
55 Thompson LU, Robb P, Serraino M, Cheung F: Mammalian lignan production from various foods. Nutr Cancer 1991;16:43–52.
56 Finlay EMH, Wilson DW, Adlercreutz H, Griffiths K: The identification and measurement of 'phyto-oestrogens' in human saliva, plasma, breast aspirate or cyst fluid, and prostatic fluid using gas chromatography-mass spectrometry. J Endocrinol 1991;129(suppl):49.
57 Adlercreutz H, Fotsis T, Bannwart C et al: Determination of urinary lignans and phytooestrogen metabolites, potential antiestrogens and anticarcinogens, in urine of women on various habitual diets. J Steroid Biochem 1986; 25:791–797.
58 Pope GS, Wright HG: Oestrogenic isoflavones in red clover and subterranean clover. Chem Ind 1954, pp 1019–1020.
59 Martin PM, Horwitz KB, Ryan DS, McGuire WL: Phytooestrogen interaction with estrogen receptors in human breast cancer cells. Endocrinology 1978;103:1860–1867.
60 Adlercreutz H, Hockerstedt K, Bannwart C et al: Effect of dietary components, including lignans and phytoestrogens on enterohepatic circulation and lier metabolism of estrogens and on sex hormone-binding globulin. J Steroid Biochem 1987;27:1135–1144.
61 Belanger A, Locong A, Noel C et al: Influence of diet on plasma steroids and sex hormone-binding globulin levels in adult men. J Steroid Biochem 1989;32:829–833.
62 Vermeulen A: Metabolic effects of obesity in men. Verh Koninkl Acad Geneesk Belgie 1993; 55:393–397.
63 Griffiths K, Eaton CL, Harper ME, Weir AMK, Evans BAJ: Some aspects of the molecular endocrinology of prostatic cancer (review); in Denis L (ed): Antiandrogens in Prostate Cancer. Berlin, Springer, 1996.
64 Evans BAJ, Griffiths K, Morton M: Inhibition of 5α-reductase and 17β-hydroxysteroid dehydrogenase in genital skin fibroblasts by dietary lignans and isoflavonoids. J Endocrinol 1995; 147:295–302.
65 Vermeulen A: Testicular hormone secretion and aging in males; in Grayshack JT, Wilson JD, Saherbenske MJ (eds); Benign Prostatic Hyperplasia. DHEW Publ No (NIH)76-1113. Washington, NIH, 1976, pp 177–182.
66 Griffiths K et al: The regulation of prostatic growth; in Cockett ATK et al (eds): Third International Consultation on BPH. Paris, SCI, 1995, pp 71–115.
67 Kellis JT, Vickery LE: Inhibition of human estrogen synthetase (aromatase) by flavones. Science 1984;225:1032–1034.
68 Kellis JT, Nesnow S, Vickery LE: Inhibition of aromatase cytochrome P-450 (estrogen synthetase) by derivatives of α-naphthoflavone. Biochem Pharmacol 1986;35:2887–2891.
69 Ibrahim AR, Abul-Hajj YJ: Aromatase inhibition by flavonoids. J Steroid Biochem Mol Biol 1990;37:257–260.
70 Adlercreutz H, Bannwart C, Wahala K et al: Inhibition of human aromatase by mammalian lignans and isoflavonoid phytoestrogens. J Steroid Biochem Mol Biol 1993;44:147–153.
71 Campbell DR, Kurzer MS: Flavonoid inhibition of aromatase enzyme activity in human preadipocytes. J Steroid Biochem Mol Biol 1993;46:381–388.
72 Aaronson S: Growth factors and cancer. Science 1991;254:1146–1153.
73 Griffiths K et al: Regulation of prostatic growth; in Denis LJ et al (eds): Fourth International Consultation on BPH. Paris, SCI, 1997, pp 85–128.
74 Akiyama T, Ishida J, Nakagawa S et al: Genistein, a specific inhibitor of tyrosine-specific protein kinases. J Biol Chem 1987;262:5592–5595.
75 Kiguchi K, Glesne D, Chubb CH, Fujiki H, Huberman E: Differential induction of apoptosis in human breast cells by okadaic acid and related inhibitors of protein phosphatases 1 and 2A. Cell Growth Differ 1994;5:995–1004.
76 Scholar EM, Toews ML: Inhibition of invasion of murine mammary carcinoma cells by the tyrosine kinase inhibitor genistein. Cancer Lett 1994;87:159–162.
77 Tiisala S, Majuri ML, Carpen O, Renkonen R: Genistein enhances the ICAM-mediated adhesion by inducing the expression of ICAM-1 and its counter-receptors. Biochem Biophys Res Commun 1994;203:443–449.
78 Spinozzi F, Pagliacci MC, Migliorati G et al: The natural tyrosine kinase inhibitor genistein produces cell cycle arrest and apoptosis in Jurkat T-leukemia cells. Leuk Res 1994;18:431–439.
79 Matsukawa Y, Marui N, Sakai T et al: Genistein arrests cell cycle progression at G2-M. Cancer Res 1993;53:1328–1331.
80 McCabe MJ Jr, Orrenius S: Genistein induces apoptosis in immature human thymocytes by inhibiting topoisomerase-II. Biochem Biophys Res Commun 1993;194:944–950.
81 Fotsis T, Pepper M, Adlercreutz H et al: Genistein, a dietary-derived inhibitor of in vitro angiogenesis. Proc Natl Acad Sci USA 1993;90: 2690–2694.
82 Folkman J, Watson K, Ingber D, Hanahan D: Induction of angiogenesis during the transition from hyperplasia to neoplasia. Nature 1989; 339:58–61.
83 Folkman J: Toward an understanding of angiogenesis: Search and discovery. Perspect Biol Med 1985;29:10–36.
84 Weidner M, Semple JP, Welch WR, Folkman J: Tumour angiogenesis and metaplasia – Correlation in invasive breast cancer. N Engl J Med 1991;324:1–8.
85 Sharma OP, Adlercreutz H, Strandberg JD, Zirkin B, Coffey DS, Ewing LL: Soy of dietary source plays a preventive role against the pathogenesis of prostatitis in rats. J Steroid Biochem Mol Biol 1992;43:557–563.
86 Lundgren R, Holmquist B, Hesselvik M, Muntzing J: Treatment of prostatitis in the rat. Prostate 1984;5:277–284.
87 Naslund MJ, Strandberg JD, Coffey DS: The role of androgens and estrogens in the pathogenesis of experimental nonbacterial prostatitis. J Urol 1988;140:1049–1053.

European
Urology

Eur Urol 1999;35:388–391

Dietary Fat and Prostate Cancer Progression and Survival

Yves Fradet   François Meyer   Isabelle Bairati   Ramak Shadmani
Lynne Moore

Laval University, Québec, Qué., Canada

Key Words
Diet · Fat · Prostate cancer · Vitamin E

Abstract
Background: The association between dietary factors and the occurrence of prostate cancer has been studied extensively, but there is, as yet, no published study on the relationship between diet and disease progression among prostate cancer patients. We studied the association between dietary fat intake and prostate cancer survival. ***Methods:*** We prospectively followed 384 men diagnosed with prostate cancer between 1990 and 1992 in the Quebec City area who participated in a case-control study of diet in relation to prostate cancer occurrence. Trained nutritionists interviewed the men on their usual diet using a diet history questionnaire. Deaths in the follow-up were documented through record linkage with the provincial mortality file and review of hospital records. The cause of death was taken as written on the death certificate. Cox proportional hazards models were used to estimate the relative risk of dying from prostate cancer associated with terciles of fat intake, expressed as percent of dietary energy, while controlling for prognostic factors and total energy. ***Results:*** The median duration of follow-up was 5.2 years. During the follow-up period, 32 patients died of prostate cancer and 39 died of other causes. The 5-year disease-specific survival was 91%. After controlling for grade, clinical stage, initial treatment, age and total energy intake, we found that saturated fat consumption was significantly associated with disease-specific survival (p = 0.008). Compared to men in the lower tercile of saturated fat, those in the upper tercile had three times the risk of dying from prostate cancer (hazards ratio 3.13, 95% confidence interval 1.28–7.67). ***Conclusion:*** Our findings suggest that, if saturated fat is causally related to disease-specific survival, a moderate reduction of its intake below 10% of energy should reduce the risk of dying from prostate cancer. This dietary goal is already recommended for health promotion and primary prevention of heart disease and cancer.

The prevalence of latent, noninfiltrating prostate cancer appears to vary little among populations, while the age-adjusted incidence of prostate cancer varies considerably among industrialized countries. This phenomenon suggests that environmental factors, such as diet, may promote or inhibit the development of prostate cancer. In the past two decades, several case-control and cohort studies have documented the relationship between food consumption and prostate cancer risk [1]. Overall, these

KARGER
Fax + 41 61 306 12 34
E-Mail karger@karger.ch
www.karger.com

0302–2838/99/0356–0388$17.50/0

Accessible online at:
http://BioMedNet.com/karger

Yves Fradet, MD, FRCSC
Laval University Cancer Research Center
CHUQ – Hôtel-Dieu de Québec
11, côte du Palais, Québec, Qué. G1R 2J6 (Canada)
Tel. +1 418 691 5575, Fax +1 418 691 5562, E-Mail yves.fradet@crhdq.ulaval.ca

studies point to an increased risk of prostate cancer with increased consumption of red meat or fat-rich animal foods. Experiments in a murine model showed that reducing fat intake slowed the growth of established prostate tumors suggesting a role of diet in cancer progression [2]. The development of life-threatening prostate cancer is the culmination of a complex series of initiation and promotional events over a period of decades. We investigated the relationship between diet and the occurrence of prostate cancer at a preclinical stage, as well as the influence of diet on cancer progression by conducting a case-control study in the Quebec City area between October 1990 and May 1993.

Total Energy Intake and Preclinical Prostate Cancer

As a first objective, we evaluated a total of 215 men with preclinical prostate cancer and 593 controls with no evidence of cancer [3]. The study population was comprised of two distinct groups. The first group consisted of men hospitalized for transurethral prostatectomy (TURP) to relieve the obstructive symptoms of benign prostatic hyperplasia hypertrophy (BPH). Cancer cases were men for whom prostate cancer was discovered in the resected prostate tissue (stage T1a and T1b). The second group consisted of men who took part in a prostate cancer screening program. Trained nutritionists interviewed the participants on their usual diet using a detailed diet history questionnaire. A positive association was observed between total energy intake and preclinical prostate cancer ($p = 0.004$). The odds ratio for prostate cancer increased with each quartile of energy intake: 1.00, 1.77, 1.9 and 2.67. Furthermore, the relationship was almost identical for patients with cancer found at TURP for BPH and those with cancer found by PSA screening. After adjusting for total energy intake, no statistically significant association was found with total fat, types of fat, selected fatty acids, and fats from animal or vegetable sources. Also no clear association was observed for β-carotene, α-carotene, lutein or lycopene or with α-tocopherol (vitamin E) and vitamin C intake. This result, together with those of previous studies, which have focused mostly on advanced prostate cancer, suggests that dietary factors could be involved not only in the progression of tumors to advanced stages but also much earlier in the occurrence of prostate cancer. However, the contribution of individual nutrients must be adjusted for total energy intake.

Dietary Fat and Advanced Prostate Cancer

We then undertook to identify dietary factors, particularly fat intake, that may be associated with advanced prostate cancer. In our study, we performed a case series analysis restricted to prostate cancer cases recruited in a hospital as part of the Quebec case-controlled study [4]. In this study, a total of 384 patients with prostate cancer completed a reliable questionnaire, including 142 patients with advanced cancer at diagnosis and 242 with local T1 and T2 prostate cancer. In the present study, advanced cancers included both clinical and pathological staging. Contrary to the results observed in clinical cancer when compared to noncancer cases, total energy intake was not associated with advanced prostate cancer when compared to localized prostate cancer. There was a moderately not statistically significant relation to total fat and monounsaturated fat. However, cases in the highest quartile of saturated fat intake had a statistically significant odds ratio of 2.15 (95% CI 1.14–4.04) for advanced cancer. In addition, the relationship between saturated fat intake and advanced prostate cancer was dose-dependent. Inverse associations of borderline significance were observed between polyunsaturated fat (trend odds ratio 0.88, 95% CI 0.73–1.07), linoleic acid and advanced prostate cancer. Saturated fat intake strongly and positively correlated with animal fat intake, while polyunsaturated fat intake strongly correlated with vegetable fat. Multivariate analyses considering the consumption of saturated and polyunsaturated fat in the same model showed that saturated fat was the factor most strongly associated with advanced prostate cancer. The results of this study suggest an association between saturated fat consumption and prostate cancer progression. They are consistent with those of two previous US cohort studies comparing men with advanced prostate cancer to healthy individuals [5, 6]. Both of those studies demonstrated increased risks with high intake of meat, fat or animal fat.

Dietary Fat and Prostate Cancer Survival

We then addressed the question of whether dietary fat is associated with disease progression among patients with prostate cancer. To this end, we prospectively followed the 384 men diagnosed with prostate cancer between 1990 and 1992. The cancer was diagnosed clinically for 169 men, was discovered through screening with digital rectal examination (DRE) and PSA for 151 men and was found incidentally after TURP for BPH in 64

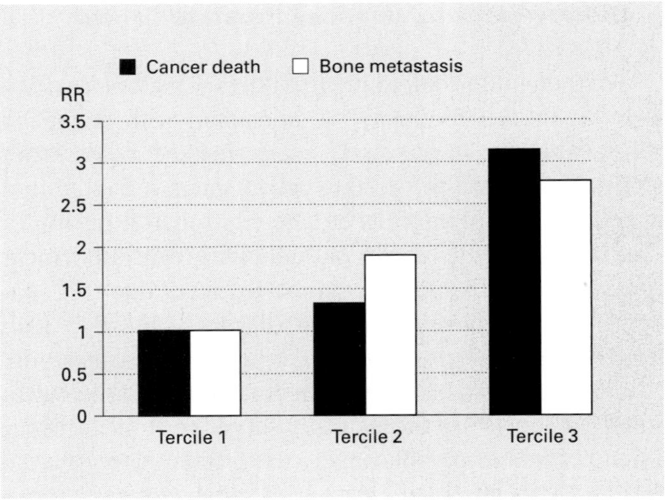

Fig. 1. Saturated fat intake is divided in terciles representing the following percent of total energy intake: tercile 1, <10.8%; tercile 2, 10.8–13.2%; tercile 3, >13.2%. Men with higher percentage of dietary energy from saturated fat had an inceased risk of dying from prostate cancer (p = 0.008) or develop bone metastasis (p = 0.03). RR = Risk ratio.

men. At diagnosis, cancer was clinically locally advanced (stage T3) in 70 men, metastatic to lymph node at exploratory laparotomy in 4 men, or metastatic to the bone (stage D2) in 14 men. The other patients had clinically localized disease of stage T1 (68 men) or T2 (228 men). Contrary to the previous study, staging was done according to clinical stage only. Initial treatment consisted of radical prostatectomy in 159 men, radiation therapy in 129, expectant management in 63 and palliative hormonal treatment in 33 patients. Information on patient follow-up was obtained from a review of hospital records between July and November 1997 which was complemented, when necessary, by information obtained from patients treating physicians. In addition, deterministic record linkage using the patient unique health insurance number was conducted with the provincial mortality file held by 'Bureau de la Statistique du Québec' for the period of January 1, 1990 to December 31, 1996 to identify men who died and to record the date and the cause of death.

The average age at diagnosis was 67.4 years (SD = 7.5). The median duration of follow-up was 5.2 years. Of the 384 men enrolled in the prospective study, 32 died of prostate cancer and 39 died of other causes during the follow-up period. The 5-year disease-specific survival was 91%. In crude analysis, advanced clinical stage, high tumor grade and elevated PSA level at diagnosis were all associated with an increased risk of dying from prostate cancer. Men with prostate cancer detected through screening or discovered after TURP and those treated by radical prostatectomy had a lower risk of dying from prostate cancer compared to men treated by radiation therapy or palliative hormonal treatment. Multivariate analyses identified the following independent determinants of the risk of dying from prostate cancer: advanced clinical stage (RR = 3.93), poorly differentiated tumor (RR = 4.49), palliative hormonal treatment (RR = 6.64), and older age (RR = 2.31). Other factors, including initial PSA level, were not statistically significant independent predictors of the risk of dying from prostate cancer.

The relation of dietary energy intake and fat consumption variables to the risk of dying from prostate cancer was assessed in Cox regression models controlling for stage, grade, initial treatment, age and for nutrients and total energy. There was no association between total energy intake and death from prostate cancer. Men with a higher percentage of dietary energy from total fat, saturated fat and monounsaturated fat had an increased risk of dying from prostate cancer, but only for saturated fat was the association statistically significant (p = 0.008) (fig. 1). Compared to men in the lower tercile of saturated fat intake (which represented <10.8% of total energy) those in the upper tercile (who had >13.2% of dietary energy from saturated fat) had three times the risk of dying from prostate cancer (RR = 3.13, 95% CI 1.28–7.67). When adjusting for other fat intake, this increased risk remained unchanged. Similarly, when adjusting for all other factors, men in the upper tercile had also three times higher risk of developing bone metastasis during the period of follow-up (RR = 3.4, 95% CI 1.2–9.2). The mode of cancer detection brought about some heterogeneity in the study population in terms of risk of dying from prostate cancer. However, when we restricted the analysis to clinically detected cases, the relative risk association with saturated fat intake remained unchanged. Finally, the specificity of the association between saturated fat intake and risk of dying from prostate cancer was confirmed by showing an absence of association between saturated fat intake and the risk of dying from other causes. The relative risk of dying from other causes associated with the second and third terciles of saturated fat intake were 1.55 and 1.04, respectively.

The results of these studies add strong support to the relationship between dietary factor and the incidence and progression of prostate cancer. Total energy intake was related to the occurrence of preclinical prostate cancer when compared to noncancer cases. When adjusting for total energy intake, no specific nutrient was found to be associated with increased or decreased risk of prostate cancer. However, results of recent randomized clinical trials have suggested that selenium supplementation and vitamin E supplementation may reduce the incidence of prostate cancer [7, 8]. These findings open new and promising avenues for the prevention of clinically detectable prostate cancer.

On the other hand, the results of our study support a strong association between saturated fat intake and prostate cancer progression and survival. The saturated fat was mostly from fat-rich animal foods and dairy products. If the association is indeed causal and received supportive evidence from other prospective studies, a dietary intervention aimed at improving prostate cancer patient survival could be initiated in patients diagnosed with prostate cancer. Our study suggests that such an intervention should focus primarily on saturated fat with the aim of reducing its contribution to 10% of dietary energy. This dietary goal is similar to that proposed by expert committees for health promotion and primary prevention of heart disease and cancer [9, 10]. Such a moderate dietary intervention among prostate cancer patients is unlikely to have adverse effects, is easily achievable and might reduce significantly the risk of dying from prostate cancer.

References

1 Clinton SK, Giovannucci E: Diet, nutrition, and prostate cancer. Annu Rev Nutr 1998;18: 413–440.
2 Wang Y, Corr JG, Thaler HT, Tao Y, Fair WR, Heston WDW: Decreased growth of established human prostate LNCaP tumors in nude mice fed a low-fat diet. J Natl Cancer Inst 1995; 87:1456–1462.
3 Meyer F, Bairati I, Fradet Y, Moore L: Dietary energy and nutrients in relation to preclinical prostate cancer. Nutr Cancer 1997;29:120–126.
4 Bairati I, Meyer F, Fradet Y, Moore L: Dietary fat and advanced prostate cancer. J Urol 1998; 159:1271–1275.
5 Giovannucci E, Rimm EB, Colditz GA, Stampfer MU, Ascherio A, Chute CC, Willett WC: A prospective study of dietary fat and risk of prostate cancer. J Natl Cancer Inst 1993;85: 1571–1579.
6 Gann PH, Hennekens CH, Sacks FM, Grodstein F, Giovannucci EL, Stampfer MJ: Prospective study of plasma fatty acids and risk of prostate cancer. J Natl Cancer Inst 1994;86: 281–286.
7 Clark LC, Dalkin B, Krongrad A, Combs GF, Turnbull BW, Slate EH, Witherington R, Herlong JH, Janosko E, Carpenter D, Borosso C, Falk S, Rounder J: Decreased incidence of prostate cancer with selenium supplementation: Results of a double-blind cancer prevention trial. Br J Urol 1998;81:730–734.
8 Heinonen OP, Albanes D, Virtamo J, Taylor PR, Huttunen JK, Hartman AM, Haapakoski J, Malila N, Rautalahti M, Ripatti S, Mäenpää H, Teerenhovi L, Koss L, Virolainen M, Edwards BK: Prostate cancer and supplementation with α-tocopherol and β-carotene: Incidence and mortality in a controlled trial. J Natl Cancer Inst 1998;90:440–446.
9 American Heart Association: Dietary guidelines for healthy American adults: a statement for physicians and health professionals by the Nutrition Committee, American Heart Association. Circulation 1988;77:721A–724A.
10 Health and Welfare Canada: Nutrition recommendations: the report of the scientific review committee 1990. Ottawa, Ministry of Supply and Services, 1990.

Molecular Targets for Chemoprevention of Prostate Cancer

European Urology

Eur Urol 1999;35:392–394

Vitamin D and Prostate Cancer Risk

Donna M. Peehl

Department of Urology, Stanford University School of Medicine, Stanford, Calif., USA

Key Words

Prostate · Cancer · Vitamin D · Chemoprevention

Abstract

Prostate cancer is a progressive, multistep disease which presents many stages for intervention. Microscopic cancer is found in the prostate beginning by age 30 in about 20% of men, and the incidence increases steadily so that by the time a man is 90 years old, he has almost a 100% chance of having cancer in his prostate. Independent, multiple foci of cancer are present in the majority of prostate specimens, and the incidence of premalignant lesions is even higher than that of cancer. Yet, despite the high incidence of microscopic cancer, only 8% of men in the US present with clinically significant disease during their lifetime. Furthermore, only 3% of men in the US die of prostate cancer. In no other human cancer is there such disparity between the high incidence of microscopic malignancy and the relatively low death rate. Thus, there are many windows of opportunity for control of prostate cancer. Evidence from diverse areas of study – epidemiologic, molecular, genetic, cellular, animal models, and clinical trials – suggests that vitamin D may be an effective preventive agent against prostate cancer.

As recently as 10 years ago, few people would have thought of the prostate as a target organ of vitamin D. Classically, vitamin D was considered to exclusively interact with bone, intestine, kidney and parathyroid to regulate calcium and phosphate homeostasis. Now, we recognize that the active metabolite of vitamin D [1,25-dihydroxyvitamin D_3 or $1,25(OH)_2D_3$] is a seco-steroid hormone that regulates growth and differentiation in a wide variety of cells by binding to the VDR, a member of the steroid hormone receptor gene superfamily.

Evidence that VDR were present in human prostatic tissues was seen in a study published in 1988, in which an immunohistochemical screen of human tissues was accomplished with antibody against VDR [1]. This study was limited in nature but positive labeling in prostatic glands was reported. The next year, an autoradiographic study of vitamin D binding described labeling of fibroblasts and epithelial cells in the mouse prostate [2].

Little was done to further explore vitamin D activity in the prostate until 1992, when Miller et al. [3] found that the human prostatic cancer cell line LNCaP expresses significant levels of VDR with an affinity for vitamin D equivalent to that reported for classic target organs. This finding was confirmed by our studies and others and was extended to six other commonly used prostatic cancer cell lines [4].

At about this time, an intriguing hypothesis linking vitamin D and prostate cancer was published which further intensified interest in exploring the interaction of vitamin D with prostate cells. Schwartz and Hulka [5] demonstrated that mortality rates from prostate cancer in the US are inversely correlated with ultraviolet radiation, the principal source of endogenous vitamin D synthesis. Although this was an indirect link, they also pointed out that vitamin D deficiency is associated with the major risk factors known for prostate cancer. Age is the strongest risk factor for prostate cancer, and the elderly are frequently vitamin D-deficient due to less exposure to ultraviolet radiation and a decline in the ability to synthesize $1,25(OH)_2D_3$ with age. Race is also a risk factor for

KARGER

Fax +41 61 306 12 34
E-Mail karger@karger.ch
www.karger.com

0302–2838/99/0356–0392$17.50/0

Accessible online at:
http://BioMedNet.com/karger

Donna M. Peehl, PhD
Department of Urology, Stanford Medical Center
300 Pasteur Drive, Stanford, CA 94305-5118 (USA)
Tel. +1 650 725 5531, Fax +1 650 723 0765
E-Mail dpeehl@leland.stanford.edu

prostate cancer, with the incidence rates of American Blacks twice those of Caucasians. This may be related to vitamin D deficiency by the fact that high melanin levels in darkly pigmented skin inhibit the formation of previtamin D. Diet has also been proposed as a risk factor for prostate cancer, and the low risk of prostate cancer for indigenous Japanese has been related to the traditional diet. This diet, among other attributes, is rich in oily fish, which are an important dietary source of vitamin D.

More direct evidence for vitamin D deficiency as a risk factor for prostate cancer came from a prospective analysis of vitamin D metabolite levels in sera. In a case-control study of serum samples collected in the San Francisco Bay area between 1964 and 1971 and matched for age, race and day of storage, Corder et al. [6] found that mean levels of serum $1,25(OH)_2D_3$ were 1.81 pg/ml lower in cases diagnosed with prostate cancer than in controls ($p = 0.002$). Interestingly, another epidemiologic study published just this year found high levels of dietary calcium were a significant risk factor for prostate cancer [7]. This may be relevant to the relationship of vitamin D and prostate cancer because high levels of calcium suppress formation of $1,25(OH)_2D_3$.

With a relationship between vitamin D and prostate cancer risk emerging from epidemiologic studies, it became imperative to investigate and define biological activity of vitamin D in prostate cells. In the initial study by Miller et al. [3] in which VDR were identified in LNCaP cells, it was observed that $1,25(OH)_2D_3$ stimulated the growth of LNCaP cells in the absence of androgen. This finding seemed at odds with the epidemiologic data indicating that vitamin D would act to limit the growth of prostate cancer cells. We subsequently determined that the stimulatory effect of vitamin D on LNCaP cells was unique to specific culture conditions and related to androgen responsiveness of this cell line [8]. The overwhelming effect of $1,25(OH)_2D_3$ on LNCaP and other prostate cancer cell lines as well as on primary cell cultures of prostatic epithelial cells from normal, benign or malignant tissues was one of growth inhibition. Vitamin D was also shown to increase the expression of prostate-specific antigen (PSA), a differentiation marker, in prostate cells [3, 4]. These observations, then, provide a biological basis for the epidemiologic findings. We hypothesize that in the prostate, normal levels of $1,25(OH)_2D_3$ act to inhibit growth and stimulate differentiation. In states of vitamin D deficiency, the balance would be tipped and growth would occur at a higher than normal rate. If initiation of cancer occurred, the faster rate of growth would presumably result in a higher incidence of diagnosis of clinical disease.

This concept of antitumor activity of vitamin D has been validated in several animal models of prostate cancer. In a study designed to test chemopreventive activity of a vitamin D analog, Lucia et al. [9] showed that the incidence of carcinogen- and androgen-promoted tumors in the Lobund-Wistar rat prostate was decreased in treated animals. Other animal models have demonstrated chemotherapeutic activity. The size of human prostate cancer xenografts of PC-3 and LNCaP in nude mice was smaller in animals treated with vitamin D or an analog than in untreated animals [10, 11]. Manipulation of vitamin D levels in normal rodents led to the observation that a diet with low levels of vitamin D resulted in increased proliferation in the dorsolateral prostate of the mouse [12], whereas elevated levels of vitamin D in rats caused the appearance of more secretory granules in the differentiated epithelium of the prostate [13]. These results parallel and extend those obtained in vitro and further support a role of vitamin D in growth regulation and differentiation in the prostate.

Based on the substantial preclinical data, investigators at Stanford University initiated a pilot clinical trial of calcitriol [$1,25(OH)_2D_3$] [14]. Seven patients with prostate cancer who recurred after radiation or radical prostatectomy were subjected to 6–15 months of therapy. The rate of rise of serum PSA (an estimation of tumor growth rate) significantly decreased in 7 of 7 individuals, providing preliminary evidence that calcitriol effectively prolongs tumor doubling time in select cases.

Recently, molecular epidemiologic studies have indicated that genetic factors may contribute to an individual's ability to respond to $1,25(OH)_2D_3$. The VDR gene has two sets of polymorphisms, one at the 3′ end of the gene involving a series of polymorphic sites [15] and the other at the 5′ end of the gene affecting the start codon and referred to as the start codon polymorphism or SCP [16, 17]. The 3′ polymorphisms are defined by the enzymes BsmI, ApaI and TaqI and a poly-A microsatellite, all of which are in linkage disequilibrium. Taylor et al. [18] tested the hypothesis that VDR gene polymorphisms are associated with prostate cancer risk and found a 3-fold increase in risk associated with the Taq allele. Similarly, Ingles et al. [19] found a relative risk of 4.6 of developing prostate cancer for men with at least one long VDR poly-A allele compared to men with two short poly-A alleles. While preliminary and apparently not found in all populations [20], these results provide yet another intriguing element in the relationship between vitamin D action and prostate cancer.

Preceding and contemporaneous with these studies on vitamin D and prostate cancer have been findings which implicate vitamin D in growth regulation and cancer control in other organs, particularly the colon and breast [21, 22]. Evidence from epidemiologic studies, molecular and cellular studies of in vitro cell cultures, and animal models have prompted pilot studies to test chemopreventive and chemotherapeutic activity of vitamin D and analogs against breast and colon cancer. These studies provide a model which can be extended to prostate cancer to fully exploit the antitumor activities of vitamin D.

Taken together, there is strong evidence supporting a role for vitamin D as a critical regulator of growth and differentiation in the prostate. Epidemiologic studies suggest the possibility that vitamin D deficiency is a risk factor for prostate cancer, and genetic studies indicate that an individual's ability to respond to vitamin D may influence his likelihood of being diagnosed with clinically significant disease. In vitro studies with prostate cell cultures provide a biological basis for these findings and show that vitamin D is a potent inhibitor of growth and induces cellular differentiation. Application of vitamin D to animal models of prostate cancer demonstrates efficacy as an antitumor agent in vivo. Finally, a pilot clinical study showed that vitamin D could slow the rate of tumor doubling in patients with early recurrence after radical prostatectomy. The combination of all of these observations at many different levels of investigation – in cultured cells, animal models, and humans – provides a strong rationale for further developing vitamin D as a preventive and therapeutic agent against prostate cancer.

References

1 Berger U, Wilson P, McClelland RA, Colston K, Haussler MR, Pike JW, Coombes RC: Immunocytochemical detection of 1,25-dihydroxyvitamin D receptors in normal human tissues. J Clin Endocrinol Metab 1988;67:607–613.

2 Schleicher G, Privette TH, Stumpf WE: Distribution of soltriol [1,25(OH)$_2$-vitamin D$_3$] binding sites in male sex organs of the mouse: An autoradiographic study. J Histochem Cytochem 1989;37:1083–1086.

3 Miller GJ, Stapleton GE, Ferrara JA, Lucia MS, Pfister S, Hedlund TE, Upadhya P: The human prostatic carcinoma cell line LNCaP expresses biologically active, specific receptors for 1α,25-dihydroxyvitamin D$_3$. Cancer Res 1992;52:515–520.

4 Skowronski RJ, Peehl DM, Feldman D: Vitamin D and prostate cancer: 1,25-Dihydroxyvitamin D$_3$ receptors and actions in human prostate cancer cell lines. Endocrinology 1993;132: 1952–1960.

5 Schwartz GG, Hulka BS: Is vitamin D deficiency a risk factor for prostate cancer? (Hypothesis). Anticancer Res 1990;10:1307–1311.

6 Corder EH, Guess HA, Hulka BS, Friedman GD, Sadler M, Vollmer RT, Lobaugh B, Drezner MK, Vogelman JH, Orentreich N: Vitamin D and prostate cancer: A prediagnostic study with stored sera (see comments). Cancer Epidemiol Biomarkers Prev 1993;2:467–472.

7 Giovannucci E, Rimm EB, Wolk A, Ascherio A, Stampfer MJ, Colditz GA, Willett WC: Calcium and fructose intake in relation to risk of prostate cancer. Cancer Res 1998;58:442–447.

8 Zhao XY, Ly LH, Peehl DM, Feldman D: 1α,25-Dihydroxyvitamin D$_3$ action in LNCaP human prostate cancer cells are androgen-dependent. Endocrinology 1997;138:3290–3298.

9 Lucia MS, Anzano MA, Slayter MV, Anver MR, Green DM, Shrader MW, Logsdon DL, Driver CL, Brown CC, Peer CW, et al: Chemopreventive activity of tamoxifen, N-(4-hydroxyphenyl)retinamide, and the vitamin D analogue Ro24-5531 for androgen-promoted carcinomas of the rat seminal vesicle and prostate. Cancer Res 1995;55:5621–5627.

10 Schwartz GG, Hill CC, Oeler TA, Becich MJ, Bahnson RR: 1,25-Dihydroxy-16-ene-23-yne-vitamin D$_3$ and prostate cancer cell proliferation in vivo. Urology 1995;46:365–369.

11 Gross C, Peehl DM, Feldman D: Vitamin D and prostate cancer; in Feldman D, Glorieux FH, Pike JW (eds): Vitamin D. San Diego, Acadmic Press, 1997, pp 1125–1139.

12 Xue L, Yang K, Newmark H, Lipkin M: Induced hyperproliferation in epithelial cells of mouse prostate by a Western-style diet. Carcinogenesis 1997;18:995–999.

13 Konety BR, Schwartz GG, Acierno JS Jr, Becich MJ, Getzenberg RH: The role of vitamin D in normal prostate growth and differentiation. Cell Growth Differ 1996;7:1563–1570.

14 Gross S, Stamey T, Hancock S, Feldman D: Treatment of early recurrent prostate cancer with 1,25-dihydroxyvitamin D$_3$ (calcitriol). J Urol 1998;159:2035–2040.

15 Morrison NA, Qi JC, Tokita A, Kelly PJ, Crofts L, Nguyen TV, Sambrook PN, Eisman JA: Prediction of bone density from vitamin D receptor alleles (see comments). Nature 1994; 367:284–287.

16 Gross C, Eccleshall TR, Malloy PJ, Villa ML, Marcus R, Feldman D: The presence of a polymorphism at the translation initiation site of the vitamin D receptor gene is associated with low bone mineral density in postmenopausal Mexican-American women (see comments). J Bone Miner Res 1996;11:1850–1855.

17 Harris SS, Eccleshall TR, Gross C, Dawson-Hughes B, Feldman D: The vitamin D receptor start codon polymorphism (FokI) and bone mineral density in premenopausal American black and white women. J Bone Miner Res 1997;12:1043–1048.

18 Taylor JA, Hirvonen A, Watson M, Pittman G, Mohler JL, Bell DA: Association of prostate cancer with vitamin D receptor gene polymorphism. Cancer Res 1996;56:4108–4110.

19 Ingles SA, Ross RK, Yu MC, Irvine RA, La Pera G, Haile RW, Coetzee GA: Association of prostate cancer risk with genetic polymorphisms in vitamin D receptor and androgen receptor (see comments). J Natl Cancer Inst 1997;89:166–170.

20 Ma J, Stampfer MJ, Gann PH, Hough HL, Giovannucci E, Kelsey KT, Hennekens CH, Hunter DJ: Vitamin D receptor polymorphisms, circulating vitamin D metabolites, and risk of prostate cancer in United States physicians. Cancer Epidemiol Biomark Prev 1998;7: 385–390.

21 Brasitus TA, Siltrin MD: Chemoprevention and colon cancer by vitamin D$_3$ and its metabolites/analogs; in Feldman D, Glorieux FH, Pike JW (eds): Vitamin D. San Diego, Academic Press, 1997, pp 1141–1154.

22 Colston K: Vitamin D and breast cancer: Therapeutic potential of new vitamin D analogs; in Feldman D, Glorieux FH, Pike JW (eds): Vitamin D. San Diego, Academic Press, 1997, pp 1107–1123.

Molecular Targets for Chemoprevention of Prostate Cancer

European Urology

Eur Urol 1999;35:395–398

Lipoxygenase Inhibition in Prostate Cancer

Charles E. Myers Jagat Ghosh

Cancer Center, University of Virginia School of Medicine, Charlottesville, Va., USA

Key Words
5-Lipoxygenase · Arachidonic acid · Dietary fat · Epidermal growth factor · Apoptosis

Abstract
Multiple population-based studies show an increased risk of prostate cancer in populations that consume large amounts of animal fat. However, the molecular mechanisms linking dietary fat to prostate cancer biology remain obscure. Animal fats are typically rich sources of arachidonic acid and this fatty acid is converted to a wide range of powerful compounds including leukotrienes, prostaglandins, etc. We have shown that PC3 and LNCaP convert arachidonic acid to the 5-lipoxygenase product, 5-HETE. When the formation of 5-HETE is blocked, human prostate cancer cells enter apoptosis in less than 1 h and are dead within 2 h. Exogenous 5-HETE can rescue these cancer cells. These findings indicate that 5-HETE is a potent survival factor for human prostate cancer cells.

Introduction

Numerous ecological studies have shown an association between diets high in animal fats and the risk of developing clinically significant prostate cancer. Nevertheless, this association remains very controversial. For example, there is no agreement as to whether it is the fat in the animal products or some other substance associated with animal fat. A high intake of animal fat is also commonly associated with a high caloric intake and it has been proposed that high caloric intake is the actual risk factor.

There are a numer of possible explanations for this confusion. First, it is possible that some fat-soluble compound may act as a promotional agent for prostate cancer and this compound is found associated with animal fat to a varying degree in different populations. Second, the promotional effects of dietary fat may reside in specific fatty acids and the fatty acid composition of food may vary over time and geography. The latter is possible because the fatty acid composition of animal fat is influenced, in part, by the fatty acid composition of the fat in the animal's food. For example, a diet high in corn will create an animal whose fat is rich in omega-6 fatty acids, while an animal fed soy will have a greater content of omega-3 fatty acids. Third, it is possible that certain dietary fatty acids play a critical role in prostate cancer biology, but that the impact of these fatty acids is commonly modulated by other dietary components, rendering the relationship difficult to detect in ecological studies.

In view of this background, we have sought to identify molecular mechanisms by which dietary fatty acids might influence the growth and survival of human prostate cancer cells.

KARGER

Fax + 41 61 306 12 34
E-Mail karger@karger.ch
www.karger.com

0302–2838/99/0356–0395$17.50/0

Accessible online at:
http://BioMedNet.com/karger

Charles E. Myers, MD
Box 334, Cancer Center
University of Virginia School of Medicine
Charlottesville, VA 22908 (USA)
Tel. +1 804 982 4190, Fax +1 804 982 0918

Points in the Natural History of Prostate Cancer Influenced by Diet

Autopsy studies have shown that clinically localized prostate cancer develops as a function of age. The first cancers appear in the second decade of life, just after the onset of puberty. With each subsequent decade, the frequency increases so that by age 80, more than 70% of all men have prostate cancer. For the United States, this leads to an estimate of more than 20 million men with prostate cancer. Despite this impressive number, only between 40,000 and 50,000 men die of prostate cancer each year. This means that the ability to grow rapidly and spread beyond the limits of the prostate are important limiting factors in prostate cancer progression.

The age-dependent appearance of localized prostate cancer appears to be relatively uninfluenced by geography or race. For example, the process appears to be quantitatively similar in the United States and Japan. In contrast, death rate for prostate cancer in Japan is much lower than it is in the United States. The death rates from prostate cancer are similarly low throughout much of Asia. These findings suggest that the major impact of diet is not on the initial development of prostate cancer, but on its subsequent progression from an indolent, local neoplasia to a metastatic cancer with lethal outcome. Thus, dietary fat seems most likely to act to promote rather than initiate the malignant process.

Signal Transduction Events That Control Growth of Epithelial Cells

A range of growth factors are known to influence the growth of epithelial cells, including those from the prostate gland. These include cytokines, such as members of the epidermal growth factor (EGF) family, that act through membrane receptors with tyrosine kinase activity. *All* cytokines that function through receptor-associated tyrosine kinases stimulate cell proliferation by activating the *ras* to MAP kinase signal transduction pathway. The importance of this pathway is also supported by the observation that a good number of the known oncogenes represent activating mutations of proteins in this pathway. These range from activation of the EGF receptor by autocrine production of EGF family members to mutational activation of *ras*.

There is a second group of cytokines that function through heterotrimeric G-protein-linked receptors. These include compounds such as bombesin, calcitonin, epinephrine and serotonin. Many carcinomas, including cancers of the lung, breast, colon and prostate, contain cells expressing markers typical of neuroendocrine cells that are known to produce and release these cytokines. Additionally, bombesin and calcitonin have been shown to act as mitogens for human prostate cancer. The signal transduction steps by which heterotrimeric G-protein-linked receptors trigger mitogenesis are not yet fully described. Nevertheless, it is clear that these mitogens also invariably activate MAP kinase. *Thus, activation of MAP kinase is a universal attribute of signal transduction pathways that foster epithelial cell growth.* Additionally, mutations of these signal transduction pathways play an important role in cancer cell biology.

Activation of either tyrosine kinase or heterotrimeric G-protein-linked receptors not only activate mitogenesis, but also promote survival of cells by blocking apoptosis or programmed cell death. While the signal transduction steps by which cytokines trigger mitogenesis are well worked out, the steps involved in antiapoptosis are less well known. Nevertheless, the ability of prostate cancer cells to survive androgen ablation, radiation therapy and chemotherapy obviously play an important role in the progression of this cancer.

Role of Dietary Fatty Acids in Epithelial Cell Signal Transduction Events

Arachidonic acid is a 20-carbon omega-6 fatty acid present in the diet, with meat being a particularly rich source. This fatty acid can undergo metabolic conversion to a series of eicosanoids with potent biological effects. These products include compounds such as prostaglandin E_2 (PGE_2), prostacyclin, and the leukotrienes. The eicosanoids are already known to play a critical role in cancer cell biology. For example, production of PGE_2 can promote the growth of colon carcinoma cells. The 12-lipoxygenase product, 12-HETE, is an important stimulus of cancer cell motility and invasion.

In epithelial cells, arachidonic acid largely exists bound to membrane phospholipids. This fatty acid is released from the cell membrane through the action of a cytoplasmic phospholipase A_2. This phospholipase A_2 is activated by serine phosphorylation followed by calcium-dependent membrane translocation and both events are necessary for optimal enzymatic activity. Under most conditions, release of arachidonic acid from the membrane is the rate-limiting step in eicosanoid formation. Activation of phospholipase A_2 by serine phosphorylation can be mediated by activated MAP kinase and protein kinase C. As we have just described, activation of MAP kinase is a universal attribute of all mitogenic cytokines. Additionally, protein kinase C is also activated by many of the same cytokines. Also, activation of protein kinase C has been repeatedly linked to the promotional phase of carcinogenesis. As you might expect, addition of many cytokines and promotional agents has been observed to trigger arachidonic acid release and eicosanoid formation through either phospholipase A_2 or protein kinase C.

The Pattern of Eicosanoid Formation Is Tissue- and Cell Lineage-Dependent

While cytokines commonly trigger the release of arachodinic acid, the subsequent transformation of this fatty acid to an eicosanoid shows striking tissue and cell lineage specificity. For example, addition of GM-CSF to myeloid cells causes the formation of 5-HETE. Addition of EGF to colon or uterine epithelia causes the formation of PGE_2. An additional level of tissue and cell lineage specificity is achieved by the expression of various eicosanoid receptors. Thus, it is possible for adjacent tissues or cells to independently control their response to selected stimuli. These observations also have important therapeutic implications. This biology is a critical reason for the promise of COX-2 inhibitors in colon cancer prevention.

Role of Eicosanoid Formation in Prostate Cancer Biology

With this background in mind, we have examined the role of eicosanoid formation in the growth and survival of the human prostate cancer cell lines, PC3 and LNCaP [1–3]. Both cell lines survive and grow slowly in serum-free media. Thus, in order to simplify our analysis, we studied the impact of first arachidonic acid and then selected eicosanoids on the growth and survival of these cell lines. We should also note that arachidonic acid and the eicosanoids are completely water-insoluble. However, in vivo fatty acids often are transported by albumin and many cells, including these prostate cells, have a cell surface receptor and transport system for albumin-bound fatty acids. For this reason, we presented these compounds to the cancer cells using fat-free albumin as a carrier. This point is ciritical, because we were unable to get reproducible results by simply adding the fatty acid to media: arachidonic acid would simply float on the top of the media.

Under serum-free conditions, arachidonic acid is an effective mitogen at concentrations between 10 and 50 μM. When endogenous phospholipase A_2 was blocked by the inhibitor, quinacrine, these prostate cancer cells underwent growth arrest and death. The lethal impact of quinacrine could be reversed by the addition of arachidonic acid.

As mentioned, arachidonic acid undergoes metabolic conversion to a range of eicosanoids. Thus, we next tried to determine the specific eicosanoids that support the growth of prostate cancer cells under serum-free conditions. As an initial step, we added a series of well-characterized inhibitors of eicosanoid formation. This experiment revealed that only inhibitors of the lipoxygenase duplicated the growth arrest and death seen following addition of the phospholipase A_2 inhibitor, quinacrine.

In mammalian cells, there are three major lipoxygenase families, the 5-, 12- and 15-lipoxygenases. Using a series of specific inhibitors, we were able to show that blockade of 5-lipoxygenase was sufficient to duplicate growth arrest and subsequent cell death. The product of 5-lipoxygenase, 5-HpETE, undergoes subsequent conversion along two distinct pathways. The best-known pathway leads to the formation of leukotrienes of the four series. A less well-known pathway involves the conversion of 5-HpETE to 5-HETE and then 5-oxoETE. Products of the latter pathway have been shown to be one of the stimuli of granulocyte migration and degranulation. We tested each of the known 5-lipoxygenase products for their ability to rescue cells from the impact of 5-lipoxygenase inhibition. The only products able to promote survival and promote growth were 5-HpETE, 5-HETE and 5-oxoETE. We were then also able to show that both cancer cell lines constitutively produce 5-HETE under serum-free conditions. Also, the production of 5-HETE was markedly increased by the addition of exogenous arachidonic acid, demonstrating that availability of arachidonic acid was rate-limiting for this pathway.

We next sought to define better the process of cell death triggered by inhibition of 5-lipoxygenase. We found that addition of the specific 5-lipoxygenase inhibitor, MK886, caused rapid onset of cell death. Under serum-free conditions, *all* of the cells in the culture entered apoptosis in less than 2 h. Since the cell cycle time for these prostate cancer cells is more than 20 h, this shows that MK866 triggers apoptosis without regard to position in the cell cycle. There are very few examples of synchronous onset of apoptosis that proceed this rapidly. For this reason, we decided to document in greater detail the nature of apoptosis in these cells.

There are two major death pathways leading to apoptosis. One involves mitochondrial permeability transition with release of cytochrome C, activation of caspase 9 and the caspase 3. The latter is at the beginning of the execution phase of apoptosis. We were able to show that addition of MK886 results in mitochondrial permeability transition beginning within 45 min and then activation of caspase 3. Other events associated with apoptosis also appear rapidly after mitochondrial permeability transition has occurred. For example, membrane bleb formation is evident beginning at 1 h. The movement of phosphatidylserine from the inner to the outer mitochondrial membrane characterizes blebs that form in association with apoptosis. This can be identified by the fact that Annexin V binds to phosphatidylserine. As expected, the blebs developing after addition of MK886 bind Annexin V in the fashion characteristic of apoptosis. Finally, DNA degradation as characterized by nucleosome formation begins at 2 h and is complete by 4–6 h.

The addition of 5-HETE or 5-oxoETE is able to delay the onset of apoptosis. The effect was both specific and potent. Concentrations of 5-HETE as low as 10 n*M* were able to protect PC3 and LNCaP cells from cell death. The product of 5-HETE metabolism, 5-oxoETE, was also active. However, leukotrienes, the other major group of 5-lipoxygenase products, were not active. Products of lipoxygenase 12 and 15 were also not active.

Androgen is a well-known survival factor for human prostate cancer cells. However, PC3 is androgen-independent. In addition, absence of androgen slows the growth, but does not trigger the death of LNCaP, even under serum-free conditions. We found that addition of the synthetic androgen, R188, did not alter cell death triggered by inhibition of 5-lipoxygenase in either cell line. Our findings document that the survival of both PC3 and LNCaP in the absence of androgen requires the presence of the arachidonic acid product, 5-HETE.

In summary: We have shown that the 5-lipoxygenase products, 5-HETE and 5-oxoETE, are potent survival factors for human prostate cancer. Constitutive formation of these eicosanoids accounts for the survival of both cell lines under serum-free conditions. Additionally, formation of 5-HETE is limited by the availability of arachidonic acid. We have shown that both prostate cancer cell lines are able to take up and convert exogenous arachidonic acid to 5-HETE in less than 1 h. These findings have led us to propose that dietary arachidonic acid might promote progression of prostate cancer by providing a potent antiapoptotic factor that allows the cells to survive androgen removal and even removal of all exogenous growth factors.

References

1 Ghosh J, Myers C: Arachidonic acid stimulates prostate cancer cell growth: Critical role of 5-lipoxygenase. Biochem Biophys Res Commun 1997;235:418–423.
2 Ghosh J, Myers C: Arachidonic acid metabolism and cancer of the prostate. Nutrition 1998; 14:48–57.
3 Ghosh J, Myers C: Arachidonic acid 5-lipoxygenase plays a role in survival of prostate cancer cells. Proc Natl Acad Sci USA 1998;95: 13182–13187.

Molecular Targets for Chemoprevention of Prostate Cancer

European Urology

Eur Urol 1999;35:399–407

Angiogenesis, p53, *bcl-2* and Ki-67 in the Progression of Prostate Cancer after Radical Prostatectomy

Judd W. Moul

Urology Service, Department of Surgery, Walter Reed Army Medical Center, Washington, D.C. and Center for Prostate Disease Research, Department of Surgery, Uniformed Services University of the Health Sciences, Bethesda, Md., USA

Key Words

Prostate · Cancer · Radical prostatectomy · p53 · bcl-2 · Ki-67 · Prognosis

Abstract

Within the past 5 years, research has increasingly addressed molecular alterations in prostate cancer (CaP). Mutations of tumor suppressor gene p53 have been found in a variety of cancers, including urologic neoplasms. Several studies have been conducted on CaP specimens, citing frequencies of p53 alterations in localized cancers ranging from 4 to 60% and with more advanced hormone refractory disease, as high as 94%. The majority of studies have revealed a low percentage of p53 abnormalities in early-stage (clinically organ-confined) CaP. The overwhelming bulk of evidence suggests that the frequency of p53 abnormalities does increase with disease progression and is highest in tissues from patients with hormone-refractory prostate cancer. More recently, our group and others have found that focal p53 expression in the primary tumor by immunohistochemistry is predictive of cancer recurrence after radical prostatectomy.

bcl-2 is an oncogene critically involved in the apoptosis, or programmed cell death. Overexpression of *bcl-2* protein by immunohistochemistry has been commonly detected in advanced hormone refractory CaP. Our group recently has also shown that *bcl-2* protein expression in primary CaP is a predictor of cancer recurrence after radical prostatectomy. Furthermore, the combination of p53 and *bcl-2* protein expression were both independent predictors of recurrence after surgery. Most recently, we have shown that even though p53 and *bcl-2* are predictive biomarkers when sampling the radical prostatectomy specimen, they are not useful to predict postoperative recurrence when sampling the pretreatment needle biopsy.

Ki-67 is an antigen of cellular proliferation. Immunohistochemical staining for Ki-67 in archival material can be performed using the MIB-1 antibody. Unlike our results with p53 and *bcl-2*, Ki-67 protein expression by immunohistochemistry using MIB-1 was not an independent prognostic marker for cancer recurrence after radical prostatectomy although it may have clinical utility in subsets of patients. Assessment of MIB-1 staining in CaP needle biopsy samples is underway.

Tumor neovascularity, or angiogenesis, is necessary for cancers to grow and metastasize. Angiogenesis in CaP as

The opinions and assertions contained herein are the private views of the author and are not to be construed as reflecting the views of the US Army or the Department of Defense.

KARGER

Fax + 41 61 306 12 34
E-Mail karger@karger.ch
www.karger.com

0302–2838/99/0356–0399$17.50/0

Accessible online at:
http://BioMedNet.com/karger

Judd W. Moul, MD
Department of Surgery, Uniformed Services University of the Health Sciences
4301 Jones Bridge Road, Bethesda, MD 20814-4799 (USA)
Tel. +1 301 295 3707, Fax +1 301 295 6396
E-Mail ltc_judd_moul@wramc1-amedd.army.mil

a prognostic marker has received recent attention. Most studies have used factor VIII immunohistochemical staining and increased angiogenesis has been suggested as a staging and prognostic marker. Our group has recently conducted a large study of radical prostatectomy patients and used CD34 antigen immunohistochemistry to assess neovascularity. We did not find that this biomarker assessment was an independent prognostic marker of cancer recurrence after radical prostatectomy. Further work is being conducted in needle biopsy samples.
More research is needed to assess new biomarkers and, most importantly, to standardize the methodology for sampling and assaying biomarkers in heterogeneous and multifocal prostate cancer.

Introduction

The elegant statement 'When treatment is possible, is it necessary, and when treatment is necessary, is it possible' by the late Dr. Willet Whitmore is as relevant today regarding prostate cancer (CaP) as it was two decades ago [1]. We are at the verge of making progress with the discovery of new molecular and cellular markers of disease progression and outcome and there is clearly a need for improved prognostic markers for CaP. The traditional prognostic markers include clinical and pathologic stage, grade, and serum acid phosphatase. More recently, pretreatment serum prostate-specific antigen (PSA) level has replaced acid phosphatase in clinical practice. In the patient who has undergone radical prostatectomy (RP), Partin et al. [2] were the first to devise a model for recurrence using stage, Gleason grade and pretreatment PSA level. More recently, our group [3] and the group from Baylor University [4] have developed similar recurrence models based on combining traditional prognostic factors. These traditional markers and combination equations are useful for men who have parameters on the extremes of 'good' and 'bad'. However, for many of those with intermediate values such as Gleason sum of 5–7, a pathologic T3a specimen-confined tumor and/or a PSA between approximately 10 and 20 ng/ml, the prognostic ability is still limited.

Molecular prognostic markers in CaP are not a new concept. Defined as the measurement of subcellular components or molecules to predict CaP outcome, DNA ploidy and nuclear roundness have been studied for over a decade [5, 6]. DNA ploidy determination by flow cytometry or image analysis in localized CaP has been found to be a significant predictor of disease course in some but not all studies [6]. It may add prognostic information in patients with intermediate grade tumors but has yet to be widely used in general clinical practice. Nuclear roundness was initially reported to be a better prognostic marker than Gleason score but later studies reported conflicting results [6–8]. As with DNA ploidy, nuclear morphometry has yet to be used in general clinical practice.

Over the last few years, the study of molecular markers in CaP and other human cancers has focused on the human genes implicated in tumorigenesis. Mutation, amplifications, or other alterations of the genes themselves or more commonly, the proteins of these genes have been measured and compared to traditional prognostic markers and outcome. Oncogenes, tumor suppressor genes and genes for other important cellular functions have been analyzed as well as their corresponding proteins. An advantage to protein analysis is the use of standard immunohistochemistry techniques, many of which can be performed in archival paraffin materials. A limiation to all these types of studies in CaP is the heterogeneity and multifocality of this human neoplasm. All molecular marker studies may have limited value if proper sampling of tumor foci is not performed. In the following sections, we will review the specific biomarkers p53, *bcl-2*, proliferation marker Ki-67, and angiogenesis or neovascularity for their value in predicting recurrence or progression in the RP patient.

p53 Tumor Suppressor Gene

The p53 gene is a tumor suppressor gene located on chromosome 17. It codes for the p53 protein centrally involved in cellular growth control. p53 mutations are now the most common genetic alterations found in human cancer. When p53 is mutated it is no longer able to suppress cellular growth and proliferation as it normally does and this contributes to the neoplastic process. The mutated p53 protein also has a prolonged half-life allowing immunohistochemical detection. The normal p53 protein has a short half-life and is not detectable by clinical immunohistochemistry.
In CaP, early studies indicated that p53 mutations were uncommon in primary CaPs and more common in metastatic CaP [9–12]. Our own results showed a progression of p53 activation in progressive stages of disease [13]. Our results showed that in needle biopsy specimens from patients with localized CaP the rate of patients with

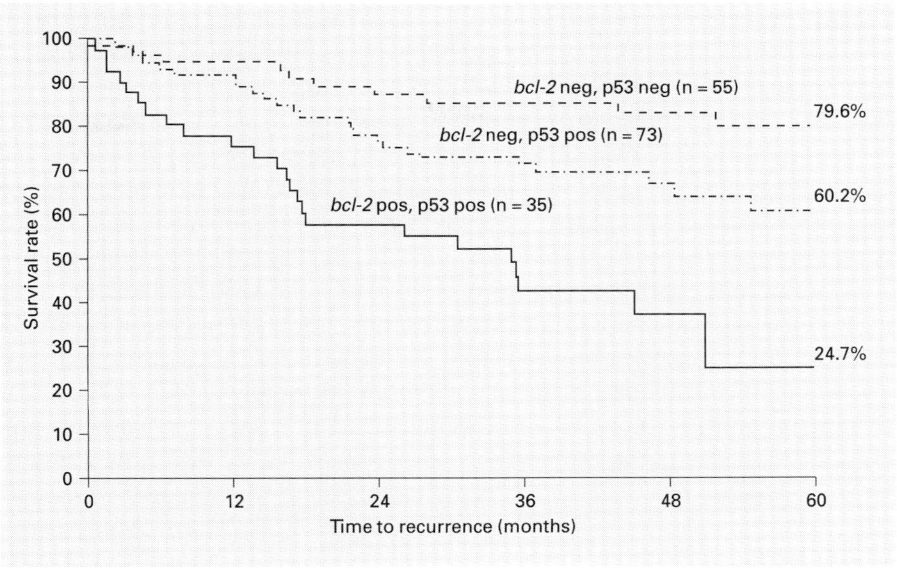

Fig. 1. Kaplan-Meier analysis of disease-free survival after RP based on expression of p53 and *bcl-2* proteins in RP surgical specimen. (No survival curve shown for *bcl-2* pos, p53 neg (n = 6)).

nuclear protein accumulation was approximately 20% [13]. In lymph node metastases from untreated patients, approximately 50% had p53 overexpression and in TURP tissue from patients with treatment-resistant disease over 75% had p53 overexpression [13]. In our follow-up work, we next extensively examined RP specimens for p53 nuclear protein expression [14]. With comprehensive sampling of multifocal clinically localized disease, we found that approximately 60% of patients have at least some p53-positive cancer cell clones in their primary tumor. Most importantly, we found that p53 overexpression was an independent prognostic marker for recurrence after surgery [14]. The research group from Baylor University also described the focal nature of p53 protein expression in primary CaP as 'clustered' p53 staining and also found that it predicted a high recurrence rate [15]. While some other groups have also found that p53 protein expression is an adverse prognostic factor [16, 17], the groups from Johns Hopkins University [18] and University of Southern California [19] have not found prognostic significance to p53 expression.

In a follow-up study, our group reassessed p53 staining in 175 RP patients having a mean 5-year follow-up [20]. In this latter study, we also performed immunohistochemistry for the *bcl-2* oncogene (see next section). p53 and *bcl-2* protein expression were both independent predictors of serologic (PSA) recurrence after RP (fig. 1). Again, it is important to point out that the biomarkers were assessed on the RP specimen with special care taken to sample multiple malignant foci and characterize the whole prostate. Under these research conditions, both of these biomarkers added unique information to the prediction of recurrence beyond pathologic stage, grade and PSA.

Most recently, we have conducted a study of p53 (and *bcl-2*) protein expression in the pre-RP diagnostic needle biopsies from the same cohort of patients [21]. We wrote to referring institutions and asked them to mail us the archival blocks from the diagnostic biopsy. In 117 cases in which material was obtained, we were able to stain the needle biopsies for p53 (and *bcl-2*) and compare them to the results we had previously obtained in their radical specimens. For p53 and *bcl-2* there was poor correlation between the needle biopsy results and the radical specimen results. In general, the needle biopsy underrepresented the biomarker expression. Furthermore, the needle biopsy p53 staining did not correlate to recurrence after the RP. In fact, the recurrence rates for biopsy p53-positive and -negative cases were virtually identical. Interestingly, in even longer follow-up (mean 6 years), the p53 protein expression in the radical specimens held up as an independent prognostic marker. These results suggest that these biomarkers are expressed heterogeneously in the multifocal primary CaP and that the needle biopsies did not sample adequately enough for prognostic ability. We are currently conducting a study of whole mounted RP specimens in which we are doing p53 immunohistochemistry at 2.5-mm intervals of the entire gland. Using computer three-dimensional reconstruction, our aim is to determine the spatial characteristics of p53 expression within the organ. We are also currently conducting another study using the laser capture microdissecting microscope to determine if p53 gene mutations are detected in the focal, clustered areas of p53 protein expression.

In summary, p53 alterations in CaP would appear to have biological significance. If one comprehensively samples a prostatectomy specimen, p53 appears to have utility as a prognostic marker. However, our current biopsy study could not confirm a clinical utility for p53 biopsy immunohistochemistry. Perhaps as more biopsy cores are taken during diagnostic transrectal ultrasound (sextant, 8, 10, 12, etc.), the biopsy material will more accurately reflect the multifocality and heterogeneity and provide clinically useful material for biomarker assessment.

bcl-2 Oncogene

The *bcl-2* proto-oncogene is a gene that encodes for a protein that has been shown to act as an inhibitor of apoptosis [22]. Studies in late stage CaP have implicated *bcl-2* in the conversion of androgen-dependent to -independent disease and have shown *bcl-2* overexpression in androgen-independent tissues [23–25]. *bcl-2* overexpression occurs in early stage CaP, however, most studies have shown lower frequencies than in advanced cancer ranging from 32 to 41% [24, 26–28].

In 1996, we published the first study analyzing *bcl-2* expression as a predictor of PSA recurrence after RP [20]. As previously noted, this study of 175 surgery patients followed for a mean of 5 years found that both p53 and *bcl-2* were both independent predictors of recurrence. *bcl-2* overexpression was a lower frequency event than p53 expression; only 47/175 (27%) patients exhibited *bcl-2* expression in their prostatectomy specimen. However, the recurrence rate was 67% at 5 years in those 47 men compared to only 30.5% in the 128 patients who did not express *bcl-2* [20]. Both p53 and *bcl-2* contributed unique prognostic information and in the 35 patients who overexpressed both p53 and *bcl-2* proteins, the recurrence rate was 100% at 6-year follow-up. Like previously noted for p53, however, *bcl-2* expression in our needle biopsy study was not predictive of recurrence presumably due to sampling and heterogeneity issues [21]. Most recently our results have been confirmed by other investigators [29–31]. Most interesting is the recent work of Huang et al. [31] who found that *bcl-2* expression predicted recurrence after radiation and was felt to be a better biomarker of radiation sensitivity than p53.

Prognostic Equation of Recurrence with p53 and *bcl-2*

Pretreatment PSA level, prostatectomy specimen Gleason sum, pathologic stage, tumor volume, endorectal coil magnetic resonance imaging (MRI), DNA ploidy, race, and more recently, molecular biomarkers (e.g., p53, *bcl-2*) have shown significant correlation to PSA recurrence after surgery. Most recently, investigators have combined prognostic variables into models or equations used to predict the likelihood of recurrence. Partin et al. [32] were the first investigators who developed a simple biostatistical model equation that categorized postradical prostatectomy patients into three risk groups (low, intermediate, and high risk) for likelihood of serological failure. Many preoperative and pathological variables were analyzed; however, after multivariate regression analysis only three variables were included in the final model to adequately select for high-risk patients after surgery. A sigmoidal transformation of PSA, prostatectomy Gleason sum, and specimen confinement (margin status) were incorporated into an equation that calculated the relative risk of recurrence, R_r, as:

$$R_r = (0.061 \times PSA_{ST}) + (0.54 \times \text{postoperative Gleason}) + (1.87 \times \text{specimen-confined})$$

Depending on the patients' calculated value of R_r, these patients could be stratified into three risk groups. This model employs traditional variables that are commonly determined at most institutions, making this form of risk assessment a practical clinical tool that can be used in decisions concerning adjuvant therapy. This model allows those patients at high risk for recurrence to be identified shortly after surgery, while their tumor burden is theoretically at a minimum.

Our research group has also been working to develop prognostic models that will predict PSA recurrence after RP. While the Hopkins model [32] has been a great start, this model did not include race or newer molecular markers as potential prognostic variables and was only developed in clinical T26(B2) patients. Employing the Hopkins model in our RP patients, we determined that it predicted disease recurrence better for Caucasian than for African-American patients [33]. Furthermore, in addition to traditional prognostic markers, work by our group as previously noted suggests that molecular biomarkers may be valuable [14, 20]. The goal of our study was to develop a model to predict recurrence after RP using the traditional clinical and pathological variables combined with the molecular biomarkers [34]. A separate model that used

Table 1. Three- and 5-year Kaplan-Meier disease-free survival rates for risk groups created from the p53 and *bcl-2* prognostic model equation [adapted from 34]

Risk groups	n (recurred)	R_r (relative risk)		Recurrence-free survival	
		mean	range	3-year	5-year
$R_r < 5.0$	44 (3)	2.6	1–4.9	97.6	92.7
$R_r > 5.0 < 15.0$	39 (14)	11.3	5–14.9	73.7	58
$R_r \geq 15.0$	49 (30)	37.7	>15.0	40.2	31.6

only the biomarkers was also developed [34]. In 132 patients who underwent RP between 1986 and 1993 having a mean follow-up of 5.4 years, we analyzed age, race, preoperative PSA, postoperative Gleason sum, postoperative nuclear grade, pathological stage (organ-confined or nonorgan-confined) and the biomarkers p53, *bcl-2*, and Ki-67 using Cox multivariable regression analysis with backward elimination of nonstatistically significant variables at the p = 0.10 level. Race (p = 0.054), PSA (p = 0.026), pathologic stage (p = 0.046), p53 (p = 0.041), and *bcl-2* (p = 0.028) stayed in the model but age, Gleason sum, nuclear grade, and Ki-67 did not. The final model, incorporating only the statically significant variables, was used to calculate the relative risk of recurrence, R_r, as:

$$R_r = \exp[(0.70 \times \text{race}) + (0.79 \times \text{PSA}\{4.1\text{–}10\}) = (1.34 \times \text{PSA}\{>10\}) + (0.91 \times \text{organ confinement}) + (0.65 \times \text{p53}\{1,2+\}) + (1.45 \times \text{p53}\{3,4+\}) + (0.70 \times bcl\text{-}2)]$$

where race was defined as '1' if the patient was African-American or '0' if Caucasian, organ-confined (no capsular penetration) was designated at '0' whereas nonorgan-confined (capsular extension and/or positive margins) was defined as '1'. The p53 variable is given a value of '1' if the protein was expressed, and *bcl-2* was given a value of '1' if the specimen exhibited protein overexpression and '0' if there was no or rare expression. PSA in the above equation was given a '1' if the preoperative PSA value was within the above stated ranges and '0' otherwise. Relative risk values were calculated for each patient using this equation and three risk groups (low, intermediate, and high risk) were created. Kaplan-Meier disease-free survival at 3 and 5 years are shown in table 1 for these risk groups. All three risk groups were statistically different from each other using the log rank test of significance ($p < 0.05$).

This p53 and *bcl-2* molecular biomarker equation is an example of how molecular markers could be used in the future to better care for patients. At present, this is a research tool that will need verification in a prospective clinical trial.

Ki-67 Proliferative Antigen

Growth potential of a tumor is one of its most important characteristics. The growth of CaP can be variable and rates of progression may vary greatly among tumors of similar stage and grade [35]. Ki-67 is a nuclear antigen present throughout the cell cycle (G1, S, G2, M) but not present at rest (G0) or early G1 phase [36]. Ki-67 nuclear staining has been related to the biological aggressiveness and prognosis in a number of cancers: the higher the proliferative index the more aggressive the carcinoma [35]. As a marker, the monoclonal antibody to Ki-67 antigen has been shown to provide a reliable method of estimating cellular proliferation correlating well with uptake of bromodeoxyuridine (BrdUrd) and thymidine labeling [37]. Statistically significant differences between mean Ki-67 indices of benign prostatic hyperplasia (BPH) and CaP have uniformly been reported [38–41]. Previous studies of Ki-67 antigen staining in CaP have shown a variable relationship with tumor stage and grade. However, significant associations have been found between Ki-67 antigen expression and time to progression, metastatic status and tumor volume [41–44]. MIB-1 is a monoclonal antibody to recombinant parts of the Ki-67 antigen and has identical nuclear staining patterns in paraffin specimens as Ki-67 monoclonal antibody in fresh sections [45].

We analyzed Ki-67 proliferative antigen using MIB-1 monoclonal antibody in archival paraffin-embedded RP specimens from 180 RP patients followed from 1 to 9 years (mean 4.4) [46]. The percentage of tumor nuclei expressing Ki-67 antigen was measured and assigned an MIB-1 score (0/rare = negative, 1+ = low, 2–4+ = high) and analyzed for PSA stage, age, race, grade and serologic recurrence following surgery. There was a significant association between higher MIB-1 score and higher nuclear grade ($p < 0.001$), Gleason score ($p < 0.001$), and pathologic stage (p = 0.01). Patients with a high MIB-1 score progressed earlier which was associated with a lower 5-year recurrence-free survival (44%) than those with low MIB-1 scores (71%) ($p < 0.001$) (table 2). In multivariate

Table 2. MIB-1 score correlation to Kaplan-Meier 5-year recurrence-free survival probability [adapted from 46]

MIB score	Total number	No progression		Progression		5-year recurrence-free survival, %
		n	%	n	%	
0/rare	18	15	12.7	3	4.8	83
1+	90	67	56.8	23	37.1	69
2–4+	72	36	30.5	36	58.1	44
Total	180	118	65.5	62	34.5	60

Cox regression analysis with backward elimination, pathologic stage ($p < 0.01$), pretreatment PSA ($p = 0.04$), and MIB-1 score ($p = 0.05$) were all statistically significant predictors of disease-free survival and patients with a high MIB-1 score were 3.1 times as likely to recur as those with a negative score. Controlling for stage, patients with organ-confined disease associated with a high MIB-1 score had a lower 5-year disease-free survival (68%) than those with a low MIB-1 score (95%) ($p < 0.01$).

Proliferative activity as measured by the Ki-67 proliferative antigen, MIB-1, appears to be a prognostic marker of recurrence for CaP patients after RP. However, this work needs to be confirmed in other large studies. Furthermore, like p53 and *bcl-2*, this work was performed in RP specimens. The clinical value of Ki-67 expression in needle biopsies has not yet been assessed.

Molecular Markers of Angiogenesis

It has been shown that both for tumor growth and for hematogeneous spread of tumor cells, the development of blood vessels toward and within a tumor is required [47, 48]. This is achieved by a multistep process referred to as tumor angiogenesis [47]. Angiogenesis promotes growth because the new vessels allow exchange of nutrients, oxygen, and waste products by a crowded cell population for which simple diffusion of these substances across its outer surfaces is no longer adequate. In addition to this perfusion effect, endothelial cells may release important paracrine growth factors for tumor cells [49]. Intratumor microvessel density (MVD) determined on histological sections by staining endothelial antigens is a quantitative measure of this process angiogenesis.

CD34, a myeloid progenitor cell antigen also present in endothelial cells, is detectable in all types of endothelium. The monoclonal antibody to CD34 (Q-bend) reacts with endothelium of arteries, venules and has been found to stain more intensely with capillary endothelium. It has been previously used in diagnosis of vascular tumors and detection of small vessel proliferation representing angiogenesis [50, 51]. von Willebrand factor (vWF, formerly called factor VIII-related antigen) is also present in endothelial cells and is one of the oldest markers applied in immunohistochemistry of vascular tumors and tumor angiogenesis [52, 53]. One of its drawbacks however is the widespread presence of this antigen in serum and body fluids creating generalized background staining making some cases uninterpretable.

Intratumor MVD in human CaP was first reported in 1993 by Bigler et al. [54]. This group reported increased density of capillaries in CaP when compared to benign prostate tissue and used a computerized image analysis system to assess factor VIII-related antigen staining in RP specimens. Later, intensity of intratumor angiogenesis or MVD using vWF was shown to be an independent predictor of pathologic stage in CaP and has been correlated with metastasis [55, 56]. More recently, Bostwick et al. [57] have used the optimized MVD developer by Bigler et al. [54], along with biopsy Gleason score and pretreatment PSA value to improve prediction of pathologic stage of RP patients. Furthermore, MVD using CD34 has been associated with progression of CaP after RP for clinically localized disease but not with pathologic stage in Gleason sum 5–7 [58].

We recently assessed the neovascularity of clinically localized CaP by immunohistochemistry using the monoclonal antibody CD34 in an attempt to identify associations between angiogenesis and disease progression following RP [59]. Microvascularity was evaluated using the CD34 monoclonal antibody in archival paraffin-embedded RP specimens from 149 RP patients followed from 3 to 10 years (mean 6.6). Vessels were quantified by counting a minimum of two selected microscopic fields (200 ×, 0.754 mm^2) from each tumor, area of PIN, and prostatic hyperplasia and given a numerical value representing the MVD count.

The mean MVD count did not vary significantly with age or race. There was a significant association between the MVD count and nuclear grade, Gleason sum, and pathologic stage. Cox survival analysis shows that MVD is significantly related to time to recurrence when considered as a continuous variable ($p = 0.03$) as well as dichotomous variable ($p = 0.007$) (MVD count <90 and ≥90). The 5-year recurrence-free survival is significantly higher in those patients with an MVD count <90 (71%) than those patients with an MVD count ≥90 (51%) ($p = 0.006$)

(table 3). The 5-year recurrence-free survival was also significantly different when MVD was used as a continuous variable (p = 0.02). Controlling for stage, Gleason sum, race, and nuclear grade, MVD remained significant in predicting recurrence (p = 0.03), however when pretreatment PSA was included in the model, MVD was no longer significant. The MVD count in the tumor area significantly increased with increasing Gleason sum and nuclear grade, however, it did not increase significantly in the adjacent benign prostate or areas of PIN in the same specimen. Microvascularity or neovascularity as measured by the CD34 antigen, may be a prognostic marker of recurrence for CaP patients after RP, however more study in PSA-era patients with sufficient follow-up will be needed.

Although MVD may be a predictor of recurrence after RP when using the surgical specimen, several practical problems may limit the effectiveness of MVD as a prognostic indicator in biopsy specimens. CaP is known to be a histopathological heterogeneous tumor and measurement of MVD, particularly in biopsy specimens, may not predict the predominant neovascularity of a tumor. Our method of searching for the 'hot spot' for MVD in the radical specimens may be difficult or impossible in biopsy samples. However in several recent preliminary abstract reports, MVD count on biopsy specimens was found to be significantly associated with recurrence after RP [60, 61]. In addition, Bostwick et al. [57] used the 'optimized' MVD in needle biopsy along with biopsy Gleason sum and pretreatment PSA value to predict pathologic stage in RP specimens. Most recently, Gettman et al. [62] from the Mayo Clinic studied 147 RP patients with a mean follow-up of 6.1 years and found that optimized MVD was also not an independent predictor of recurrence for PSA-era patients.

Table 3. CD34 angiogenesis MVD cut-point to predict recurrence after RP [adapted from 59]

MVD categories	Patients	PSA recurrence	
		n	%
<90	45	12	26.7
≥90	104	50	48.1

Other Potential Molecular Biomarkers

A variety of other markers have received some study as prognostic markers in CaP including chromosomal anomalies [63], oncogenes such as *c-erbB-2* [64], growth factors such as epidermal growth factor receptor [65], proteins implicated in metastases such as cathepsin-D [65] and others [66]. In particular, our group has analyzed *c-erbB-2* protein [64], epidermal growth factor receptor [65], and cathepsin-D protein expression [65] in RP specimens. These biomarkers were not predictive of recurrence after surgery in our hands. In addition, we have analyzed peripheral blood for PSA-expressing cells by reverse transcriptase-polymerase chain reaction and it also was not predictive of recurrence after RP [67].

In summary: Of the many new molecular prognostic markers being evaluated in CaP, p53 and *bcl-2* appear to have promise. These biomarkers appear useful in RP specimens but not in needle biopsy. Undoubtedly, we are still in the infancy of molecular biomarker study in CaP. In the future, we will be able to determine the genetic pedigree of individuals with CaP and will be able to answer the questions posed by Dr. Whitmore.

Acknowledgment

The author is supported by a grant from the Center for Prostate Disease Research, a program of the Henry M. Jackson Foundation for the Advancement of Military Medicine (Rockville, Md.), funded by the US Army Medical Research and Materiel Command.

References

1 Whitmore WF: The natural history of prostate cancer. Cancer 1973;32:1104.

2 Partin AW, Piantodosi S, Sanda MG, et al: Selection of men at high risk for disease recurrence for experimental adjuvant therapy following radical prostatectomy. Urology 1995; 45:831–838.

3 Bauer JJ, Connelly RR, Sesterhenn IA, et al: Biostatistical modeling using traditional preoperative and pathological prognostic variables in the selection of men at high risk for disease recurrence after radical prostatectomy for prostate cancer (abstract). J Urol 1997;157(suppl): 298.

4 Kattan MW, Eastham JA, Stapleton AMF, Wheeler TM, Scardino PT: A preoperative nomogram for disease recurrence following radical prostatectomy for prostate cancer. J Nat Cancer Inst 1998;90:766–771.

5 Shanky TV, Kallioniema OP, Koslowskim HM, Lieber ML, Mayall BH, Miller G, Smith GJ: Consensus review of the clinical utility of DNA content cytometry in prostate cancer. Cytometry 1993;14:497–500.

6 Diamond DA, Berry SJ, Jewett HJ, Eggleston JC, Coffey DS: A new method to assess metastatic potential of human prostate cancer: Relative nuclear roundness. J Urol 1982;128:729–734.

7 Mohler JL, Partin AW, Epstein JI, Lohr WD, Coffey DS: Nuclear roundness factor measurement for assessment of prognosis of patients with prostatic carcinoma. II. Standardization of methodology for histologic sections. J Urol 1988;139:1085–1090.

8 Veltri RW, Partin AW, Epstein JE, Marley GM, Miller CM, Singer DS, Patton KP, Criley SR, Coffey DS: Quantitative nuclear morphometry, Markovian texture descriptors, and DNA content captured on a CAS-200 image analysis system, combined with PCNA and HER-2/neu immunohistochemistry for prediction of prostate cancer progression. J Cell Biochem Suppl 1994;19:249–258.

9 Bookstein R, MacGrogan D, Hilsenbeck SG, Sharkey F, Allred DC: p53 is mutated in a subset of advanced-stage prostate cancer. Cancer Res 1993;53:3369–3373.

10 Navone NM, Troncoso P, Pisters LL, Goodrow TL, Palmer JL, Nichols WW, von Eschenbach AC, Conti CJ: p53 protein accumulation and gene mutation in the progression of human prostate carcinoma. J Natl Cancer Inst 1993; 85:1657–1669.

11 Effert PJ, McCoy RH, Walther PJ, Liu ET: p53 gene alterations in human prostate carcinoma. J Urol 1993;150:257–261.

12 Hall MC, Navone NM, Troncoso P, Pollack A, Zagars GK, von Eschenbach AC, Conti CJ, Chung LW: Frequency and characterization of p53 mutations in clinically localized prostate cancer. Urology 1995;45:470–475.

13 Heidenberg HB, Sesterhenn I, Gaddipati J, Weghorst C, Buzard G, Moul J, Srivastava S: Alteration of the tumor suppressor gene p53 in a high fraction of treatment-resistant prostate cancer. J Urol 1995;154:414–421.

14 Bauer JJ, Sesterhenn IA, Mostofi FK, McLeod DG, Srivastava S, Moul JW: p53 nuclear protein expression is an independent prognostic marker in clinically localized prostate cancer patients undergoing radical prostatectomy. Clin Cancer Res 1995;1:1295–1300.

15 Yang G, Stapleton AMF, Wheeler TM, Truong LD, Timme TL, Scardino PT, Thompson TC: Clustered p53 immunostaining: A novel pattern associated with prostate cancer progression. Clin Cancer Res 1996;2:399–401.

16 Thomas DJ, Robinson M, King P, Hasan T, Charlton R, Martin J, Carr TW, Neal DE: p53 expression and clinical outcome in prostate cancer. Br J Urol 1993;72:778–781.

17 Shurbaji MS, Kalbfleisch JH, Thurmond TS: Immunohistochemical detection of p53 protein as a prognostic indicator in prostate cancer. Hum Pathol 1995;26:106–109.

18 Brooks JD, Bova GS, Ewing CM, Piantadosi S, Carter BS, Robinson JC, Epstein JI, Issacs WB: An uncertain role of p53 gene alterations in human prostate cancer. Cancer Res 1996;56: 3814–3822.

19 Salem CE, Tomasic NA, Elmajian DA, et al: p53 protein and gene alterations in pathological stage C prostate carcinoma. J Urol 1997; 158:510–514.

20 Bauer JJ, Sesterhenn IA, Mostofi FK, McLeod DG, Srivastava S, Moul JW: Elevated levels of apoptosis regulator proteins p53 and *bcl-2* are independent prognostic biomarkers in surgically treated clinically localized prostate cancer patients. J Urol 1996;156:1511–1516.

21 Stackhouse GB, Sesterhenn IA, Mostofi FK, McLeod DG, Moul JW: Immunohistochemical staining for p53 and *bcl-2* in needle biopsies of the prostate does not appear to predict clinical recurrence rate after radical prostatectomy. Proc Am Assoc Cancer Res 1997;38:256.

22 Hockenbury D, Nunez G, Milliman C, Schreiber RD, Korsmeyer SJ: *Bcl-2* is an inner mitochondrial membrane protein that blocks programmed cell death. Nature 1990;348:334.

23 Colombel M, Olsson CA, Ng PY, Buttyan R: Hormone-regulated apoptosis results from reentry of differentiated prostate cells onto a defective cell cycle. Cancer Res 1992;52:4313.

24 McDonnell TJ, Tumcoso P, Brisbay SM, Logothetis C, Chung LW, Hsieh JT, Tu SM, Cambell ML: Expression of the proto-oncogenes *bcl-2* in the prostate and its association with emergence of androgen-independent prostate cancer. Cancer Res 1992;52:6940–6944.

25 Colombel M, Symmans F, Gil S, O'Toole KM, Chopin D, Benson M, Olsson CA, Vorsmeyer S, Battyou R: Detection of the apoptosis-suppressing onco-protein *bcl-2* in hormone refractory prostate cancers. Am J Pathol 1993;143: 390–400.

26 Kallakury BVS, Figgie J, Leihovich B, Rifkin M, Kaufman R, Figgie HL, Nazeer T, Ross JS: Increased *bcl-2* protein levels in prostatic adenocarcinomas are not associated with rearrangements in the 2.8 kb major breakpoint region or with p53 protein accumulation. Mod Pathol 1995;8:78,abstr447.

27 Aprikian I, Robinson M, Fuller C, Boyds J, Neal DE, Hamdy FC: *bcl-2* protein combined with p53 mutant expression correlates with hormone refractory disease and poor prognosis in human prostatic adenocarcinoma. J Urol 1995;153:283,abstr217.

28 Galli S, Gaboardi F, Rozzola A, Ferrari A: Immunohistochemical expression of *bcl-2*, p53, Ki-67 and chromograms in prostate carcinoma. Correlation with stage and grade. J Urol 1995;153:483,abstr1018.

29 Bubendorf L, Sauter G, Moch H, et al: Prognostic significance of *bcl-2* in clinically localized prostate cancer. Am J Pathol 1996;148: 1557.

30 Furuya Y, Krajewski S, Epstein JI, Reed JC, Isaacs JT: Expression of *bcl-2* and the progression of human and rodent prostatic cancers. Clin Cancer Res 1996;2:389–398.

31 Huang A, Gandour-Edwards R, Rosenthal SA, et al: p53 and *bcl-2* immunohistochemical alterations in prostate cancer treated with radiation therapy. Urology 1998;51:346–351.

32 Partin AW, Piantadosi S, Marshall FF, et al: Selection of men at high risk for disease recurrence for experimental adjuvant therapy following radical prostatectomy. Urology 1995; 45:831–837.

33 Douglas TH, McCarthy WF, McLeod DG, Moul JW: Patient selection for experimental adjuvant therapy after radical prostatectomy (letter to editor). Urology 1996;47:284–285.

34 Bauer JJ, Connelly RR, Sesterhenn IA, Bettencourt MC, McLeod DG, Srivastava S, Moul JW: Biostatistical modeling using traditional variables and genetic biomarkers for predicting risk for prostate cancer recurrence after radical prostatectomy. Cancer 1997;79:952–962.

35 Brown DC, Gatter KC: Monoclonal antibody Ki-67: Its use in histopathology. Histopathology 1990;17:489–503.

36 Gerdes J, Lemke H, Baisch H, Wacker H, Schwab U, Stein H: Cell cycle analysis of a cell proliferation-associated human nuclear antigen defined by the monoclonal antibody Ki-67. J Immunol 1984;133:1710–1715.

37 Cher ML, Chew K, Werner R, Carroll PR: Cellular proliferation in prostatic adenocarcinoma as assessed by bromodeoxyuridine uptake and Ki-67 and PCNA expression. Prostate 1995;26: 87–93.

38 Gallee MPW, Visser-DeJong E, Ten Kate FJW, Schroder FH, Van Der Kwast THH: Monoclonal antibody Ki-67 defined growth fraction in benign prostatic hyperplasia and prostatic cancer. J Urol 1989;142:1342–1346.

39 Raymon WA, Leong ASY, Bolt JW, Milios J, Jose JS: Growth fraction in human prostatic carcinoma determined by the Ki-67 immunostaining. J Pathol 1988;156:161–167.
40 Oomens EHGM, Van Steenbrugge GJ, Van Der Kwast THH, Schroder FH: Application of the monoclonal antibody Ki-67 on prostate biopsies to assess the proliferative cell fraction of human prostatic carcinoma. J Urol 1991; 145:81–85.
41 McLoughlin J, Foster CS, Price P, Williams G, Abel PD: Evaluation of Ki-67 monoclonal antibody as prognostic indicator for prostate carcinoma. Br J Urol 1993;72:92–97.
42 Sadi MV, Barrack ER: Determination of growth fraction in advanced prostate cancer by Ki-67 immunostaining and its relationship to the time to tumor progression after hormonal therapy. Cancer 1991;67:3065–3071.
43 Harper ME, Goddard L, Wilson DW, Matanhelia SS, Conn IG, Peeling WB, Griffiths K: Pathological and clinical associations of Ki-67 defined growth fractions in human prostatic carcinoma. Prostate 1992;21:75–84.
44 Van Weerden WM, Moerings E, Van Kreuningen A, DeJong FH, Van Steenbrugge GJ, Schorder FH: Ki-67 expression and BrdUrd incorporation as markers of proliferative activity in human prostate tumor models. Cell Prolif 1993;26:67–75.
45 Cattoretti G, Becker MHG, Key G, Duchrow M, Schluter C, Galle J, Gerdes J: Monoclonal antibody against parts of the Ki-67 antigen (MIB-1 and MIB-3) detect proliferating cells in microwave-processed formalin-fixed paraffin sections. J Pathol 1992;168:357–363.
46 Bettencourt MC, Bauer JJ, Sesterhenn IA, Mostofi FK, McLeod DG, Moul JW: Ki-67 expression is an independent prognostic marker of recurrence in patients with organ confined prostate cancer after radical prostatectomy. J Urol 1996;156:1064–1068.
47 Folkman J: What is the evidence that tumors are angiogenesis-dependent? J Natl Cancer Inst 1990;82:4–6.
48 Folkman J: Tumor angiogenesis: Therapeutic implications. N Engl J Med 1971;285:1182–1186.
49 Folkman J: Angiogenesis and breast cancer. J Clin Oncol 1994;12:441–443.
50 Miettinen M, Lindenmayer A, Chaubal A: Endothelial cell markers CD31, CD34, and BNH9 antibody to H- and Y-antigens. Evaluation of their specificity and sensitivity in the diagnosis of vascular tumors and comparison with von Willebrand factor. Mod Pathol 1994; 7:82–90.
51 Fina L, Molgaard H, Robertson D, Bradley J, Monaghan P, Delia D, Sutherland DS, Baker M, Greaves M: Expression of the CD34 gene in vascular endothelial cells. Blood 1990;75: 2417–2426.
52 Reinders J, de Groot P, Sixma J, van Mouik J: Storage and secretion of von Willebrand factor b endothelial cells. Hemostasis 1988;18:246.
53 Burgord W, Mukai K, Rosai J: Immunohistochemical identification of factor VIII-related antigen in vascular endothelial cells of cutaneous lesions of alleged vascular nature. Am J Clin Pathol 1981;75:167.
54 Bigler SA, Deering RE, Brawer MK: Comparison of microscopic vascularity in benign and malignant prostate tissue. Hum Pathol 1993; 24:220–226.
55 Brawer M, Deering R, Brown M, Preston S, Bigler S: Predictors of pathologic stage in prostatic carcinoma: The role of neovascularity. Cancer 1994;73:678–687.
56 Weidner N, Carrol P, Flax J, Blumenfeld W, Folkman J: Tumor angiogenesis correlates with metastasis in invasive prostate carcinoma. Am J Pathol 1993;143:401–409.
57 Bostwick DG, Wheeler TM, Blute M, et al: Optimized microvessel density analysis improves prediction of cancer stage from prostate needle biopsies. Urology 1996;48:47–57.
58 Silberman M, Partin A, Veltri R, Epstein J: Tumor angiogenesis correlated with progression after radical prostatectomy but not with pathologic stage in Gleason sum 5 to 7 adenocarcinoma of the prostate. Cancer 1997;79: 772–779.
59 Bettencourt MC, Bauer JJ, Sesterhenn IA, Connelly RR, Moul JW: CD34 immunohistochemical assessment of angiogenesis as a prognostic marker for prostate cancer recurrence after radical prostatectomy. J Urol 1998;160:459–465.
60 Spitz A, Bochner B, Groschen S, Young L, Skinner D, Nichols P, Lieskovsky G, Cote R: Prostate angiogenesis: Correlation of microvessel density of needle biopsies and prostatectomy specimens. J Urol 1997;157:A470.
61 Miles B, Katten M, Scardino P, Wheeler T, de Vere White R, Gandour-Edwards R, Humphrey P, Hudson M, Fradet Y, Mahan H, Bostwick D: Optimized microvessel density is associated with recurrence. J Urol 1997;157: A1157.
62 Gettman MT, Bergstralh EJ, Blute M, Zincke H, Bostwick DG: Prediction of patient outcome in pathologic stage T2 adenocarcinoma of the prostate: Lack of significance for microvessel density analysis. Urology 1998;51:79–85.
63 Takahashi S, Qian J, Brown JA, Alcaraz A, Bostwick DG, Lieber MM, Jenkins RB: Potential markers of prostate cancer aggressiveness detected by fluorescence in situ hybridization in needle biopsies. Cancer Res 1994;54:3574–3579.
64 Kuhn EJ, Kurnot RA, Sesterhenn IA, Chang EH, Moul JW: Expression of the *c-erbB-2* oncoprotein in prostate cancer. J Urol 1993;150: 1427–1433.
65 Moul JW, Maygarden SJ, Ware JL, Mohler JL, Maher PD, Schenkman NS, Ho CK: Cathepsin-D and epidermal growth factor receptor immunohistochemistry does not predict recurrence of prostate cancer patients undergoing radical prostatectomy. J Urol 1996;155:982–985.
66 Bostwick DG, Qian J: Current and proposed biologic markers in prostate cancer (review). J Cell Biochem Suppl 1994;19:197–210.
67 Gao C, Maheshwari S, Dean RC, et al: Blinded multi-evaluation of reverse-transcriptase chain reaction prostate-specific antigen peripheral blood assay for molecular staging of prostate cancer. Urology 1999, in press.

Molecular Targets for Chemoprevention of Prostate Cancer

European Urology

Eur Urol 1999;35:408–412

Changes in Gene Expression and Targets for Therapy

Marion J.G. Bussemakers

Urology Research Laboratory, University Hospital, Nijmegen, The Netherlands

Key Words

Gene expression · Prostate cancer · Marker · Therapy

Abstract

A better understanding of the molecular changes associated with the onset and progression of prostate cancer may provide us with a rational basis for the development of new diagnostic and therapeutic tools. Likewise, the recent identification of critical biochemical pathways, including angiogenesis, programmed cell death, cell adhesion and signal transduction, provide us with promising targets for therapeutic approaches. Furthermore, the identification and characterization of new tumor-specific antigens or prostate-cancer-specific gene promoters could be instrumental for the development of new treatment modalities. Many research groups are trying to identify genes that are involved in prostate cancer development and which may serve as new tumor markers and potential targets for therapy. In addition to prostate-specific antigen, prostate-specific membrane antigen and human kallikrein-2, the recently identified prostate stem cell antigen may also provide us with a new tool for the diagnosis and treatment of prostate cancer. Our own studies led to the identification of DD3, a gene that is strongly overexpressed in human prostatic cancers and the expression of which appears to be restricted to the prostate. Further studies are necessary to establish the clinical usefulness of these new prostate-cancer-specific genes for the management of prostate cancer patients.

Introduction

Prostate cancer is increasingly recognized as a major health problem; it is the most frequently diagnosed cancer in the Western male population and the second leading cause of male cancer deaths in this population [1]. Over the past decades, tremendous efforts have been made in various fields of prostate cancer research to improve the early diagnosis of prostate cancer, when it is still locally confined and potentially curable, and to develop new treatment modalities for advanced prostate cancer, for which currently no effective treatment is available. Also studies concerning the chemoprevention of prostate cancer have been in the focus of many research projects.

Theoretically, characterization of the molecular differences between prostatic tumors and normal prostate tissues will provide us with more insight into the process of tumorigenesis. Furthermore, it can lead to the identification of new candidate tumor markers and potential targets for the treatment of prostate cancer patients. In order to identify changes that are etiologically related to pros-

KARGER

Fax + 41 61 306 12 34
E-Mail karger@karger.ch
www.karger.com

0302–2838/99/0356–0408$17.50/0

Accessible online at:
http://BioMedNet.com/karger

M.J.G. Bussemakers, PhD
Urology Research Laboratory (814 URL)
University Hospital Nijmegen, Geert Grooteplein 16
PO Box 9101, NL–6500 HB Nijmegen (The Netherlands)
Tel. +31 24 3615157, Fax +31 24 3541222, E-Mail m.bussemakers@uro.azn.nl

tate tumorigenesis, molecular genetics is an accepted approach. Loss of heterozygosity studies, for instance, have given indications for chromosomal regions that harbor putative tumor suppressor genes. However, many genetic alterations that are frequently observed in other solid tumors (e.g., alterations affecting the tumor suppressor genes p53 and Rb or the oncogene *ras*), do not play a prominent role in prostate cancer development, although they may be involved in a subset of prostatic tumors [2].

Changes in Gene Expression

Genetic alterations, regardless of the mechanisms by which they occur (allelic gain or loss, translocations, mutations or hypermethylation), often result in changes in mRNA expression, which will subsequently affect the protein expression pattern of cells, leading to a change in phenotype. Therefore, genetic alterations associated with prostate cancer can be identified by studying the changes in gene expression that occur during the onset and progression of this disease. A straightforward approach is to study the expression of genes that are known for their involvement in the process of tumorigenesis like oncogenes, tumor suppressor genes, growth factors and their receptors, molecules involved in signal transduction pathways, cell adhesion molecules, detoxifying enzymes, and DNA-repair genes. Analysis of the expression of these genes in prostatic tumors revealed, amongst others, that decreased expression of the cell adhesion molecule E-cadherin is associated with loss of differentiation and correlates with a poor survival of the prostate cancer patient [3]. Although the mechanisms involved in the loss of E-cadherin-mediated adhesion are not fully understood, recently evidence was provided that it is caused by downregulation of gene transcription [4]. E-cadherin is a cell-cell adhesion molecule that has been implicated in terminal differentiation [5] and is considered to be an invasion suppressor protein [6]. Upregulation of E-cadherin expression, e.g., by stimulating the E-cadherin gene promoter, in patients that show loss of expression of this molecule, may restore terminal differentiation in the tumor cells and thereby prevent progression to metastatic disease [7]. Another important finding was the loss of expression of glutathione S-transferase pi-1 (GSTP1), due to hypermethylation of the regulatory sequences of the GSTP1 gene promoter, in all prostate cancer specimens examined [8]. Loss of GSTP1 expression also occurs in prostatic intraepithelial neoplasia (PIN) [9]. Considering that GSTs have been proposed to play a critical role in defending normal cells against electrophilic carcinogens and that loss of expression of this detoxifying enzyme may confer a higher risk of acquiring genetic mutations, a possible prostate cancer prevention strategy might be the augmentation of GST activity by GST inducers [10]. Furthermore, the hypermethylation of the regulatory region of GSTP1 can be used as an important molecular genetic marker [11].

Besides studying the expression of known genes, one can try to identify new genes that have not previously been associated with the process of tumorigenesis, using techniques like differential or subtraction hybridization or the more recently described differential display analysis [12]. Differential display allows the simultaneous comparison of 'steady-state' mRNA levels of multiple RNA samples, up- as well as downregulated expression of genes can be studied in one experiment, and only small amounts of RNA are required for this technique, thus allowing the use of rare and/or small human tissue samples. Although differential display analysis is hampered by a large number of false-positives, the technique is widely used to search for changes in gene expression. For prostate cancer, this technique has been applied to study changes in gene expression occurring during prostate cancer development in general or more specifically in searching for genes involved in the transition from hormone-dependent to hormone-independent disease or to gain more insight into the process of invasion and metastasis. The studies have been performed using mRNA extracted from human prostate tissue specimens, human prostate cancer cell lines, xenografts and mouse model systems. Many differentially expressed genes have been identified this way, however, their number is too large to mention all of them and, furthermore, their usefulness for the management of prostate cancer patients, either as a marker or as a tool or target for therapy, remains to be determined.

Recently, representational differential analysis which was used to compare androgen-dependent and -independent tumors of the LAPC-4 xenograft model of human prostate cancer, resulted in the identification of prostate stem cell antigen (PSCA), a cell surface antigen that is highly overexpressed in prostate cancer [13] and the expression of which seems to be prostate-specific. It is hypothesized that PSCA plays a role in prostate cancer progression and that it may serve as a potential new target for prostate cancer diagnosis and treatment, however, further investigations are required.

Differential display analysis performed in our own laboratory resulted in the identification of DD3, a gene that is highly overexpressed in 53 of 56 human prostatic tumors studied whereas no (or very low levels of) expression is found in normal prostate or BPH tissue from the same patients. The level of overexpression of DD3 in prostatic cancers shows a trend towards a positive correlation with tumor grade, an observation that is different from what is reported for prostate-specific antigen (PSA), since PSA expression levels decrease with loss of differentiation [14]. Furthermore, there is at least 10- to 100-fold overexpression of DD3 in prostatic carcinomas in comparison to normal prostate or BPH tissues, which is also distinctly different from the mRNA expression of PSA which is reported to be decreased in malignant versus benign tissues [14]. DD3 expression is also detected in metastatic lesions. RT-PCR analysis using DD3-specific primers showed that DD3 expression is very prostate-specific since no product could be amplified in 18 different normal human tissues that were tested. Characterization of the DD3 transcription unit and subsequent computer analysis revealed that DD3 has no homology to any other gene described in the computer databases. These data suggest that DD3 is one of the most prostate-cancer-specific genes described today and make DD3 an interesting candidate to be used both as a diagnostic and/or prognostic marker for prostate cancer as well as a tool for new treatment modalities: i.e., the DD3-encoded protein can be used for strategies of immunotherapy and the DD3 gene promoter may be useful for gene therapy strategies since the elements that regulate the prostate-cancer-specific expression of DD3 can be utilized to selectively drive the expression of therapeutic agents in prostate cancer cells.

Targets and Tools for Therapy

The identification and characterization of changes in gene expression associated with cancer development and progression not only provide us with new insights into the process of prostate tumorigenesis but also with potential new markers and new targets and tools for the management of prostate cancer patients. Several recently identified critical biochemical pathways, including angiogenesis, programmed cell death, the E-cadherin/catenin cell adhesion complex, telomerase activity, and receptor kinases, represent promising targets for therapeutic approaches [7, 15–19]. Also the previously mentioned GSTP1 gene is an interesting target for (chemoprevention) therapy [8, 10].

Even if the biological function of differentially expressed genes is unknown, these genes can still prove to be useful targets and tools for therapy. Especially, prostate-(cancer-)specific genes offer approaches for new treatment modalities such as immuno- and gene therapy strategies. The immunotherapy of cancer, based on eliciting or enhancing the body's own capacity to mount an effective antitumor response, has produced encouraging results in the areas of melanoma and renal cell carcinoma. The development of many current immunotherapy approaches is based on the assumption that cancers contain unique antigens which are preferably not expressed in normal tissues and can serve as targets for immune destruction. The validity of this assumption was shown by the identification of tumor-specific T lymphocytes that specifically recognize cancer cells in vitro [20] and by the observation that passive immune therapy reduces tumor recurrence when administered as adjuvant [21]; e.g., in melanoma, various T-cell epitopes of melanoma-associated antigens (MAGE) have been identified [22]. Dendritic cells, immune cells that are excellent antigen presenters, can be pulsed with peptides derived from tumor-specific antigens and subsequently can be administered to patients to evoke an immune response. For melanoma, MAGE-derived peptides are currently tested in clinical trials [22]. For prostate cancer, dendritic cells loaded with prostate-specific membrane (PSM)-derived peptides are being used for vaccine therapy trials: phase I/II clinical trials showed that the administration of dendritic cells pulsed with PSM-derived peptides induces no significant toxicity in the prostate cancer patients. Decreasing PSA levels, enhanced cellular responses and partial clinical responses in some patients suggest that dendritic cell therapy with PSM peptides has potential as a new prostate cancer therapy [23, 24]. Another candidate target for such therapeutical approaches is the previously mentioned cell surface antigen PSCA. Also DD3 fulfills all essential requirements of a tumor-associated antigen: homogeneous expression in the vast majority of prostatic tumors and absence of expression in all normal tissues. Although very low expression of DD3 can be observed in normal prostate tissue, it is highly unlikely that this will intervene with the use of DD3 as a therapeutic target. Clinical studies with melanoma-associated gene products have shown that expression in normal tissue does not interfere with their use as immunotherapeutics [20, 22].

Also gene therapy offers new hope and can prove to be a very powerful approach to treat cancer, once we are able to selectively deliver the therapeutic gene to the target cancer cells [25]. Such cancer-cell-specific gene delivery is necessary not only for the treatment of locoregional or organ-confined disease, but also for the treatment of disseminated disease. Furthermore, it is important to achieve a high efficiency of gene transfer and to select the optimal therapeutic agent; for instance, suicide genes that convert inactive prodrugs into cytotoxic compounds, genes encoding cytokines and stimulatory markers to enhance immunogenicity against tumors, tumor suppressor genes which can block tumor cell proliferation, or agents that can induce apoptosis. The intrinsic heterogeneity and multifocality of prostatic tumors may hamper the alteration of cell behavior by a single genetic manipulation. However, specific deliverance of a gene to a tumor cell (sub) population and invoking a 'bystander' effect may potentially overcome this problem [25]. To establish selective gene targeting of therapeutic agents to the prostate, the usefulness of prostate-specific promoters is currently under investigation: the PSA gene promoter has already been studied extensively and is being tested [26, 27]. Furthermore, the osteocalcin promoter is being studied to determine its usefulness for the treatment of prostate cancer bone metastases [28]. However, none of these promoters are specific for prostate cancer cells: PSA is expressed in both normal as well as in malignant prostatic cells and osteocalcin is expressed in osteoblasts. Therefore, the identification and characterization of other prostate-cancer-specific promoters is important to selectively target therapeutic agents to tumor cells of the prostate. One candidate would be the PSCA-gene promoter. Also the DD3 gene promoter is a very promising tool to selectively express therapeutic genes in prostate cancer cells, especially when considering that in contrast to PSA and PSM, the level of overexpression of DD3 in prostatic cancers appears to increase with tumor grade and DD3 is at least 10- to 100-fold overexpressed in prostatic carcinomas in comparison to normal or BPH tissues.

Conclusion

Molecular genetics, and molecular and cell biology have provided a rapid increase in our knowledge about tumorigenesis: genes predisposing for (prostate) cancer are being identified; genes and proteins involved in invasion and metastasis are characterized; networks of protein interactions and signal transduction pathways are being elucidated; new diagnostic and prognostic markers are becoming available, and new targets for therapy are being identified. And although this, by itself, is not sufficient for progress in the prevention and treatment of (prostate) cancer, it is a necessary part of such advances since the ultimate success of a (prostate) cancer therapy strategy will rely on comprehensive studies of the biology of the tumor and careful planning of an effective intervention.

References

1 Parker SL, Tong T, Bolden S, Wingo PA: Cancer statistics, 1997. CA Cancer J Clin 1997;47:5–27.

2 Isaacs WB, Bova GS, Morton RA, Bussemakers MJG, Brooks JD, Ewing CM: Molecular genetics and chromosomal alterations in prostate cancer. Cancer 1995;75:2004–2012.

3 Umbas R, Isaacs WB, Bringuier PP, Schaafsma E, Karthaus HF, Oosterhof GON, Debruyne FMJ, Schalken JA: Decreased expression of E-cadherin is associated with poor prognosis in patients with prostate cancer. Cancer Res 1994;54:3929–3933.

4 Giroldi LA, Bringuier PP, De Weijert M, Jansen C, Van Bokhoven A, Schalken JA: Role of E-boxes in the repression of E-cadherin expression. Biochem Biophys Res Commun 1997;241:453–458.

5 Takeichi M: Cadherin cell adhesion receptors as a morphogenetic regulator. Science 1991;251:1451–1455.

6 Behrens J, Mareel MM, Van Roy FM, Birchmeier W: Dissecting tumor cell invasion: Epithelial cells acquire invasive properties after the loss of uvomorulin-mediated cell-cell adhesion. J Cell Biol 1989;108:2435–2447.

7 Schalken JA: New perspectives in the treatment of prostate cancer. Eur Urol 1997;31 (suppl 2):20–23.

8 Lee WH, Morton RA, Epstein JI, Brooks JD, Campbell PA, Bova GS, Hsieh WS, Isaacs WB, Nelson WG: Cytidine methylation of regulatory sequences near the pi-class glutathione-S-transferase gene accompanies human prostate cancer carcinogenesis. Proc Natl Acad Sci USA 1994;91:11733–11737.

9 Brooks JD, Weinstein M, Lin X, Sun Y, Pin SS, Bova GS, Epstein JI, Isaacs WB, Nelson WG: CG island methylation changes near the GSTP1 gene in prostatic intraepithelial neoplasia. Cancer Epidemiol Biomarkers Prev 1998;7:531–536.

10 Wilkinson J, Clapper ML: Detoxication enzymes and chemoprevention. Proc Soc Exp Biol Med 1997;216:192–200.

11 Lee WH, Isaacs WB, Bova GS, Nelson WG: CG island methylation changes near the GSTP1 gene in prostatic carcinoma cells detected using the polymerase chain reaction: A new prostate cancer biomarker. Cancer Epidemiol Biomarkers Prev 1997;6:443–450.

12 Liang P, Pardee AB: Differential display of eukaryotic messenger RNA by means of the polymerase chain reaction. Science 1992;257:967–971.

13 Reiter RE, Zhennen G, Watabe T, Thomas G, Szigeti K, Davis E, Wahl M, Nisitani S, Yamashiro J, Le Beau MM, Loda M, Witte ON: Prostate stem cell antigen: A cell surface marker overexpressed in prostate cancer. Proc Natl Acad Sci USA 1998;95:1735–1740.

14 Hakalahti L, Vihko P, Henttu P, Autio-Harmainen H, Soini Y, Vihko R: Evaluation of PAP and PSA gene expression in prostatic hyperplasia and prostatic carcinoma using Northern blot analysis, in situ hybridization and immunohistochemical stainings with monoclonal and bispecific antibodies. Int J Cancer 1993;55:590–597.

15 Battegay EJ: Angiogenesis: Mechanistic insights, neovascular diseases, and therapeutic prospects. J Mol Med 1995;73:333–346.

16 Dorai T, Olsson CA, Katz AE, Buttyan R: Development of a hammerhead ribozyme against bcl-2: Preliminary evaluation of a potential gene therapeutic agent for hormone-refractory human prostate cancer. Prostate 1997;32:246–258.

17 Furuya Y, Lundmo P, Short AD, Gill DL, Isaacs JT: The role of calcium, pH and cell proliferation in the programmed (apoptotic) death of androgen-independent prostatic cancer cells induced by thapsigargin. Cancer Res 1994;54:6167–6175.
18 Blackburn EH: Structure and function of telomeres. Nature 1991;350:569–573.
19 Camoratto AM, Jani JP, Angeles TS, Maroney AC, Sanders CY, Murakata C, Neff NT, Vaught JL, Isaacs JT, Dionne CA: CEP-751 inhibits TRK receptor tyrosine kinase activity in vitro OFF exhibits anti-tumor activity. Int J Cancer 1997;72:673–679.
20 Van den Eynde BJ, Boon T: Tumor antigens recognized by T lymphocytes. Int J Clin Lab Res 1997;27:81–86.
21 Riethmuller G, Schneider-Gadicke E, Schlimok G, Schmiegel W, Raab R, Hoffken K, Gruber R, Pichlmaier H, Hirche H, Pichlmayr R: Randomised trial of monoclonal antibody for adjuvant therapy of resected Dukes' C colorectal carcinoma. German Cancer Aid 17-1A Study Group. Lancet 1994;343:1177–1183.
22 Kawakami Y, Robbins PF, Wang RF, Parkhurst M, Kang X, Rosenberg SA: The use of melanosomal proteins in the immunotherapy of melanoma. J Immunother 1998;21:237–246.
23 Tjoa BA, Erickson SJ, Bowes VA, Ragde H, Kenny GM, Cobb OE, Ireton RC, Troychak MJ, Boynton AL, Murphy GP: Follow-up evaluation of prostate cancer patients infused with autologous dendritic cells pulsed with PSMA peptides. Prostate 1997;32:272–278.
24 Tjoa BA, Simmons SJ, Bowes VA, Ragde H, Rogers M, Elgamal A, Kenny GM, Cobb OE, Ireton RC, Troychak MJ, Salgaller ML, Boynton AL, Murphy GP: Evaluation of phase I/II clinical trials in prostate cancer with dendritic cells and PSMA peptides. Prostate 1998;36:39–44.
25 Boulikas T: Gene therapy of prostate cancer: p53, suicidal genes, and other targets. Anticancer Res 1997;17:1471–1506.
26 Rodriguez R, Schuur ER, Lim HY, Henderson GA, Simons JW, Henderson DR: Prostate attenuated replication competent adenovirus (ARCA) CN706: A selective cytotoxic for prostate-specific antigen-positive prostate cancer cell. Cancer Res 1997;57:2559–2563.
27 Gotoh A, Ko SC, Shirakawa T, Cheon J, Kao C, Miyamoto T, Gardner TA, Ho LJ, Cleutjens CB, Trapman J, Graham FL, Chung LW: Development of prostate-specific antigen promoter-based gene therapy for androgen-independent human prostate cancer. J Urol 1998;160:220–229.
28 Ko SC, Cheon J, Kao C, Gotoh A, Shirakawa T, Sikes RA, Karsenty G, Chung LW: Osteocalcin promoter-based toxic gene therapy for the treatment of osteosarcoma in experimental models. Cancer Res 1996;56:4614–4619.

Molecular Targets for Chemoprevention of Prostate Cancer

European Urology

Eur Urol 1999;35:413–419

Mechanism of Androgen Receptor Activation and Possible Implications for Chemoprevention Trials

Helmut Klocker[a] Zoran Culig[a] Iris E. Eder[a] Claudia Nessler-Menardi[a] Alfred Hobisch[a] Thomas Putz[a] Georg Bartsch[a] Heike Peterziel[b] Andrew C.B. Cato[b]

[a]Department of Urology, University of Innsbruck, Austria and [b]Institute of Genetics, Research Center, Karlsruhe, Germany

Key Words

Androgen receptor · Transcriptional activity · Ligand-independent activation · Androgen withdrawal · LNCaP · Du-145 · Reporter gene · PSA

Abstract

Androgens are pivotal regulators of prostate cell growth, differentiation and function, and their actions are believed to be involved in prostate cancer development. The androgen-signaling pathway in the prostate gland is therefore one of the possible sites of intervention in prostate cancer prevention efforts. The central element of androgen signaling in the cell is the androgen receptor (AR), a member of the superfamily of nuclear receptors. Binding of androgen to its ligand-binding domain transforms the receptor to an active transcription factor that regulates gene expression by interacting with specific regulatory elements in the promoters of genes. In addition to this genomic action, the AR also interacts with other signaling pathways through protein-protein interaction, for example with AP-1 or Ets transcription factors. It is not only the action of androgenic hormones, but also the interactions with growth factor and protein kinase A-signaling pathways that can induce activation of AR. Moreover, these ligand-independent activators act synergistically together with low concentrations of androgens. The effects of long-term androgen deprivation on androgen signaling have been investigated in the LNCaP cell culture system. Long-term culture in a steroid-free medium results in a subline showing a hyperreactive AR characterized by increased AR expression and enhanced AR transcriptional activity in an environment with low levels of androgen hormones. It is not yet clear if similar changes also occur in normal or premalignant prostate epithelial cells and are thus relevant for prevention trials which interfere with androgen hormone signaling.

Introduction

The dependence of the developing and mature prostate gland on androgens is well documented [1, 2] and is the basis for treatment of nonorgan-confined prostatic carcinoma by androgen ablation and/or androgen receptor (AR) blockade [3–5]. Androgenic stimulation also plays a pivotal role in the development of prostate cancer. Therefore, strategies to reduce androgenic stimulation are discussed and pursued in chemoprevention trials as a means

Dr. Helmut Klocker
Department of Urology, University of Innsbruck
Anichstrasse 35, A–6020 Innsbruck (Austria)
Tel. +43 512 504 4818, Fax +43 512 504 4817
E-Mail helmut.klocker@uibk.ac.at

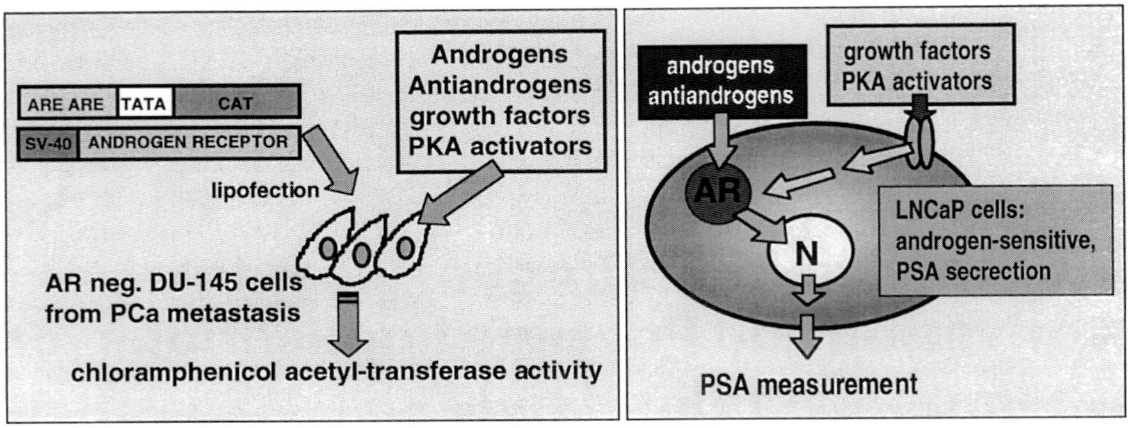

Fig. 1. Investigation of AR activation in prostate cancer cell lines. Receptor-negative Du-145 prostate cancer cells were transfected with an AR expression vector and an androgen-regulated chloramphenicol acetyltransferase reporter gene (ARE_2TATA-CAT). After stimulation with AR activators and/or inhibitors for 2 days, reporter gene activity was determined in the cell lysates. In the AR-positive, androgen-sensitive LNCaP cells, stimulation with AR activators results in stimulation of expression and secretion of PSA, which was then measured in the cell supernatant by an ELISA technique.

to prevent or slow down prostate carcinogenesis. A chemoprevention trial performed in the United States used an inhibitor of the enzyme 5α-reductase to reduce the intracellular level of dihydrotestosterone (DHT), the most potent androgen in the prostate [6,7].

DHT and other androgens stimulate prostatic cells through activation of the AR. In the last few years the knowledge of the molecular mechanism of AR activation has steadily improved and it became clear that it is also activated by ligand-independent mechanisms. In addition, cell culture model systems showed that androgen deprivation selects for tumor cells, which are adapted to low androgen levels. This contribution intends to give an overview of these findings and to discuss possible consequences for chemoprevention strategies.

The AR is a member of the large superfamily of nuclear receptors; it is most closely related to the glucocorticoid and the progesterone receptor [8]. The gene is located on the long arm of the X chromosome, the 110-kDa protein shows the typical structure of a nuclear receptor: an N-terminal transactivation domain, a central DNA-binding domain consisting of two zinc finger elements, and a C-terminal ligand-binding domain. The receptor must be activated to become a transcription factor that is able to regulate the expression of androgen-sensitive genes by interaction with the hormone-responsive elements in the promoters of these genes [9, 10]. Binding of an agonist to the AR ligand-binding domain is the classical route of AR activation. It triggers a cascade of molecular events including dissociation of heat-shock proteins, phosphorylation, conformational changes, dimerization and interaction with other proteins [11].

Ligand-Dependent and Ligand-Independent AR Activation

We investigated ligand-dependent and ligand-independent activation of the AR in two cell systems (fig. 1). The first one was the LNCaP tumor cell line derived from a prostate cancer lymph node metastasis. These cells express an AR containing a point mutation in the ligand-binding domain [12]. After AR activation they produce and secrete prostate-specific antigen (PSA), which can be measured in the cell supernatant. The second cell system used was the Du-145 cell line derived from a prostate cancer brain metastasis. These cells do not contain an endogenous AR [13]. They were cotransfected with an AR expression vector and a second vector containing a chloramphenicol acetyltransferase (CAT) reporter gene driven by an androgen-inducible promoter (two androgen-responsive elements arranged in tandem in front of a minimal promoter). After transfection the Du-145 cells were treated with various AR activators and the reporter gene activity was measured after 2 days in the cell extracts.

In the Du-145 cell system, insulin-like growth factor-I (IGF-I) stimulated AR-mediated reporter gene transcription – in the absence of androgens – to the same extent as

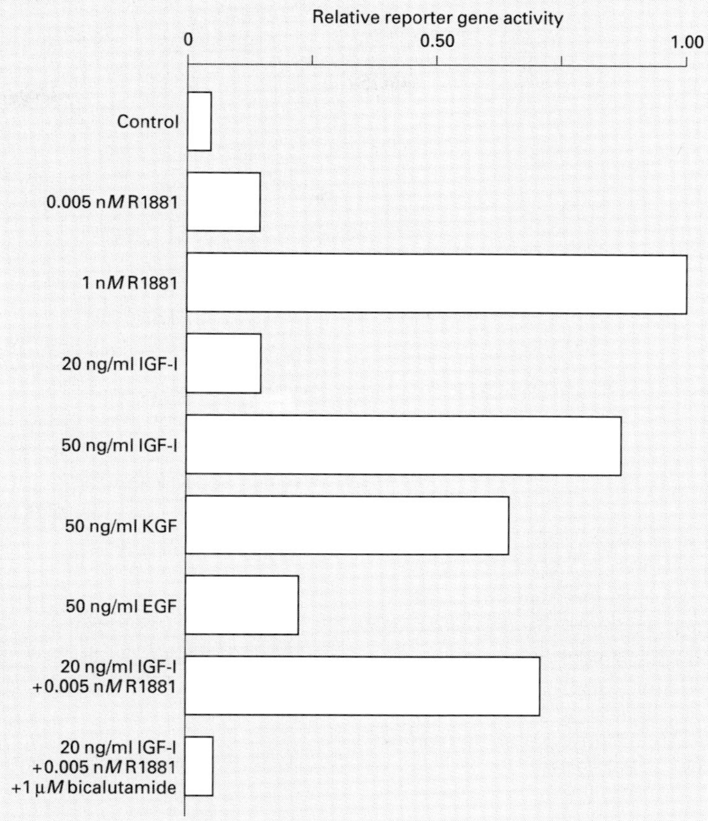

Fig. 2. AR activation by growth factors. Transiently cotransfected Du-145 cells were stimulated with the indicated concentrations of the synthetic androgen methyltrienolone (R1881), the growth factors insulin-like growth factor (IGF-I), keratinocyte growth factor (KGF) and epidermal growth factor (EGF), and the antiandrogen bicalutamide (Casodex). After 2 days, reporter gene activity was measured in the cell lysates.

the synthetic androgen methyltrienolone (R1881). Keratinocyte factor (KGF) and epidermal growth factor (EGF) also activated reporter gene transcription in the absence of androgen although the potency of these two growth factors was smaller than that of IGF-I (fig. 2) [14, 15]. None of the growth factors stimulated reporter gene activity in control experiments when added to cells cotransfected with the CAT gene and an empty expression vector. AR activation by IGF-I, KGF and EGF was completely inhibited by the pure AR antagonist bicalutamide (Casodex), showing that these effects are AR-mediated. In LNCaP cells grown in steroid-stripped culture medium, IGF-I increased the PSA level in the supernatant 5-fold (fig. 3). Again, the IGF-I effect on PSA secretion was blocked by bicalutamide. When low concentrations of IGF-I or EGF were combined with very low concentrations of androgens (in the p*M* range) a strong synergistic effect was observed in cotransfection experiments as well as in the LNCaP cell system (fig. 2, 3).

Another ligand-independent activator of AR transactivation function that was identified recently is interleukin-6 (IL-6). IL-6 is a pleiotropic cytokine, which regulates antigen-specific immune responses and inflammatory reaction [16]. It is implicated in the modulation of growth and differentiation in several tumors and is frequently elevated in the sera of prostate cancer patients with advanced tumors [17–19]. IL-6 receptors are expressed in prostate cancer cell lines, as well as in benign prostate hyperplasia and prostate cancer tissue specimens [20–22]. We tested the effects of this cytokine on AR transcriptional activity in cotransfected Du-145 cells. IL-6 up-regulated AR activity in a ligand-independent manner, as well as synergistically with very low doses of the synthetic androgen methyltrienolone (fig. 4) [23]. The nonsteroidal antiandrogen bicalutamide (Casodex) nearly completely inhibited AR activation by IL-6 showing that this IL-6 effect is AR-mediated. In LNCaP cells, IL-6 treatment induced a small but significant increase of PSA secretion and this induction was prevented by bicalutamide.

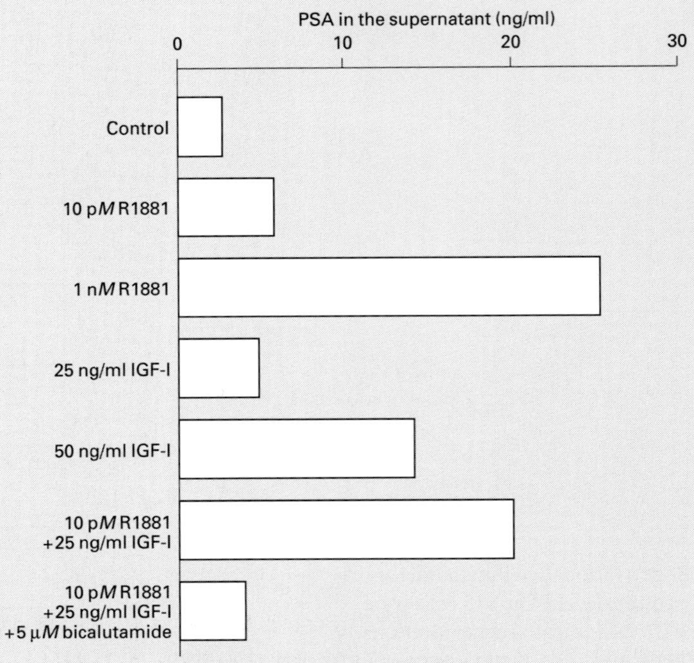

Fig. 3. Growth factor induction of PSA secretion in LNCaP cells. LNCaP cells were stimulated by the synthetic androgen methyltrienolone or IGF-I or combinations of both. The concentrations used are indicated in the figure. After 3 days the PSA concentrations were measured in the supernatants using an ELISA technique and the values were corrected for cell mass.

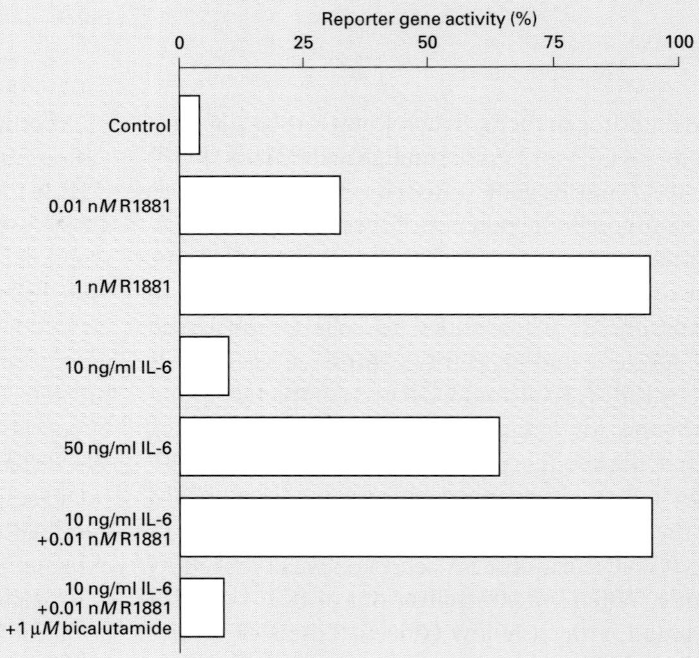

Fig. 4. AR activation by IL-6. Stimulation of reporter gene activity in Du-145 cells transfected with the reporter plasmid ARE_2TATA-CAT and the AR expression vector pSG5AR. Cotransfected cells were treated with either R1881, IL-6 or R1881 and IL-6. In a control sample, induction of reporter gene activity induced by R1881 and IL-6 was blocked with the nonsteriodal antiandrogen bicalutamide.

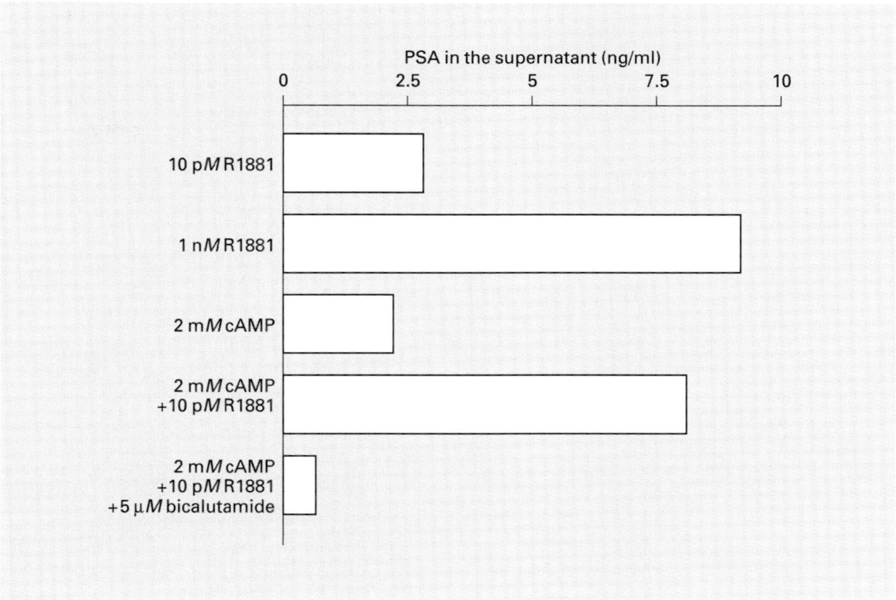

Fig. 5. AR activation by the pKA activator cAMP. LNCaP cells were treated with either R1881 or cyclic adenosine monophosphate or a combination of both. After 3 days the PSA concentration in the cell supernatant was measured and corrected for cell mass.

Besides growth factors, activators of protein kinase A (pKA) also activate the AR. pKA activators are for example forskolin and the second messenger cyclic adenosine monophosphate (cAMP). When a cAMP analogue is applied at a concentration of 2 m*M* in cotransfection-transactivation experiments in Du-145 cells, about 20% of the maximal reporter gene activity is induced in the absence of androgen (fig. 5) [24]. Again, there is a distinct synergistic effect of cAMP with very low doses of androgen. Application of cAMP and 10 p*M* of R1881 maximally induced reporter gene activity. Thus, activation of pKA by increasing the intracellular cAMP level dramatically reduced the androgen concentration needed for maximal AR activation. Many cellular regulators use cAMP as a second messenger system and increase intracellular cAMP levels. In prostate cancer cells, LHRH, that is used for endocrine therapy of prostate cancer, is such a peptide. In fact all the effects on the AR seen with a synthetic cAMP derivative can also be triggered by treatment with an LHRH agonist in Du-145 and LNCaP cells [24].

These results provide evidence that growth factors, IL-6 and pKA activate the AR. There is full or partial activation in the absence of androgen, and, more important for physiological conditions, there is a strong functional synergism between low doses of androgen and ligand-independent activators. This is of particular importance in an androgen-depleted or androgen-reduced environment. In prostate cancer treatment, androgen ablation therapy results in very low abundance of androgens. We postulate that tumor cells compensate the loss of androgens by increasing ligand-independent AR stimulation. In these tumor cells very low concentrations of androgens in combination with growth factors, IL-6 or elevated cAMP levels are most likely sufficient to activate the androgen-signaling cascade. Theoretically a similar mechanism may also compensate reduced androgen stimulation expected to result from a chemoprevention treatment. However, this question has not been addressed so far and has to be investigated in the future. The situation is further complicated by interaction of the AR with other transcriptional regulators by protein-protein interaction and by modulation of AR activity by a group of proteins that are called coactivators and corepressors [25]. AR gene regulation by protein-protein interaction was shown for the collagen I promoter. In that example the AR interacts with Ets transcription factors and attenuates their activity on the promoter [26]. This property of the AR is called transrepression and was also demonstrated for the transcription factor AP-1 [27, 28]. Coactivators such as SRC-1 (steroid receptor coactivator), AIB-1 (amplified in breast cancer), ARA-70 (androgen receptor activator), CBP (CREB-binding protein) and corepressors like N-CoR (nuclear receptor corepressor) and SMRT (silencing mediator of retinoic acid and thyroid hormone receptors) enhance or repress AR transcriptional activity on target gene promoters. Their relevance for androgenic stimulation of prostate cells and in prostate tumor progression has yet to be established.

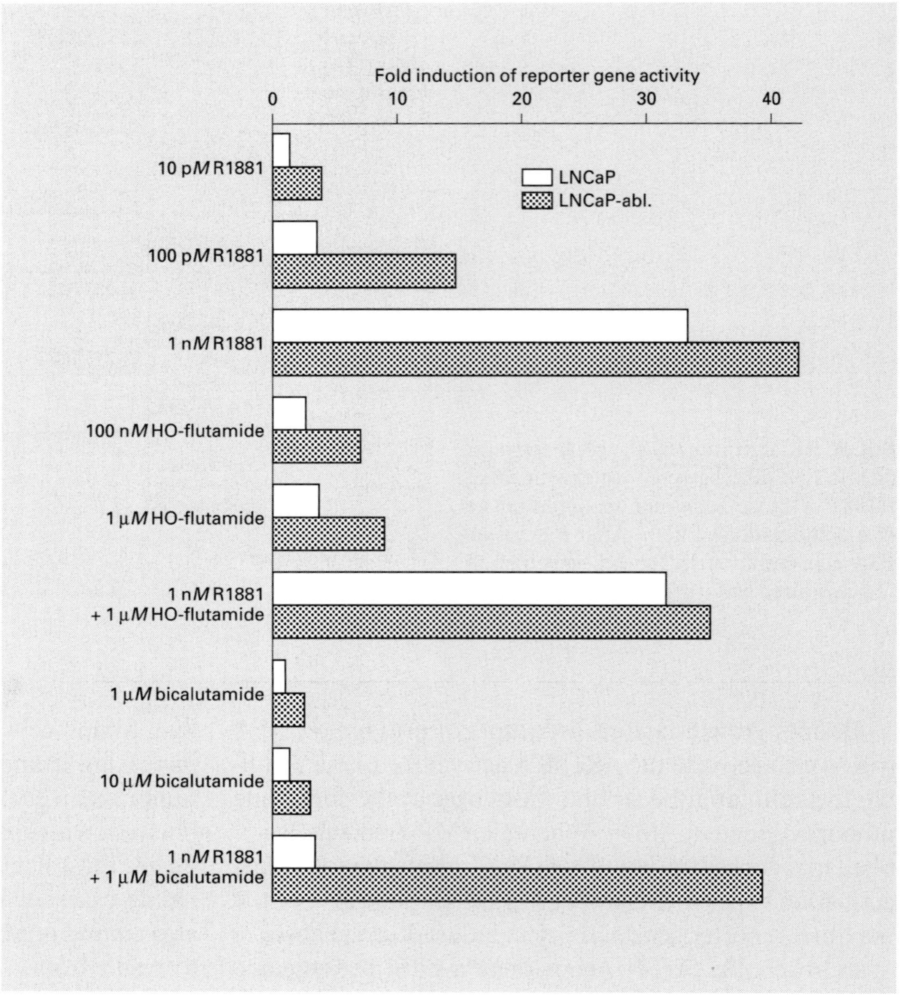

Fig. 6. Hypersensitive AR activation in long-term androgen-ablated LNCaP cells. LNCaP and long-term androgen-ablated LNCaP cells (LNCaP-abl) were transfected with the androgen-inducible reporter plasmid ARE_2TATA-CAT and treated for 40 h with androgens and/or antiandrogens. Thereafter, CAT reporter gene activity was measured in the cell extracts.

Effects of Long-Term Androgen Ablation on LNCaP Cells

How do androgen-sensitive cells respond to androgen deprivation? We simulated androgen withdrawal in LNCaP cells by long-term growth of these cells in steroid-depleted medium. The androgen-sensitive LNCaP cells were kept in medium containing charcoal-treated serum for more than 80 passages. After several months in culture, a subline, LNCaP-abl, was established, which showed alterations of androgen signaling, which resemble those observed during prostate cancer progression. The AR protein level in LNCaP-abl cells was increased 3 times over those in the parental cells. They displayed a hypersensitive biphasic proliferative response to androgen. Maximal proliferation was observed with 1 p*M* of the synthetic androgen methyltrienolone, whereas 10 p*M* of this compound induced the same effect in parental cells. The nonsteroidal antiandrogen bicalutamide slightly stimulated proliferation of LNCaP-abl cells but inhibited the parental cell line.

Basal AR transcriptional activity (in the absence of androgen), determined by means of a reporter gene assay, was 30 times (in the presence of serum) and 6 times (in serum-free medium), respectively, higher in LNCaP-abl than in LNCaP cells. Similar to the stimulation of proliferation, an androgen-inducible gene was activated at lower androgen concentrations in LNCaP-abl cells as compared to parental LNCaP cells (fig. 6). Bicalutamide that acts as a pure antagonist in parental LNCaP cells showed small agonistic effects on AR transactivation activity in LNCaP-abl cells and was not able to block the effects of androgen in these cells. Hydroxyflutamide, another nonsteroidal antiandrogen, exerted stimulatory effects on AR activity in both LNCaP and LNCaP-abl cells; however, AR activation was up to 4-fold more efficient in the LNCaP-abl subline. The results show that androgen deprivation can induce alterations of the androgen-signaling cascade in prostate tumor cells that result in androgen hypersensitivity and allow the tumor cells to maintain androgen stimulation in a low-androgen environment. Moreover, in long-term ablated cells the nonsteroidal antiandrogen bicalutamide is no longer able to block AR activation. These findings may have implications on the treatment of prostate cancer as well as on chemopreventive interventions, which intend to reduce androgenic stimulation in the prostate by reducing androgen levels.

Acknowledgement

The work summarized here was made possible by support of the Austrian Science Foundation (SFB 002, project F203).

References

1 Coffey DS, Isaacs JT: Control of prostate growth. J Urol 1981;1.
2 Cunha GR, Donjacour AA, Cooke PS, Mee S, Bigsby RM, Higgins SJ, Sugimur Y: The endocrinology and developmental biology of the prostate. Endocr Rev 1987;8:338–362.
3 Vogelzang NJ, Kennealey GT: Recent developments in endocrine treatment of prostate cancer. Cancer 1992;70:966–976.
4 Labrie F: Endocrine therapy for prostate cancer. Endocrinol Metab Clin North Am 1991; 20:845–872.
5 Labrie F, Belanger A, Simard J, Labrie C, Dupont A: Combination therapy for prostate cancer. Endocrine and biologic basis of its choice as new standard first-line therapy. Cancer 1993;71:1059–1067.
6 Brawley OW, Thompson IM: The chemoprevention of prostate cancer and the Prostate Cancer Prevention Trial. Cancer Treat Res 1996;88:189–200.
7 Thompson IM, Coltman CA Jr, Crowley J: Chemoprevention of prostate cancer: The Prostate Cancer Prevention Trial. Prostate 1997;33:217–221.
8 Tenbaum S, Baniahmad A: Nuclear receptors: Structure, function and involvement in disease. Int J Biochem Cell Biol 1997;29:1325–1341.
9 Roy AK, Chatterjee B: Androgen action. Crit Rev Eukaryot Gene Expr 1995;5:157–176.
10 Kallio PJ, Pakvimo JJ, Janne OA: Genetic regulation of androgen action. Prostate Suppl 1996;6:45–51.
11 Jänne OA, Palvimo JJ, Kallio P, Mehto M: Androgen receptor and mechanism of androgen action. Ann Med 1993;25:83–89.
12 Veldscholte J, Berrevoets CA, Ris Stalpers C, Kuiper GG, Jenster G, Trapman J, Brinkmann AO, Mulder E: The androgen receptor in LNCaP cells contains a mutation in the ligand binding domain which affects steroid binding characteristics and response to antiandrogens. J Steroid Biochem Mol Biol 1992;41:665–669.
13 Culig Z, Klocker H, Eberle J, Kaspar F, Hobisch A, Cronauer MV, Bartsch G: DNA sequence of the androgen receptor in prostatic tumor cell lines and tissue specimens assessed by means of the polymerase chain reaction. Prostate 1993;22:11–22.
14 Culig Z, Hobisch A, Cronauer MV, Hittmair A, Radmayr C, Bartsch G, Klocker H: Activation of the androgen receptor by polypeptide growth factors and cellular regulators. World J Urol 1995;13:285–289.
15 Culig Z, Hobisch A, Cronauer MV, Radmayr C, Trapman J, Hittmair A, Bartsch G, Klocker H: Androgen receptor activation in prostatic tumor cell lines by insulin-like growth factor-I, keratinocyte growth factor, and epidermal growth factor. Cancer Res 1994;54:5474–5478.
16 Kishimoto T, Akira S, Taga T: Interleukin-6 and its receptor: A paradigm for cytokines. Science 1992;258:593–597.
17 Twillie DA, Eisenberger MA, Carducci MA, Hseih WS, Kim WY, Simons JW: Interleukin-6: A candidate mediator of human prostate cancer morbidity. Urology 1995;45:542–549.
18 Seymour JF, Kurzrock R: Interleukin-6: Biologic properties and role in lymphoproliferative disorders. Cancer Treat Res 1996;84:167–206.
19 Seymour JF, Talpaz M, Cabanillas F, Wetzler M, Kurzrock R: Serum interleukin-6 levels correlate with prognosis in diffuse large-cell lymphoma. J Clin Oncol 1995;13:575–582.
20 Siegall CB, Schwab G, Nordan RP, FitzGerald DJ, Pastan I: Expression of the interleukin-6 receptor and interleukin-6 in prostate carcinoma cells. Cancer Res 1990;50:7786–7788.
21 Siegsmund MJ, Yamazaki H, Pastan I: Interleukin-6 receptor mRNA in prostate carcinomas and benign prostate hyperplasia. J Urol 1994;151:1396–1399.
22 Borsellino N, Belldegrun A, Bonavida B: Endogenous interleukin-6 is a resistance factor for cis-diamminedichloroplatinum and etoposide-mediated cytotoxicity of human prostate carcinoma cell lines. Cancer Res 1995;55:4633–4639.
23 Hobisch A, Eder IE, Putz T, Horninger W, Bartsch G, Klocker H, Culig Z: Interleukin-6 regulates prostate-specific protein expression in prostate carcinoma cells by activation of the androgen receptor. Cancer Res 1998;58:4640–4645.
24 Culig Z, Hobisch A, Hittmair A, Cronauer MV, Radmayr C, Zhang J, Bartsch G, Klocker H: Synergistic activation of androgen receptor by androgen and luteinizing hormone releasing hormone in prostatic carcinoma cells. Prostate 1997;32:106–114.
25 Shibata H, Spencer TE, Onate SA, Jenster G, Tsai SY, Tsai MJ, O'Malley BW: Role of co-activators and co-repressors in the mechanism of steroid/thyroid receptor action. Recent Prog Horm Res 1997;52:141–164.
26 Schneikert J, Peterziel H, Defossez PA, Klocker H, Launoit Y, Cato AC: Androgen receptor-Ets protein interaction is a novel mechanism for steroid hormone-mediated down-modulation of matrix metalloproteinase expression. J Biol Chem 1996;271:23907–23913.
27 Kallio PJ, Poukka H, Moilanen A, Janne OA, Palvimo JJ: Androgen receptor-mediated transcriptional regulation in the absence of direct interaction with a specific DNA element. Mol Endocrinol 1995;9:1017–1028.
28 Sato N, Sadar MD, Bruchovsky N, Saatcioglu F, Rennie PS, Sato S, Lange PH, Gleave ME: Androgenic induction of prostate-specific antigen gene is repressed by protein–protein interaction between the androgen receptor and AP-1/c-Jun in the human prostate cancer cell line LNCaP. J Biol Chem 1997;272:17485–17494.

European Urology

Eur Urol 1999;35:420–423

New Agents for Chemoprevention of Prostate Cancer

Michael B. Sporn

Department of Pharmacology, Dartmouth Medical School, Hanover, N.H., USA

Key Words

Chemoprevention · Retinoids · Tamoxifen · Deltanoids

Abstract

The magnitude of the problem of prostate cancer, and the failure of conventional chemotherapy and surgery to effect a marked diminution in the total number of deaths from this disease, now indicate that chemoprevention of prostatic carcinogenesis must be seriously considered. We describe the development of a new system for quantitating the process of prostatic carcinogenesis in an experimental animal, and the use of this system to demonstrate that the retinoid, 4-hydroxyphenylretinamide, the deltanoid, Ro24-5531, and the estrogen analog, tamoxifen, all are effective agents for prevention of experimental prostate cancer.

Morbidity and mortality from prostate cancer continues to be a major problem throughout the Western world. In spite of aggressive surgical and chemotherapeutic approaches to this problem, there has not been a truly significant decrease in mortality rates from prostate cancer during the past 25 years. In spite of our having accumulated so much basic knowledge about the molecular biology of cancer, this has not translated into a reduction in mortality statistics for prostate cancer.

Elsewhere, I have suggested that there are several principal reasons for this dismal situation [1]. First of all, we have not had a realistic understanding of the natural history and genesis of invasive and metastatic prostatic carcinoma. This is particularly important in the prostate, an organ in which epithelial-mesenchymal interactions are so important in determining the ultimate differentiation and fate of epithelial cells [2]. Epithelium and stroma are in constant reciprocal communication with each other throughout life, and carcinogenesis should be viewed as a defect in this communication, rather than the exclusive result of excessive cell proliferation [3]. Invasive prostate carcinoma is not the primary and exclusive result of uncontrolled multiplication of prostatic epithelium. Ultimately, it is local invasion and distant metastasis that kill the patient, rather than excessive cell proliferation per se. In the past, insufficient effort has been devoted to the study of the biochemical and cellular parameters that determine invasion and metastasis.

Secondly, there has been an obsession with the concept of 'cure' of advanced disease, as opposed to prevention of early disease; this is particularly true of many well-intentioned efforts to support research in prostate cancer (some foundations insist that proposals must be relevant to treatment of advanced disease and do not even consider funding research on prevention). The concept of chemoprevention [4, 5] has been very slow in coming to the field of prostate cancer. Thus, there has been inadequate effort devoted to the pharmacology of arrest of preneoplastic

KARGER

Fax + 41 61 306 12 34
E-Mail karger@karger.ch
www.karger.com

0302–2838/99/0356–0420$17.50/0

Accessible online at:
http://BioMedNet.com/karger

M.B. Sporn
Department of Pharmacology, Dartmouth Medical School
Remsen 524, Hanover, NH 03755 (USA)
Tel. +1 603 650 6557, Fax +1 603 650 1129
E-Mail michael.sporn@dartmouth.edu

Table 1. Effects of Ro24-5531, 4-HPR, and tamoxifen on development of prostate and seminal vesicle carcinomas in rats initiated with NMU (30 mg/kg) and promoted with TP (10 mg every 2 months)[a]

	Stage	Control	5531 high[b]	5531 low[c]	4-HPR high[d]	4-HPR low[e]	Tam high[f]	Tam low[g]
Number of rats		18	18	18	18	18	18	18
DLP	0	72	78	67	83	72	61	67
	1–2	6	0	0	17	6	39	28
	3–4	0	6	0	0	0	0	0
	5–6	22	17	33	0	22	0	6
AP	0	22	56	17	22	50	72	44
	1–2	6	6	0	6	12	6	6
	3–4	50	17	50	61	28	22	39
	5–6	22	22	33	11	11	0	11
P1[h]			0.05			0.04	0.001	0.05
P2[i]						0.05	0.003	
SV	0	17	28	28	56	50	94	33
	1–2	11	6	0	0	0	0	17
	3–4	11	17	6	11	0	0	6
	5–6	61	50	67	33	50	6	44
P1[h]					0.02		0.0001	
P2[i]							0.0001	
Total % with invasive tumor		83	72	100	83	72	22	78

DLP = Dorsolateral prostate; AP = anterior prostate; SV = seminal vesicle.
Staging of tumors is defined in reference 6. Data are described in detail in reference 7.
[a] Numbers in the table are the percentages of rats with lesions of any defined stage. Duration of the experiment was 11 months;
[b] Ro24-5531, 2.5 nmol/kg diet; [c] Ro24-5531, 1.25 nmol/kg diet; [d] 4-HPR, 2 nmol/kg diet; [e] 4-HPR, 1 nmol/kg diet;
[f] tamoxifen, 5.0 mg/kg diet; [g] tamoxifen, 0.5 mg/kg diet; [h] P1 = Wilcoxon's rank sum test (stage-for-stage);
[i] P2 = Fisher's exact test [invasive (stages 3–6) versus noninvasive (stages 0–2)].

states and prevention of the development of invasive and metastatic disease. We have inadequate animal models to study carcinogenesis in the prostate, and very poor biomarkers to evaluate the efficacy of potential chemopreventive agents.

With this as background, several years ago we began serious efforts directed at chemoprevention of prostate cancer. Since animal models that can be quantitated are essential for this effort, we established a new grading system for the evaluation of the histogenesis of neoplastic lesions in the prostate and seminal vesicle of the laboratory rat [6]. Carcinomas were induced in Lobund-Wistar rats by initiation with intravenous nitrosomethylurea (NMU) and promotion with subcutaneous testosterone propionate (TP) implants. A large number of animals was analyzed in a serial sacrifice study, and a system of staging was created which allowed three different categories (in situ change, invasion, desmoplasia) of tumor development to be ranked progressively in a manner conducive to nonparametric analysis. Each category was then further subdivided to create a system of 6 stages: stage 0 represents histologically normal tissue; stages 1 and 2 are lesions with intraepithelial neoplastic changes (stage 1, one or two foci; stage 2, three or more foci); stages 3 and 4 are lesions characterized by stromal invasion (stage 3, one or two foci; stage 4, two or more foci); stage 5 lesions are characterized by a marked scirrhous reaction confined to the gland of origin, and stage 6 lesions are characterized by a markedly invasive scirrhous tumor that can no longer be traced to a particular organ of origin (prostate or seminal vesicle).

We then evaluated the ability of several chemopreventive agents to suppress prostatic carcinogenesis in this animal model, and some of our important results are shown in tables 1 and 2. Three agents, all of a different chemical nature, but all belonging to families of molecules that are ligands of nuclear receptors of the steroid receptor superfamily, were found to be active molecules [7]. These

Table 2. Effects of Ro24-5531, 4-HPR, and tamoxifen on development of prostate and seminal vesicle carcinomas in rats initiated with NMU (15 mg/kg) and promoted with TP (10 mg every 2 months)[a]

	Stage	Control	5531 high[b]	5531 low[c]	4-HPR high[d]	4-HPR low[e]	Tam high[f]	Tam low[g]
Number of rats		18	17	18	17	18	17	17
DLP	0	78	71	72	65	67	71	76
	1–2	22	29	28	29	33	29	24
	3–4	0	0	0	0	0	0	0
	5–6	0	0	0	6	0	0	0
AP	0	28	65	61	47	28	82	71
	1–2	22	6	6	12	39	0	6
	3–4	50	18	33	35	33	18	24
	5–6	0	12	0	6	0	0	0
P1[h]				0.05			0.002	0.011
P2[i]							0.05	
SV	0	11	35	28	35	61	94	41
	1–2	6	24	28	18	0	0	12
	3–4	44	24	44	41	28	6	47
	5–6	39	18	0	6	11	0	0
P1[h]			0.01	0.0004	0.0005	0.003	0.0001	0.0003
P2[i]			0.01	0.02	0.03	0.01	0.0001	0.03
Total % with invasive tumor		100	59	61	65	61	18	53

DLP = Dorsolateral prostate; AP = anterior prostate; SV = seminal vesicle.
Staging of tumors is defined in reference 6. Data are described in detail in reference 7.
[a] Numbers in the table are the percentages of rats with lesions of any defined stage. Duration of the experiment was 11 months;
[b] Ro24-5531, 2.5 nmol/kg diet; [c] Ro24-5531, 1.25 nmol/kg diet; [d] 4-HPR, 2 nmol/kg diet; [e] 4-HPR, 1 nmol/kg diet;
[f] tamoxifen, 5.0 mg/kg diet; [g] tamoxifen, 0.5 mg/kg diet; [h] P1 = Wilcoxon's rank sum test (stage-for-stage);
[i] P2 = Fisher's exact test [invasive (stages 3–6) versus noninvasive (stages 0–2)].

include the vitamin D analog ('deltanoid'), Ro24-5531, the retinoid, 4-hydroxyphenylretinamide (4-HPR, fenretinide), and the estrogen analog, tamoxifen. The concept of using an estrogen analog to prevent prostate cancer, which at first glance might seem quite strange, has taken on a new significance with the discovery and cloning of a new estrogen receptor, ER-β, in the prostate [8].

The data in tables 1 and 2, taken from independent long-term experiments involving several hundred animals [7], show that while all three agents have chemopreventive activity, tamoxifen has a particularly marked ability to suppress prostate carcinogenesis. Tamoxifen caused a dramatic inhibition in the extent and number of invasive lesions. Histologic evaluation of the prostate glands also showed that tamoxifen caused a marked decrease in the height of prostatic secretory epithelium and the amount of secretory material in the lumina of glandular units.

Additional animal studies are now indicated to evaluate the effect of other retinoids, deltanoids, and estrogen analogs for prevention of prostate cancer. In particular, it will be of interest to determine the chemopreventive effects of retinoids that bind selectively to the RXR receptor ('rexinoids'), as well as newer estrogen analogs, such as raloxifene, which have a spectrum of action somewhat different than that of tamoxifen. Furthermore, the mechanisms of action of the above chemopreventive agents need to be determined. In this regard, the development of a new non-neoplastic prostatic epithelial cell line, NRP-152, now offers the opportunity to study such problems [9]. It has already been shown that retinoids and deltanoids can inhibit the growth of these cells; moreover, they are also sensitive to the growth-inhibitory actions of TGF-β [9].

References

1 Sporn MB: The war on cancer. Lancet 1996;347:1377–1381.
2 Cunha GR, Hayward SW, Dahiya R, Foster BA: Smooth muscle-epithelial interaction in normal and neoplastic development. Acta Anat 1996;155:63–72.
3 Clark WH: The nature of cancer: Morphogenesis and progressive (self)-disorganization in neoplastic development and progression. Acta Oncol 1995;34:3–21.
4 Sporn MB, Dunlop NM, Newton DL, Smith JM: Prevention of chemical carcinogenesis by vitamin A and its synthetic analogs (retinoids). Fed Proc 1976;35:1332–1338.
5 Hong WK, Sporn MB: Recent advances in chemoprevention of cancer. Science 1997;278:1073–1077.
6 Slayter MV, Anzano MA, Kadomatsu K, Smith JM, Sporn MB: Histogenesis of induced prostate and seminal vesicle carcinoma in Lobund-Wistar rats: A system for histologic scoring and grading. Cancer Res 1994;54:1440–1445.
7 Lucia MS, Anzano MA, Slayter MV, Anver M, Green DM, Shrader MW, Logsdon DL, Driver CL, Brown CC, Peer CW, Roberts AB, Sporn MB: Chemopreventive activity of tamoxifen, *N*-(4-hydroxyphenyl)retinamide, and the vitamin D analogue Ro24-5531 for androgen-promoted carcinomas of the rat seminal vesicle and prostate. Cancer Res 1995;55:5621–5627.
8 Kuiper GGJM, Enmark E, Pelto-Huikko M, Nilsson S, Gustafsson JA: Cloning of a novel estrogen receptor expressed in rat prostate and ovary. Proc Natl Acad Sci USA 1996;93:5925–5930.
9 Danielpour D, Kadomatsu K, Anzano MA, Smith JM, Sporn MB: Development and characterization of non-tumorigenic and tumorigenic epithelial cell lines from rat dorsal-lateral prostate. Cancer Res 1994;54:3413–3421.

Congress Calendar

(Continued from page 354)

2.9.–4.9.1999 **Fribourg** Switzerland	55th Assembly of the Swiss Society for Urology	**Information:** Prof. H.-J. Leisinger, Service d'Urologie, CHUV BH-10, CH–1011 Lausanne (Switzerland), Tel. +41 21 314 29 81, Fax +41 21 314 29 82, E-Mail: hans-jurg.leisinger@chuv.hospvd.ch
2.9.–5.9.1999 **Rhodes** Greece	17th World Congress on Endourology and SWL	**Information:** Erasmus Conference Center, 227 Kifisias Avenue, 14561 Kifisia, Athens (Greece), Tel. +30 1 61 25022/3, Fax +30 1 61 25021, E-Mail: erasmus@netit.gr
24.9.1999 **Padua** Italy	3rd International Symposium on Bladder Cancer Invasive Bladder Cancer – The State of the Art	**Information:** Dr. P.F. Bassi (Scientific Coordinator), Department of Urology, University of Padova, I–35122 Padova (Italy), Fax +39 049 8212721, E-Mail: bassipf@tin.it
1.10.–2.10.1999 **Varese** Italy	XXIII International Meeting and XIV Surgical Course on Pediatric Urology	**Information:** Dr. G.A. Manzoni, Section Pediatric Urology, Ospedale di Circolo, Varese (Italy), Fax +39 0332 260 520, E-Mail: urolva@ats.it Omnia Meeting & Congress: Via Torino, 29, I–00184 Rome (Italy), Fax +39 06 481 5339, E-Mail: omnia.meeting@interbusiness.it
14.10.–15.10.1999 **Munich** Germany	27th Munich Endourological Symposium	**Information:** Prof. Leyh, Department of Urology, Technische Universität München, Klinikum rechts der Isar, Ismaninger Str. 22, D–81675 München (Germany), Tel. +49 89 41 40 25 07, Fax +49 89 41 40 25 85, E-Mail: http://www.med.tu-muenchen.de/uro/endo.html
5.11.–6.11.1999 **Marburg** Germany	3rd International Symposium on Uro Oncology Advances in Diagnosis and Therapy of Bladder Cancer	**Information:** Dr. A. Heidenreich, Dr. V. Knobloch, Department of Urology, Philipps Universität Marburg, Baldingerstrasse, D–35033 Marburg (Germany) Tel. +49 6421 286239, Fax +49 6421 285590
6.11.–7.11.1999 **Vienna** Austria	Update in Prostatic Disease 2nd International Galician Urological Meeting in conjunction with the 1st Congress of the Central European Association of Urology	**Information:** Prof. Z. Dobrowolski, Department of Urology, Collegium Medicum Jagiellonian University, Cracow (Poland), Fax +48 12 42 29 44

European Urology

Eur Urol 1999;35:424–428

Retinoids in Chemoprevention

Peter Whelan

Pyrah Department of Urology, St. James's University Hospital, Leeds, UK

Key Words
Retinoids · Chemoprevention · Prostate cancer · Breast cancer · Cervical cancer · Lung cancer · Head and neck cancer

Abstract
Over several decades, in vitro experimental studies have demonstrated that retinoids effect the process of carcinogenesis and tend towards the alteration of cells back to more normal differentiation. This hypothesis has formed the basis of several chemopreventive studies in breast cancer, cervical cancer, head and neck cancer and lung cancer. Experimental evidence exists to suggest that chemoprevention with retinoids may well have a beneficial effect in patients at high risk of acquiring prostate cancer. None of the studies, however, in any of the cancers have yet been definitive, but opportunities exist with newer retinoids that appear to be able to be given on a long-term basis with minimal toxic side effects, to explore this exciting potential treatment pathway.

Introduction

Vitamin A and its products, retinoic acid (RA), and the retinoids, are essential in the normal control of epithelial cell growth and cellular differentiation. They appear to act in a hormone-like way being targeted against specific organs, the eye and the liver being the best documented. They have been known for a long time to be important for the maintenance of normal germal epithelium [1] and to be necessary for the normal differentiation of prostate glandular epithelium [2].

There is an interdependence between vitamin A and zinc, as clearly demonstrated in patients with poor dark adaptation in whom full night vision is not restored until both elements are replaced, the presence of either one alone being insufficient. A reciprocal relationship between serum zinc and serum vitamin A in patients with prostate cancer has been demonstrated [3], suggesting that this interdependence may be disrupted in patients with prostate cancer.

It is believed that the effects of retinoids are mediated by two families of receptors. The first family comprises the RA receptors (RARS) α, β and γ, all of which bind all-trans-RA, with high affinity. The second family consists of retinoid X receptors (RXRS), α, β and γ which bind 9-cis-RA with high affinity [4–6]. RARS and RXRS are members of a super family of nuclear proteins, that include the receptors for steroid hormones, vitamin D, and thyroid hormones. These hormones bind to specific DNA elements situated in the promoter region of the genes and, upon hormone binding, regulate the expression of these genes [6–8]. Accordingly, RARS and RXRS, similar to other hormone receptors, are master regulators of various physiological processes.

Because retinoids and particularly RA are capable of inducing terminal differentiation in cultured cancer cell lines [9, 10], there has been a longstanding interest in their use in differentiating therapy [11]. One of the most

KARGER

Fax + 41 61 306 12 34
E-Mail karger@karger.ch
www.karger.com

0302–2838/99/0356–0424$17.50/0

Accessible online at:
http://BioMedNet.com/karger

Dr. Peter Whelan
Pyrah Department of Urology
St. James's University Hospital
LS9 7TF Leeds (UK)
Fax +44 1 13 242 6496

impressive effects of retinoids is on acute promyelocyte leukaemia that is caused by a chromosomal translocation, resulting in formation of a fusion gene between RAR α and another gene that encodes a transcription factor known as promyelocytes [12–14]. Treatment of acute promyelocyte leukaemia patients with high doses of RA result in a complete remission [15, 16].

There is abundant in vitro experimental evidence demonstrating that vitamin A has a beneficial effect in preventing carcinogenesis. In 1955, Lasnitzki [18] showed that the carcinogen 3-methylcholanthrene induced a premalignant phenotype in cultured mass prostate gland, and excess of retinoids was able to restore a more normal cell morphology in the atypical cells resulting from carcinogen treatment. She also noted that vitamin A-deficient prostate epithelium and prostate epithelium treated with 3-methylcholanthrene were morphologically similar, but that this histological type appeared to show squamous differentiation, rather than adeno-differentiation which we see in human prostate cancer.

Recent studies by Pollard et al. [19] using Lobund-Wistar rats in which primary and secondary prostate cancers were induced by injection of methylnitrosourea, with a diet containing N-hydroxyphenaline retinomide (a synthetic retinoid), a significant reduction of both primary and secondary tumours was demonstrated.

Studies of Retinoids in Cancer Chemoprevention

Breast Cancer

It is antioestrogens and principally the nonsteroidal antioestrogen tamoxifen citrate that has demonstrated its effectiveness as a chemopreventative agent in breast cancer, with reported reductions in second primary tumours of between 30 and 50%. After antioestrogens, the retinoids including natural vitamin A and its synthetic analogues are the furthest along in clinical development. More than 4,000 retinoids have been described and several dozen are currently being studied in preclinical models or within clinical trials. Several retinoids have already demonstrated significant chemopreventative effects against carcinogen-induced mammary carcinoma in animal models [20, 21]. The retinoids, as stated above, bind to RARS and RXRS, and the complexes act as transcription factors, binding to retinoid-response elements of multiple target genes, one of which is TGF-β, an antiproliferative molecule for mammary epithelium. Another retinoid, 4-hydroxyphenylretinamide, or fenretinide, has been shown to decrease circulating levels of IGF-1 [21], a potent breast cancer mitogen, to also induce the expression of RAR-β, a putative growth factor receptor, and to decrease the expression of EHR-2LNEU-a putative tumor suppressor gene, on breast cancer cells [22].

The Eastern Cooperative Oncology Group is currently evaluating tamoxifen versus tamoxifen plus fenretinide as adjuvant therapy for patients older than 65 years with oestrogen receptor-positive, node-positive breast cancer. There are currently no results from this study. In a protocol by the National Tumour Institute in Milan, Italy, DePoalo et al. [23] have randomized nearly 3,000 node-negative patients with breast cancer to receive 200 mg/day of fenretinide versus placebo for 5 years. A recent report from an early interim analysis of this study suggests that women who receive the retinoid have a decreased incidence of primary ovarian cancer, and the results of the incidents of second primary breast cancers are due to be reported in an interim fashion in the near future.

Prototype breast cancer tissue-based chemoprevention trials involving surrogate biomarkers as study endpoints are being developed. In a pilot study conducted by Zujewski et al. at the National Cancer Institute (NCI), women with ADH and a family history of breast cancer (1 or 2 first-degree relatives), women with LCIS or a history of treated DCIS, or women with a strong family history of breast cancer (2 first-degree relatives), undergo a baseline stereotactic 14-gauge core needle biopsy of normal appearing glandular breast tissue and a mammogram, as well as fine needle aspiration of other breast tissue. The women are then treated with 20 mg/day of tamoxifen for 2 years and with 200 mg/day of fenretinide for 4 months. Repeated core biopsies and fine needle aspirations are performed at 6 and 24 months to study modulation of biomarker expression. Endometrial monitoring and monitoring of dark adaptation changes takes place at several time points. The object of this trial is to study the frequency and possible modulation of several biomarkers in these high-risk women's breast tissue. The surrogate biomarkers of interest in this study include nuclear morphometric, proliferative markers – including cycline D1 – and TGF-β, P53, oestrogen and RARS, and serum and tissue oestrogen metabolites.

Ratko et al. [21] have demonstrated that second primary breast tumours were greatly reduced with a combination of tamoxifen and fenretinide in rat models. Several studies including that of Butta et al. [24] have shown upregulation of TGF-β which may explain the observed synergism between tamoxifen and fenretinide.

In an ongoing study, Dhingra et al. at M.D. Anderson Cancer Center are conducting a randomized chemopreventive study of tamoxifen versus fenretinide versus the combination in high-risk patients and using similar surrogate endpoints as those to the study from the NCI. The hope is by use of surrogate endpoints early information as to the possible effectiveness of these chemopreventative strategies will become available.

Cervical Cancer

Chemoprevention trials in cervical cancer have tended to look at high-risk cohorts, and particularly patients with high-grade lesions. The rationale for using patients with high-grade lesions is that such lesions are more likely to progress to invasive cancer; up to 35% of (CIS) lesions progressed in a series of studies in which 353 patients were followed without treatment over a period of 3 months to 30 years [25]. Patients with high-grade lesions are therefore suitable for all types of trials including phase I, II and III. The cervix has, in addition, been thought by pathologists to be a model for the progression from mildly dysplastic lesions through severely dysplastic lesions to invasive cancer. The ability of clinicians, therefore, to observe cervical lesions over time with colposcopy and PAP smears, should make the cervix a unique organ for chemopreventative action that can be closely monitored.

In cervical cancer nutritional data demonstrates that vitamin A deficiency increases the relative risk of squamous preneoplastic and neoplastic lesions. Romney et al. [26] reported on the phase I/II trial using retinyl acetate gel applied topically in patients with CIN-1 to 2. No serious side effects were noted in this study and there was a high compliance rate, but a phase III trial awaits reporting. Meyskens et al. [27] recently reported the results of a randomized phase III trial of topical 0.375% all-trans RA in 141 patients with CIN-2 lesions and 160 patients with CIN-3 lesions, patients with CIS being excluded from the study. There was a statistically significant regression in the CIN-2 lesions, but not in the CIN-3 lesions. Sporn and Roberts [28] speculated in an editorial that the CIN-2 responded and CIN-3 did not, because lesions further along the line towards neoplasia may be harder to turn round, as they require both higher doses and longer exposure to the chemopreventative agent. It was also felt that combination therapy rather than single therapy may have been indicated with these severe lesions. The ease of accessibility to the cervix, however, and the fact that this is a squamous dysplasia that is being corrected does lend support to its use as a model for long-term chemopreventative therapy with retinoids being currently the most logical therapy [29].

Head and Neck Cancer

Several studies [30, 31] have demonstrated beneficial effects with administration of retinoids in preventing as well as treating oral leukoplakia. The original observation of Hong et al. [31] that retinoid treatment could reduce the incidence of early second primaries in oral cancer has been substantiated by longer follow-up of the treatment groups [33]. After more than 4 years of follow-up the treatment group did appear to be deriving continual benefits, in that the incidence of second primaries continue to be less than one half that of the placebo group [33]. Bolla et al. [32], however, using etretinate (a synthetic retinoid) showed the equivalent rates of both second primaries and equivalent times to relapse in the original tumours in a randomized trial of retinoid versus placebo. It was felt, however, because of the significant toxicity associated with etretinate, that patient compliance and a high dropout rate may have been factors in the outcome of this particular study.

Lung Cancer

Studies using retinyl palmitate did decrease the incidence of second primaries in non-small cell lung cancer patients [38]. However, similar response in lung cancer patients using intermediate endpoints such as sputum atypia reversal, were not seen in long-term smokers with the use of either etretinate or retinol treatment [34, 35]. And patients with definitive squamous metaplasia treated by retinoids have shown a mixed response [36, 37].

These results suggest that sputum atypia and squamous metaplasia may be either too nonspecific or too insensitive to be used as biomarkers for a response to chemopreventive agents in lung cancer. Other molecular and biochemical intermediate endpoints have been looked at in patients with lung cancer, and accumulation of the P53 protein has been found to accelerate as bronchial epithelium progresses from dysplasia to invasive carcinoma [39], and the loss of the alleles in the short arm of both chromosomes 3 and 9 have been reported to occur in dysplastic airway lesions [40, 41].

As β-carotene is known to be a precursor of retinol, chemopreventive trials in lung cancer have been carried out using this agent. This was based on the fact that β-carotene decreased the frequency of micronuclei in a study of long-term smokers [42], although it did not alter sputum atypia [35]. A large trial using α-tocopherol and β-carotene carried out in Finland gave β-carotene to 29,000 male smokers who received this therapy for between 5 and 8 years. Worryingly, an 18% increase in lung cancer incidents was seen in the group receiving β-carotene. And thus no protection, rather the adverse, was seen with regard to lung cancer [43].

The unexpected results with β-carotene could have resulted from several causes: the period of treatment may have been too short to have protective effect, β-carotene may not be the compound that produces protective effects in individuals who consume large amounts of fruits and vegetables, or the higher β-carotene serum levels that protect against cancer may be a nonspecific indicator of some other protective factor. It is also possible the primary effect of β-carotene is as an antioxidant and not as a precursor of retinol. Antioxidants may have unexpected side effects, or may not have the same ability as retinoids to interfere with carcinogenesis in the respiratory tract. It reemphasizes again that the move from laboratory bench to bedside often brings about unexpected effects. This negative effect with β-carotene, however, has negated the studies that show apparent beneficial effects with other retinoids in lung cancer prevention.

The Role of Retinoids in Chemoprevention in Prostate Cancer

At present the physiological role of retinoids in the prostate is still poorly understood. As well as any possible effect towards terminal differentiation mediated by retinoid receptors, RA appears to have a varying effect on the activity of 5α-reductase, the enzyme involved in the conversion of testosterone to dihydrotestosterone. This has been shown in in vitro studies using prostatic cell lines [44], and demonstrated that RA suppressed the activity of 5α-reductase. Similar findings in the reduction of 5α-reductase activity by retinoids were also demonstrated by Jutley et al. [45]. There is also an apparent interdependence between retinoid and androgen physiology, not dissimilar to that hypothesized for oestrogens and retinoids. There is more clinical basis and evidence, however, for the interrelation between androgens and retinoids as exemplified in the treatment of the androgen-dependent skin disease, acne. In the last decade or more, significant benefits to the treatment of acne have been demonstrated by the use of antiandrogens such as cyproterone acetate and use of the synthetic retinoid atretinate which has greatly enhanced the control of this disease [46].

Recent studies by Pasquali et al. [47] have demonstrated low levels of retinoid receptors in prostate cancer, possibly indicating that this has contributed to the malignant transformation of prostate epithelium. They found encouragement in the confirmation of these findings, as they were able to demonstrate that all prostate cancer cells investigated expressed RARS, and that these appeared able to respond to exogenously provided natural or synthetic retinoids. Their studies have also demonstrated that retinol, a component of a normal diet, is present in the prostate and can readily be converted to the biologically active RA. This again suggested that supplementation with retinoids could have a modifying effect upon the process of carcinogenesis within the prostate. How this occurs and to what extent it may be dependent on the provision of zinc supplements, remain questions to be answered by future research.

References

1 Wolbach SB, Howe PR: Tissue changes following deprivation of fat-soluble vitamin. J Exp Med 1925;42:753–777.
2 Chopra DP, Wilkoff DF: Effects of retinoids and oestrogens on testosterone-induced hyperplasia of mouse prostate explants in organ culture. Proc Soc Exp Biol Med 1979;162:229–234.
3 Whelan P, Walker BCG, Kelleher J: Zinc, vitamin A and prostate cancer. Br J Urol 1983;55: 525–528.
4 Heyman R, Mangelsdorf DJ, Dyck JA, et al: 9-cis-Retinoic acid is a high affinity ligand for the retinoid X receptor. Cell 1992;68:397–406.
5 Levin AA, Sturzenbecker LJ, Kazmer S, et al: 9-cis-Retinoic acid stereoisomer binds and activates the nuclear receptor RAR alpha. Nature 1992;355:359–361.
6 Allenby G, Bocquel MT, et al: Retinoic acid receptors and retinoid X receptors: Interactions with endogenous retinoic acids. Proc Natl Acad Sci USA 1993;90:30–34.
7 Evans MR: The steroid and thyroid hormone receptor superfamily. Science 1988;240:889–895.
8 Beato M: Gene regulation by steroid hormones. Cell 1989;56:335–344.
9 Strickland S, Mahdavi M: The induction of differentiation in teratocarcinoma stem cells by retinoic acid. Cell 1978;15:393–403.
10 Collins SJ, Robertson KA, LeMoyne M: Retinoic acid-induced granulocytic differentiation of HL-60 myeloid leukemia cells is mediated directly through the retinoic acid receptor (RAR-alpha). Mol Cell Biol 1990;10:2154–2163.
11 Lotan R: Differentiation therapy. Cancer Res 1990;50:3453–3464.
12 Borrow J, Goddard AD, Sheer D, Solomon E: Molecular analysis of acute promyelocytic leukemia breakpoint cluster region on chromosome 17. Science 1990;249:1577–1580.
13 Kakizuka A, Miller WH Jr, Umesone K, et al: Chromosomal translocation t(15;17) in human acute promyelocytic leukemia fuses RAR-alpha with a novel putative transcription factor, PML. Cell 1991;66:675–684.
14 De The H, Lavau C, Marchio A, Chomienne C, Degos L, Dejan A: The PML-RAR-alpha fusion MRNA gene t(15;17) translocation in acute promyelocytic leukemia encodes and functionally altered RAR. Cell 1991;66:675–684.
15 Huang ME, Yu-Chen Y, Shu-Rong C, et al: Use of all-trans-retinoic acid in the treatment of acute promyelocytic leukaemia. Blood 1998; 72:567–572.

16 Castigne S, Chomienne C, Daniel MT, et al: All-trans-retinoic acid as differentiation therapy for acute promyelocytic leukaemia. I. Clinical results. Blood 1990;76:1704–1709.
17 Boring CC, Squires TS, Tong T: Cancer statistics: 1991. CA Cancer J Clin 1991;41:19–36.
18 Lasnitzki I: The influence of A hypervitaminosis on the effect of 20-methylcholanthrene on mouse prostate glands grown in vitro. Br J Cancer 1955;9:434–441.
19 Pollard M, Luckert PH, Sporn MB: Prevention of primary prostate cancer in Lobund-Wistar rats by N-(4-hydroxyphenyl)retinamide. Cancer Res 1991;51:3610–3611.
20 Anzano MA, Byers SW, Smith J, et al: Prevention of breast cancer in the rat with 9-cis-retinoic acid as a single agent and in combination with tamoxifen. Cancer Res 1994;54: 4610–4614.
21 Ratko TA, Detrsac CJ, Dinger NM, et al: Chemopreventive efficacy of combined retinoid and tamoxifen treatment following surgical excision of a primary mammary cancer in female rats. Cancer Res 1989;49:4472–4476.
22 Bacus SS, Kiguchi K, Chin D, et al: Differentiation of cultures of human breast cancer cells (AU-585 and MCF-7) associated with loss of cell surface. HER-2/neu antigen. Mol Carcinog 1990;3:350–365.
23 DePualo G, Veronesi U, Camerini T, et al: Can fenretinide protect women against ovarian cancer? J Natl Cancer Inst 1995;87:146–147.
24 Butta A, MacLennon K, Flanders KC, et al: Induction of transforming growth factor-beta-1 in human breast cancer in vivo following tamoxifen treatment. Cancer Res 1992;52:4261–4264.
25 Mitchell MF, Hittelman WN, Hong WK, Lotan R, Schottenfeld D: The natural history of cervical intraepithelial neoplasia: An argument for intermediate endpoint biomarkers. Cancer Epidemiol Biomarkers Prev 1994;3:619–626.
26 Romney SL, Dwyer A, Slagle S, Duttagupta C, Palan PR, Basu J, et al: Chemoprevention of cervix cancer: Phase I–II: a feasibility study involving the typical vaginal administration of retinyl acetate gel. Gynecol Oncol 1985;20: 109–119.
27 Meyskens FL, Surwit EA, Moon TE, Childers JM, Davis JR, Dorr RT, et al: Enhancement of regression of cervical intraepithelial neoplasia II (moderate dysplasia) with topically applied all-trans-retinoic acid: A randomised trial. J Natl Cancer Inst 1994;86:539–543.
28 Sporn MB, Roberts AB: Cervical dysplasia regression induced by all-trans-retinoic acid. J Natl Cancer Inst 1994;86:476–477.
29 Current Clinical Trials Oncology. National Cancer Institute PDQ, vol 1, No 2. March–April 1994 (protocol 09088).
30 Stich HF, Hornby AP, Mathew B, et al: Response of oral leukoplakias to the administration of vitamin A. Cancer Lett 1988;40:93–101.
31 Hong WK, Endicott J, Itri LM, et al: 13-cis-Retinoic acid in the treatment of oral leukoplakia. N Engl J Med 1986;315:1501–1505.
32 Bolla M, LeFur R, Ton Van J, et al: Prevention of second primary tumours with etretinate in squamous cell carcinoma of the oral cavity and oropharynx: Results of a multicentric double-blind randomised study. Eur J Cancer 1994;30: 767–772.
33 Benner SE, Lippman S, Hong WK: Current status of retinoid chemoprevention of lung cancer. Oncology 1995;9:205–209.
34 Arnold AM, Browman GP, Levine MN, et al: The effect of the synthetic retinoid etretinate on sputum cytology: Results from a randomised trial. Br J Cancer 1992;65:737–743.
35 McLarty JW, Holiday DB, Girard WM, et al: Beta-carotene, vitamin A, and lung cancer chemoprevention: Results of an intermediate end point study. Am J Clin Nutr 1995;62(suppl): 1431–1438.
36 Misset JL, Homasson JP, Santelli G, et al: Regression of bronchial epidermoid metaplasia in heavy smokers with etretinate treatment. Cancer Detect Prev 1986;9:167–170.
37 Lee JS, Lippman SM, Benner SE, et al: Randomised placebo-controlled trial of isotretinoin in chemoprevention of bronchial squamous metaplasia. J Clin Oncol 1994;12:937–945.
38 Pastorino U, Infante M, Maioli M, et al: Adjuvant treatment of stage 1 lung cancer with high-dose vitamin A. J Clin Oncol 1993;11:1216–1222.
39 Bennett WP, Colby TV, Travis WD, et al: p53 protein accumulates frequently in early bronchial neoplasia. Cancer Res 1993;53:4817–4822.
40 Kishimoto Y, Sugio K, Hung JY, et al: Allele-specific loss in chromosome 9p loci in preneoplastic lesions accompanying non-small cell lung cancers. J Natl Cancer Inst 1995;87:1224–1229.
41 Rabbitts P: Somatic genetic changes in lung cancer and precancerous lesions (abstract). CCPC-93: Second International Cancer Chemoprevention Conference, Berlin, April 28–30, 1993.
42 Van Poppel G, Kok FJ, Hemus RJ: Beta-carotene supplementation in smokers reduces the frequency of micronuclei in sputum. Br J Cancer 1992;66:1164–1168.
43 The Alpha-Tocopherol, Beta-Carotene Cancer Prevention Group: The effect of vitamin E and beta-carotene on the incidence of lung cancer and other cancers in male smokers. N Engl J Med 1994;330:1029–1035.
44 Halgunset J, Sunde A, Lundmo PI: Retinoic acid (AA): An inhibitor of 5-alpha-reductase in Luman prostatic cancer cells. J Steroid Biochem 1987;28:731–738.
45 Jutley JK, Meaney S, Kelleher J, Whelan P: Interactions of retinoic acid and androgens in human prostatic tissue. Prostate 1990;16:229–304.
46 Landon K: Dispelling myths about acne. Postgrad Med 1997;102:94–99, 103–104, 110–112.
47 Pasquali D, Thaller C, Eichele G: Abnormal level of retinoic acid in prostate cancer tissues. J Clin Endocrinol Metab 1996;81:2186–2191.

Molecular Targets for Chemoprevention of Prostate Cancer

European Urology

Eur Urol 1999;35:429–438

Evaluation of Biomarker Modulation by Fenretinide in Prostate Cancer Patients

D. Urban[a] R. Myers[a] U. Manne[a] H. Weiss[a] J. Mohler[b] D. Perkins[a] M. Markiewicz[a] R. Lieberman[c] G. Kelloff[c] M. Marshall[a] W. Grizzle[a]

[a]University of Alabama at Birmingham, Ala., [b]University of North Carolina at Chapel Hill, N.C., and [c]Chemoprevention Branch of the National Cancer Institute, Bethesda, Md., USA

Key Words

Prostate cancer · Chemoprevention · (4-Hydroxyphenyl)retinamide · Fenretinide · Surrogate endpoint biomarker

Abstract

An NCI-sponsored, phase II trial of N-(4-hydroxyphenyl)-retinamide (4-HPR) in patients with organ-confined prostate cancer in the period prior to radical prostatectomy was carried out. Thirty-seven men with the histologic diagnosis of prostate cancer planning to have radical prostatectomy entered the study after informed consent and were given 4-HPR (or matching placebo) as a single daily dose (two 100-mg capsules of 4-HPR or two capsules of placebo daily) for 3 weeks prior to surgery. Four men dropped out for unrelated reasons. Thirty-three men completed the study. At the time of surgery, repeat biopsies of the prostate were performed to study the effects of the drug on potential surrogate endpoint biomarkers (SEBs) of malignancy within the tissue. The panel of potential SEBs of malignancy include p53, cytomorphometric indices, ploidy, PNCA, erbB-2, erbB-3, EGF receptor, TGF-α tumor-associated glycoprotein-72, fatty acid synthetase and Lewis Y antigen. Twenty-three patients had matching pre- and posttherapy lesions and were considered informative. Results from the patients indicate significant differential expression of biomarkers in pretreatment specimens of uninvolved prostatic tissue (normal-appearing epithelia) prostatic intraepithelial neoplasia (PIN) and prostate cancer. The mean erbB-2 expression was 0.58 in uninvolved vs. 1.04 in PIN ($p = 0.002$); while the mean erbB-2 expression was 1.35 in prostate cancer ($p = 0.0007$, uninvolved vs. prostate cancer). A similar pattern of increased biomarker expression between uninvolved and PIN or prostate cancer tissues can be observed for EGF receptor (mean = 1.21, 1.87 and 1.76 for uninvolved, PIN and prostate cancer, respectively) and erbB-3 (mean = 0.81, 1.59 and 1.30 for uninvolved, PIN and prostate cancer, respectively). There were no statistically significant differences in biomarkers observed in the 4-HPR-treated patients when compared with placebo-treated control patients. There was a posttreatment up-regulation of biomarkers observed in both groups of patients. This observation is most likely explained by an effect due to the diagnostic sextant biopsy equally affecting both groups of patients. Results from this study do not demonstrate a chemoprevention effect of 4-HPR on tissue-based SEBs at the dose given.

Introduction

Carcinoma of the prostate is a major health problem among American men. In 1998, there were over 184,500 newly diagnosed cases and over 39,000 deaths [1]. Because there is no curative therapy for advanced prostate

KARGER

Fax +41 61 306 12 34
E-Mail karger@karger.ch
www.karger.com

0302–2838/99/0356–0429$17.50/0

Accessible online at:
http://BioMedNet.com/karger

Donald Urban, MD
Division of Urology, MEB 603, Department of Surgery
University of Alabama at Birmingham
Birmingham, AL 35294 (USA)
Tel. +1 205 934 1421, Fax +1 205 934 4933, E-Mail durban@urology.uab.edu

cancer, recent interest has focused on chemoprevention of prostate cancer. Chemoprevention is the administration of nontoxic compounds to prevent cancer by blocking the progression of precancerous cells to malignancy or by preventing the formation of carcinogens or halting the interaction of an active carcinogen with target tissue [2].

We carried out a short-term, phase II, double-blind, randomized, placebo-controlled chemoprevention trial, administering fenretinide (4-HPR) or a matching placebo as a single daily dose (two 100-mg capsules of 4-HPR or two capsules of placebo daily) for 3 weeks prior to surgery in men with localized prostate cancer who selected radical prostatectomy as their therapy. Diagnostic needle biopsy material was compared with needle biopsies taken from the prostatectomy specimen at the time of surgery. A panel of surrogate endpoint biomarkers (SEBs) was used to evaluate the chemopreventive effects of 4-HPR.

Background

4-HPR

4-HPR is a member of a large group of structurally related substances known as retinoids that include vitamin A and its natural and synthetic analogs. Vitamin A has been shown to be necessary for normal growth and maintenance of differentiation in epithelial tissues and for normal vision and reproduction [3]. Diets deficient in vitamin A, when fed to experimental animals, resulted in hyperkeratinization, squamous metaplasia and the appearance of tumors in multiple tissus [4]. Studies in laboratory animals have shown that various retinoids can inhibit carcinogenesis in several different organs, primarily of epithelial origin.

The development of drugs with chemopreventive potential for chronic administration to healthy humans requires the identification of drugs with minimal toxicity. One of the major obstacles to the development of retinoids for human use has been the significant toxicity associated with these agents at pharmacological doses. Thus, efforts have been made to alter the basic structure of retinoids in order to reduce their toxicity while simultaneously retaining their chemopreventive properties. 4-HPR is a synthetic amide of all-*trans*-retinoic acid. The terminal carboxyl group of retinoic acid has been replaced by an N-substituted carboxyamide group. Because 4-HPR does not accumulate in the liver to the same extent as natural retinoids, it is less toxic. Furthermore, 4-HPR appears to have chemopreventive activity comparable to, or better than the natural retinoids [4].

Retinoids appear to act at the promotion and/or progression stages of carcinogenesis, since they are most effective when administered subsequent to a carcinogenic agent. Activities of the retinoids have been postulated to be due to their effects on tissue differentiation, influences on regulation of growth factors implicated in preneoplastic development and immune modulation [5].

In human clinical trials, 4-HPR has been well tolerated in doses up to 400 mg/day. In clinical studies extenting 1–2 years, 4-HPR doses ranging from 100 to 300 mg produced side effects such as nyctalopia (dark adaptation) and skin rash, both of which are reversible upon discontinuation of drug. Other side effects in humans include headaches, dizziness, vertigo, diarrhea, nausea, visual disturbances (dry eyes and light sensitivity), dermatologic toxicity such as pruritis, dry skin, exfoliation of the hands and feet, erythema multiforme, alopecia, abnormal bone metabolism and abnormal liver function tests. 4-HPR administration results in a significant reduction in the plasma levels of retinol and retinol-binding protein. The levels recover between 3 and 7 days after cessation of drug. 4-HPR may also interfere with the absorption of vitamin A and block mobilization of vitamin A from the liver [6, 7].

Biomarkers

Chemoprevention studies which utilize the endpoint of cancer incidence require large numbers of subjects followed for many years. An example is the phase III, Prostate Cancer Prevention Trial (PCPT) which completed patient accrual in 1996, comparing finasteride (Proscar) to placebo in over 18,000 men followed for 7 years with the incidence of biopsy-proven prostate cancer as the primary endpoint. These are very expensive clinical studies which require thousands of patients and many years to reach meaningful results that will allow the science of cancer chemoprevention to advance. An alternative approach has been to use biochemical, molecular and morphologic tissue markers to both help establish a potentially effective but nontoxic dose range in phase I trials as well as to monitor response in placebo-controlled phase II trials, reserving the endpoint of cancer for larger phase III trials [8–11].

There are three classes of biomarkers with potential utility in chemoprevention trials. Biochemical activity markers (BAM) are quantitative measures of a drug's activity and are useful for establishing a dose response, finding a dose range and monitoring patient compliance.

Risk biomarkers (RBs) are biochemical or biological markers whose existence or expression is directly correlated with cancer but vary in latency and strength of linkage to invasive cancer. SEBs are RBs used as indicators of efficacy of chemoprevention that correlate with cancer incidence reduction. Candidate chemoprevention agents can be tested in a shorter time frame by assessing their ability to alter the expression of validated SEBs [11–15].

The ideal SEB for prostate cancer is the marker which is biologically plausible and differentially expressed in normal, high-risk tissue (high-grade prostatic intraepithelial neoplasia; PIN) and prostate cancer. It needs to be present in the population of men at risk, easy to sample and quantitative, and potentially reversible or modulated with successful chemoprevention. In addition, the expression should not be significantly affected by normal physiologic processes. The panel of potential SEBs of malignancy in this study include p53, cytomorphometric indices, ploidy, proliferating cell nuclear antigen (PNCA), $p185^{erbB-2}$, $p180^{erbB-3}$, epidermal growth factor receptor (EGF-R), transforming growth factor-α (TGF-α), tumor-associated glycoprotein-72 (TAG-72), fatty acid synthetase (FASE) and Lewis Y antigen [16].

Materials and Methods

Description of Study

The study was initiated December 1995, after obtaining an investigational new drug (IND) approval for 4-HPR and protocol approval from the University of Alabama at Birmingham (UAB) Institutional Review Board. Men of any race, ethnic origin and age (>18 years old) were eligible if they had sextant biopsy of the prostate establishing a diagnosis of adenocarcinoma of the prostate, paraffin-embedded material was available for biomarker studies and patients were planning to undergo a radical prostatectomy within 6–8 weeks of study entry.

Eligible subjects had a good performance status (ECOG >3), normal or satisfactory baseline laboratory values and were free of symptomatic cardiovascular disease, congestive heart failure, cardiomyopathy, uncontrolled hypertension, uncontrolled cardiac arrhythmia, or prior coronary artery bypass surgery or acute myocardial infarction within the previous year. In addition, they could not have an untreated or active secondary malignancy or chemotherapy within the previous 5 years. They were excluded for concurrent immunotherapy, radiation therapy or steroids for any clinical indication. Finasteride (Proscar) for benign prostatic hyperplasia (BPH) and total androgen deprivation therapy prior to surgery were also a cause for exclusion. Patients could not take concurrent vitamin A or any other vitamins (single vitamins of any type or multivitamin preparations). Personal or family history of tapetoretinal degeneration was also cause for exclusion.

At baseline (3–4 weeks before surgery), the day before surgery and 3 weeks postoperatively, approximately 10 ml blood was collected. The blood was spun down and the plasma was separated and collected from the red-top tube and the serum was separated and collected from the purple-top tubes. The serum and plasma were divided into aliquots in cryovials, frozen to –70 °C and stored until batched analyses were performed for 4-HPR levels and PSA.

4-HPR and PSA Assay

4-HPR and 4-MPR were assayed by HPLC using a Hitachi Model L6200 Intelligent Pump with a L4200 UV-VIS Detector and a 02000 Chromato-Integrator. All HPLC analyses were performed at ambient temperature under yellow light. Plasma samples (250 µl) were deproteinized with 750 µl ethanol and then extracted with 4 ml hexane. After evaporation, 120 µl of the HPLC mobile phase (methanol:water, 90:10) were added. 100 µl were then injected into a Spherisorb ODS-2 3-µm HPLC column. The retinoid peaks were monitored by absorption at 362 nm (flow rate 1.0 ml/min). The amount of the compounds was determined by internal standardization (using 4-ethoxyphenylretinamide). The retention times for 4-HPR and 4-MPR were approximately 5.9 and 8.6 min, respectively [17]. Serum PSA concentrations were measured using the Abbott AXSYMPSA assay [18].

Prostate Sampling

Pretreatment prostatic tissue was available from the paraffin-embedded diagnostic biopsy material. Sextant biopsies were preferred, but adequate pretreatment material with sufficient remaining tissue in the block was accepted. Posttreatment tissue was taken from sextant biopsies of the prostate following its removal at the time of prostatectomy. These biopsies were fixed and paraffin-embedded.

Choice of Biomarkers

If a biomarker is characteristic of a neoplastic lesion, there should be differential expression of the biomarker between uninvolved glandular epithelium and specific neoplastic lesions. To determine if the biomarkers selected for evaluation are characteristic of a specific neoplastic lesion, uninvolved glandular epithelium is compared with specific neoplastic lesions. Our initial choice of biomarkers was based upon our prior studies of biomarker expression in the neoplastic process of the prostate [16]. The biomarkers chosen included PCNA, p53, $p185^{erbB-2}$, $p180^{erbB-3}$, TGF-α, EGF-R, FASE, TAG-72 and Lewis Y.

Statistical Analysis

Descriptive statistics such as mean, standard error and median immunohistochemistry scores were calculated for each biomarker at baseline and posttreatment. In order to determine whether there is differential expression of biomarkers in the normal-appearing and PIN tissues, we calculated the difference in immunohistochemistry scores between these tissues for each patient. The Wilcoxon signed-ranks test was performed to determine whether there is a significant difference between normal and PIN tissues for each biomarker. A similar analysis was performed to determine differential expression of each biomarker between normal and tumor tissues.

The change in biomarker expression between pre- and posttreatment biopsies was calculated for each patient. The Wilcoxon rank-sum test was used to determine whether there was a significant difference in the change in biomarker expression between 4-HPR and placebo groups.

Table 1. Adverse effects by treatment group

	Regimen					
	4-HPR (n = 20)		placebo (n = 16)		total (n = 36)	
	n	%	n	%	n	%
Patients with at least one adverse effect	2/20	10.0	3/16	18.8	5/36	13.9
Events						
Total number	3	15.0	6	38.0	9	25.0
Dryness and soreness in mouth	1	5.0	0		1	2.8
Headache	0		1	6.2	1	2.8
Cold symptoms	0		1	6.2	1	2.8
Hypertension	0		1	6.2	1	2.8
Bad taste in mouth	1	5.0	0		1	2.8
Dehydration	0		1	6.2	1	2.8
Elevated blood pressure	0		1	6.2	1	2.8
Pulmonary embolism	0		1	6.2	1	2.8
Surgery canceled progressive DZ	1	5.0	0		1	2.8
Grade						
Mild	2	10.0	1	6.2	3	8.3
Moderate	1	5.0	2	12.5	3	8.3
Severe	0		0		0	
Life-threatening	0		0		0	
Fatal	0		1[1]	6.2	1	2.8
Missing	0		2	12.5	2	5.6
Relation						
Unrelated	0		3	18.8	3	8.3
Unlikely	0		2	12.5	2	5.6
Possible	1	5.0	1	6.2	2	5.6
Probable	0		0		0	
Definite	0		0		0	
Missing	2	10.0	0		2	5.6

[1] Death due to pulmonary embolism.

Results

Subjects

The subjects in this study were 37 men, median age 60.8 (range 49–71), median height 70.6 inches (range 66–76), median weight 189.8 lb (127.5–279), 68% white and 32% black, with the histologic diagnosis of adenocarcinoma of the prostate. The subjects were in good health and appropriate candidates for radical prostatectomy. Prior diagnosis of nonprostate cancer more than 5 years before enrollment was present in 38%. Among the subjects, 36% had cardiovascular disease, 6% had bronchopulmonary disease, 3% had gastrointestinal disease, 3% had dermatologic disease, none had hepatobiliary disease, diabetes or hematologic disease. Thirty-one percent had a family history of cancer. Baseline laboratory results were normal or satisfactory for radical prostatectomy in all subjects. Thirty-three men completed the study. Four dropped out of the study, 1 chose not to take the study medication, 2 decided not to undergo surgery, 1 experienced sore mouth and inability to wear dentures and discontinued the study medication.

Patient Accrual and Interim Analysis

Patient accrual was initially slow with less than 1 patient accrued per month. The poor accrual was attributed to the initial study design of a 6- to 8-week presurgery treatment period. Eligible patients refused to participate in this study because they did not want to delay their surgical procedure. The protocol was modified to a 3-week presurgery treatment period in October 1996 and four affiliate study sites began to actively recruit patients

Table 2. Epithelial compartments in 25 cases evaluated

Prostatic epithelial compartment	Cases[1] pretherapy	Cases[1] posttherapy	Informative[1]
Uninvolved glands			
Basal cells	23	25	23
Luminal cells	23	25	23
Low-grade PIN			
Basal cells	8	10	7
Luminal cells	8	10	7
High-grade PIN			
Basal cells	7	7	7
Luminal cells	7	7	7
Adenocarcinomas	17	19	15

[1] Maximum number for any one antigen; some antigens may have fewer cases available for analysis and/or may be less informative due to loss or unavailability of specific sections.

resulting in improved accrual. The distribution of subjects was UAB, 23 (62%), Birmingham Veterans Administration Medical Center, 1 (3%), Norwood Clinic, 1 (3%), Urology Associates, 2 (5%) and University of North Carolina at Chapel Hill, 10 (27%). To faciliate monitoring of progress and expedite the data analysis, a bayesian sequential monitoring scheme was employed. This method provides an efficient approach for early stopping of a trial with a relatively small sample size [15].

Compliance and Adverse Events

The patients entered into this study were compliant with taking their study medication and completing the presurgical treatment (88–100%). No patients reported visual disturbance of any kind including decreased visual acuity, dark adaptation of diminished night vision. Dryness, soreness and bad taste in the mouth was reported in 5% of patients taking 4-HPR and none taking placebo (table 1). At least one adverse event was experienced by 10% of patients on 4-HPR and 18% of patients on placebo while on the study medication ($p > 0.05$). These events were mild to moderate in severity and were self-limited in duration.

There was one serious adverse event that was not related to the study medication. One patient completed taking the study medication (placebo) for 3 weeks prior to prostatectomy surgery. Seventeen days after taking the last dose of placebo and 16 days after surgery, this patient suffered a pulmonary embolism which was fatal. The pulmonary embolism was attributed to the prostatic surgery which has a known risk of embolic complications.

4-HPR and PSA Levels

The median baseline PSA was 6.5 ng/ml and 9.0 ng/ml in the 4-HPR-treated and placebo patients respectively. PSA values were not changed by treatment with 4-HPR or placebo when baseline values were compared to PSA levels after treatment and before prostatectomy (6.4 ng/ml 4-HPR, $p = 0.0895$ and 9.2 ng/ml, $p = 0.625$ placebo). The 4-HPR plasma levels during therapy taken within 8 h of the last dose ranged from 6.6 to 161 ng/ml in those patients for whom values were available.

Informative Cases

The specific aim of the protocol was to compare epithelial compartments and lesions in the pretherapy biopsy with the same epithelial compartments and lesions in posttherapy biopsies obtained from the radical prostatectomy specimens after therapy. The following epithelial compartments were evaluated: uninvolved prostatic glandular epithelium, basal cells and luminal cells; low-grade PIN, basal cells and luminal cells; high-grade PIN, basal cells and luminal cells; prostatic adenocarcinoma. For a case to be informative, the same epithelial compartment/lesion must be in both the pre- and posttherapy biopsies from the same patient. Of the 25 cases evaluated, the epithelial compartments that were informative are shown in table 2.

In general, the postbiopsy sample (3 biopsies from each lobe) represented a better sample than the prebiopsy sample because much of the prebiopsy sample had been utilized in diagnosis. Also, uninvolved glands are the most common features found in all biopsies. Informative samples may be less than the lowest number of pre- or posttherapy cases respectively because, for example, not all pretherapy cases with adenocarcinomas will have matching adenocarcinoma with posttherapy specimens and vice versa.

Biomarker Expression

In our study, we evaluated the effect of the retinoid, 4-HPR, on the epithelial compartments of the prostate. As would be predicted, the epithelial compartment for which there were the most matches pre- and posttherapy was the uninvolved glandular epithelium. The results indicate significant differential expression of biomarkers in pretreatment specimens of uninvolved prostatic tissue, PIN and prostate cancer (table 3). The mean erbB-2 expression was 0.58 in uninvolved vs. 1.04 in PIN (p =

Table 3. Comparison of SEB expression in prostate biopsy tissue

	Uninvolved glandular epithelium		Low-grade PIN		High-grade PIN		Adeno-carcinoma
	basal	luminal	basal	luminal	basal	luminal	
PCNA, %	2.84±1.23	2.70±1.52	3.31±2.14	5.24±4.20	5.0±3.82	5.4±3.82	6.61±3.52*(l)
$p185^{erbB-2}$							
Cytoplasmic	1.61±0.12	0.58±0.07	1.24±0.21	1.04±0.15	1.44±0.10	1.51±0.09	1.35±0.15**(l)
Membrane	NM	0.61±0.08	NM	1.12±0.24***(l)	NM	1.40±0.12*(l)	1.13±0.17**(l)
$p180^{erbB-3}$							
Cytoplasmic	0.98±0.16	0.81±0.13	1.51±0.27	1.59±0.26**(l)	1.17±0.26	1.27±0.27*(l)	1.30±0.21***(l)
Membrane	NM	0.82±0.13	NM	1.60±0.25**(l)	NM	1.06±0.24	1.15±0.21**(l)
EGF-R							
Cytoplasmic	1.78±0.14	1.21±0.12	1.56±0.20	1.87±0.14*(l)	1.47±0.10	1.67±0.20	1.76±0.18
Membrane	NM	1.25±0.14	NM	1.86±0.27*(l)	NM	1.27±0.22	1.58±0.17**(l)
TGF-α	1.22±0.15	0.97±0.10	1.21±0.34	1.30±0.28*(l)	1.66±0.27	1.93±0.23*(l)	1.54±0.20**(l)
TAG-72	0.01±0.01	0.13±0.06	0.10±0.06	1.06±0.27*(l)	0.02±0.02	1.20±0.28	2.38±0.23***(l)
FASE	0.10±0.04	0.62±0.11	0.16±0.09	1.01±0.26	0.11±0.08	1.03±0.27	1.13±0.14*(l)
Lewis Y	0.61±0.35	0.21±0.05	0.58±0.29	0.68±0.14*(l)	0.08±0.05	0.44±0.11	0.71±0.22
p53	0	0	0	0	0	0	0

NM = Not measured. * $p < 0.05$ compared to uninvolved glandular epithelium (b = basal; l = luminal).
** $p < 0.01$ compared to uninvolved glandular epithelium (b = basal; l = luminal).
*** $p < 0.005$ compared to uninvolved glandular epithelium (b = basal; l = luminal).

0.002), while the mean erbB-2 expression was 1.35 in prostate cancer (p = 0.0007, uninvolved vs. prostate cancer). A similar pattern of increased biomarker expression between uninvolved and PIN or prostate cancer tissues was observed for EGF-R (mean 1.21, 1.87 and 1.76 for uninvolved, PIN and prostate cancer, respectively) and erbB-3 (mean 0.81, 1.59 and 1.30 for uninvolved, PIN and prostate cancer, respectively). None of the 25 cases that were evaluated had observable nuclear accumulation of p53 either in uninvolved glandular epithelium, in PIN or in adenocarcinoma. Thus, p53 was not an informative biomarker in these studies. In these studies, we also observed essentially no expression of TAG-72 or FASE in the basal or luminal cells of uninvolved prostatic epithelium; however, both TAG-72 and FASE were expressed in PIN and in adenocarcinoma. A pattern of differential phenotypic expression of TGF-α, PCNA and Lewis Y was also observed in this study.

Biopsy Effect

Our results indicate that following multiple sextant biopsies (n = 6) of the prostate, there is a generalized activation of the prostatic epithelium. This can be observed in the placebo group in which indices of proliferation (PCNA) increase significantly (fig. 1, 2) as well as biomarkers such as TGF-α and EGF-R for which one would expect a correlation with increased stimulation toward proliferation of the various epithelial compartments (table 4). The results of the pre- and postbiopsies in the placebo group indicate that in this study most biomarkers were affected by the original diagnostic biopsies. In the placebo group, statistically significant increases were noted in the normal uninvolved tissue for erbB-2 and TGF-α, and a trend for increased postbiopsy for PCNA and erbB-3 (not statistically significant).

Fig. 1. The change from pretherapy to posttherapy in the basal and luminal cells of uninvolved prostate glands in patients receiving 4-HPR.

Fig. 2. The change from pretherapy to posttherapy in the basal and luminal cells of uninvolved prostate glands in patients receiving placebo. This result together with figure 1 indicates an activation of the cells of uninvolved glands between the beginning and end of the study period. The prevalues circled are from patients who had a biopsy of the prostate before they had the pretherapy biopsy.

Table 4. Effect of biopsy on PCNA in epithelial compartments

PCNA	Placebo group	4HPR Rx group	P (placebo vs. 4HPR)
Uninvolved – basal			
Pretherapy	3.61±2.16	2.47±1.59	0.49
Posttherapy	13.80±4.55	16.57±4.89	0.888
Δ (post-pre)	10.19±5.29	14.34±5.43	0.925
p for Δ	p = 0.156	p = 0.012	
Uninvolved – luminal			
Pretherapy	3.71±3.00	2.12±1.70	0.970
Posttherapy	8.10±2.78	8.57±3.55	0.977
Δ (post-pre)	4.39±4.59	7.7±3.58	0.900
p for Δ	p = 0.281	p = 0.039	
Low-grade PIN – luminal[1]			
Pretherapy	0.05±0.05	0.06±0.06	
Posttherapy	34.0±11.37	12.62±6.09	
Δ (post-pre)	30.95±19.05	13.14±9.65	
High-grade PIN – luminal[1]			
Pretherapy	0±0	9.0±5.69	
Posttherapy	15.5±14.5	25.67±7.22	
Δ (post-pre)	15.5±14.5	16.67±2.85	
Adenocarcinoma			
Pretherapy	7.2±3.67	6.29±5.26	0.487
Posttherapy	13.31±5.57	15.32±6.06	0.933
Δ (post-pre)	10.1±4.68	11.13±5.47	0.935
p for Δ	p = 0.125	p = 0.094	

[1] No comparisons were made due to small samples in the PIN tissue.

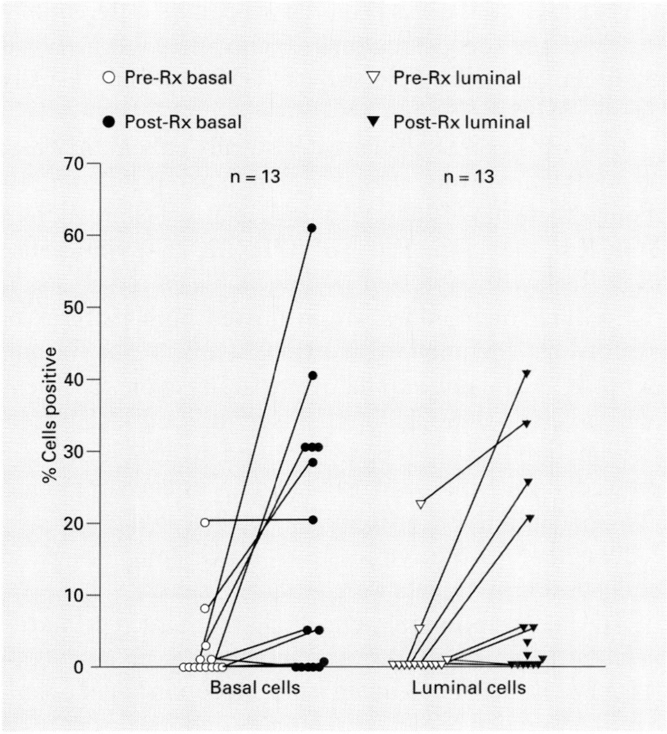

1

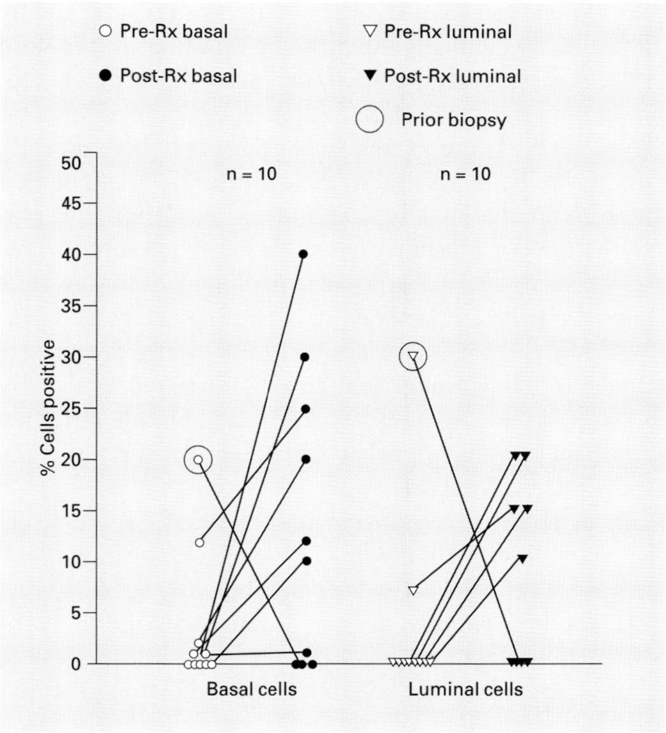

2

In one case the biomarkers were noted to decrease. The same pattern of response were noted in the group treated by 4-HPR with statistically significant increases in PCNA, erbB-2, EGF-R, erbB-3 and TGF-α. The same increasing trend was observed in tumor and PIN tissues, but none achieved statistical significance due to small number of informative cases available for these samples. When the change in the placebo group was compared with the change in the 4-HPR treated group, no statistical differences in any biomarker in any epithelial compartment was identified.

As an example, consider the changes in PCNA, membrane or cytoplasmic expression of EGF-R and expression of TGF-α in the various epithelial compartments. An increase in PCNA would be correlated with an increase in proliferative activity of cells of the epithelial compartment evaluated. Similarly, an increase in the membrane or cytoplasmic expression of EGF-R might indicate the potential for an increased signal from EGF-Rs and increased phenotypic expression of TGF-α could correlate with the potential for the ligand, TGF-α, to react with its receptor, EGF-R ($p > 0.05$).

Discussion

A number of concurrent factors had a significant impact on patient accrual and acceptance of this chemoprevention presurgical study. Patient accrual was greatly impacted by changing the protocol duration from 6–8 to 3 weeks presurgical therapy. There were other factors that could not be controlled that impacted on number of eligible patients. These factors were relevant to how prostate cancer was being treated in the community and included the use of neoadjuvant total androgen ablation and brachytherapy for prostate cancer. Neoadjuvant total androgen ablation became a popular presurgical therapy after being reported by Soloway in 1996. Prostate cancer brachytherapy, a treatment modality for localized prostatic cancer utilizing implanted iodine-125, was reported on by Blasco in 1996 and quickly became a popular alternative to radical prostatectomy because of its comparable results and limited side effects.

The majority of patients participating in this study were compliant with the daily dose of two capsules taken before breakfast. The toxicity attributed to 4-HPR (dryness, soreness and bad taste in mouth) occurred in 5% of patients, was mild to moderate in grade and reversible upon discontinuation of the study medication. The patients were willing to continue the study medication beyond surgery, however, this was not done. Our experience would support a longer treatment phase in patients if the timing for prostate cancer treatment allowed for a longer time interval between diagnosis and definitive therapy such as brachytherapy.

Following the biopsy of any tissue, an inflammatory reparative change occurs in the vicinity of the site of the biopsy. The time and area involved in the completion of the reparative process is likely to be variable, including variable responses secondary to the specific type of tissue, size of the biopsied area, the location of the biopsy within the specific organ, and specific characteristics of the patient (i.e., how rapidly the patient heals). Similarly the direction and magnitude of the change in specific antigens expressed by uninvolved or neoplastic epithelial cells within the area affected by the biopsy initially cannot be predicted and may be equally variable as are the time and area of the inflammatory response to the biopsy. In addition, systemic stresses associated with the diagnosis of prostate cancer may affect various tissues as could the agent used as the placebo.

PCNA was chosen as an index of proliferation because uninvolved prostatic epithelium, PIN and prostatic adenocarcinomas characteristically have relatively low rates of proliferation [19–21]. Thus, PCNA is preferable to Ki-67/MIB-1 because the expression of Ki-67/MIB-1 is likely to be less than 1% in epithelial compartments of the prostate. For studies involving the prostate, TGF-α was chosen because TGF-α has been reported to be differentially expressed in adenocarcinomas compared to uninvolved glandular epithelium in which TGF-α is not usually expressed [22–25].

EGF-R is expressed characteristically only in the basal cells of uninvolved prostatic glandular epithelium, although there may be lateral and basolateral expression of EGF-R in the luminal cells of BPH [22, 26–29]. Because EGF-R may be expressed in the cytoplasm as well as on the cellular membranes, we evaluated both patterns of expression. The phenotypic expression of $p185^{erbB-2}$ and of $p180^{erbB-3}$ are limited characteristically to the basal cells of uninvolved glandular epithelium with minimal expression in luminal cells; $p185^{erbB-2}$ and $p180^{erbB-3}$ are expressed differentially in PIN and in adenocarcinomas [29–35]. Both these antigens may be detected at the subcellular level in the cytoplasm or on cell membranes so both subcompartments were evaluated separately.

The nuclear accumulation of p53 is observed primarily in late stage prostatic adenocarcinomas (i.e., about 50% of stage IV lesions), but a much smaller proportion of organ-confined prostatic adenocarcinomas and low proportion of cases of PIN [36–42] typically show nuclear accumulation of p53. TAG-72 is an oncofetal tumor biomarker which has not been observed in either the basal or luminal cells of uninvolved prostatic glandular epithelium; however, it is observed in benign glands in the setting of prostatitis as well as in neoplastic lesions (e.g., PIN or adenocarcinoma). Expression of TAG-72 is increased in low-grade PIN, in high-grade PIN and in adenocarcinomas [43–46]. FASE is similar to TAG-72 in that it usually is not expressed in the basal or luminal cells of uninvolved prostatic glandular epithelium [16, 47]. Our results [16] and those of others have found that FASE shows increased phenotypic expression in PIN [48], and in prostatic adenocarcinomas [49]. Lewis Y, as recognized by the antibody BR96, usually is not expressed in the luminal cells of uninvolved prostatic epithelium but Lewis Y frequently is expressed strongly in a proportion of basal cells. There also is phenotypic expression in basal cells or in luminal cells of low-grade PIN and of high-grade PIN or in prostatic adenocarcinoma [25].

Because there was increased expression of specific biomarkers in the placebo group for which high expression would be expected to correlate with tumor aggressiveness (e.g., PCNA, TGF-α), no change in the 4-HPR-treated group suggests that the dosage of 4-HPR was ineffective as a chemopreventive agent. This is demonstrated by increases in PCNA in the placebo and 4-HPR groups in table 3.

Because multiple sextant biopsies stimulated the proliferation of both benign and neoplastic epithelium of the prostate, one would expect that an effective dose of a chemopreventive agent would decrease such a stimulatory signal. It is possible that this type of stimulus to epithelial growth might not be affected by a specific dose of 4-HPR even though a stimulus related to neoplastic growth would be decreased by this same dose of 4-HPR. However, this is unlikely and such differences in responses are unlikely to be detected by protocols similar to that used in this study.

Our finding that the dose of 4-HPR used in this study was ineffective is consistent with our in vitro studies of the effect of 4-HPR on three cell lines of prostate cancer, i.e., LNCaP, DU145, and PC-3 [50]. Only a high dose of 4-HPR (10^{-6} M or approximately 400 ng/ml), consistently reduced the growth of the three cell lines. A concentration of 10^{-7} M did however exert a small inhibitory effect on the growth of the DU145 cell line after 3–7 days of exposure. These in vitro studies are consistent with previous studies which have demonstrated that concentrations of 10^{-6}–10^{-5} M 4-HPR typically are required to inhibit the growth of prostate cancer cells in vitro [51, 52]. Thus, based on the inability of this dose of 4-HPR to modulate the phenotypic expression of multiple selected biomarkers in any of the epithelial compartments evaluated, we conclude that the dose of 200 mg of 4-HPR a day for 3 weeks is ineffective for chemoprevention. Future clinical trials of 4-HPR in patients with early prostate cancer should consider using higher doses or 4-HPR in combination with other agents which may be given intermittently so as to increase efficacy and minimize toxicity.

Acknowledgments

This study was funded by an NCI Chemoprevention Contract (N01CN35577-01) to the University of Alabama at Birmingham Comprehensive Cancer Center. The affiliated study sites at Norwood Clinic, Urology Associates and Veterans Administration are acknowledged for patient accural and follow-up.

References

1 Parker SL, Tong T, Bolden S, Wingo PA: Cancer statistics, 1996. CA Cancer J Clin 1996;65: 5–27.
2 Kelloff GJ, Crowell JA, Boone CW et al: Strategy and planning for chemopreventive drug development: Clinical development plans. J Cell Biochem 1994;20:55–62.
3 Goodman DS: Overview of current knowledge of metabolism of vitamin A and carotenoids. J Natl Cancer Inst 1984;73:1375–1379.
4 Moon RC, McCormick DL, Mehta RG: Inhibition of carcinogenesis by retinoids. Cancer Res 1983;43:2469–2475.
5 Thompson HJ, Herbst EJ, Meeker LD: Chemoprevention of mammary carcinogenesis: A comparative review of the efficacy of a polyamine antimetabolite, retinoids and selenium. J Natl Cancer Inst 1986;77:595–598.
6 Investigator's Brochure: Fenretinide. Springhouse, Pa., RW Johnson Pharmaceutical Research Institute, 1990.
7 Modiano MR, Dalton WS, Lippman SM, Joffe L, Booth AR, Meyskens FL: Ocular toxic effect of fenretinide. J Natl Cancer Inst 1990;82: 1063.
8 Kelloff GJ, Boone CW, Steele VE et al: Mechanistic considerations in chemopreventive drug development. J Cell Biochem 1994; 20(suppl G):1–24.
9 Goodman GE: The clinical evaluation of cancer chemoprevention agents: Defining and contrasting phase I, II and III objectives. Cancer Res 1992;52:2752S–2757S.
10 Freedman LS, Schatkin A, Shiffman MH: Statistical validation of intermediate markers of precancer for use as endpoints in chemoprevention trials. J Cell Biochem 1992;16(suppl G):27–32.
11 Kelloff GJ, Boone CW, Steel VE, et al: Progress in cancer chemoprevention: Perspectives on agent selection and short-term clinical intervention trials. Cancer Res 1994;54(suppl): 2015S–2024S.

12 Kelloff GJ, Lieberman R, Brawer MK, Crawford ED, Labrie F, Miller G: Strategies for chemoprevention of prostate cancer. Prostate Cancer Prostate Dis 1998;5:1–7.

13 Schatzkin A, Freedman LS, Dorgan J et al: Surrogate end points in cancer research: A critique. Cancer Epidemiol Biomarkers Prev 1996;5:947–953.

14 Lieberman R, Crowell JA, Hawk ET, Boone CW, Segman C, Kelloff GJ: Development of new cancer chemoprevention agents: Role of pharmacokinetic/pharmacodynamic and intermediate endpoint biomarker monitoring. Clin Chem 1998;44:420–427.

15 Cronin KA, Lieberman R, Freedman LS, Weiss H, Beenken SW, Kelloff GJ: Bayesian sequential analysis of intermediate endpoints in cancer prevention trials. Proc Am Assoc Cancer Res 1998;39:642.

16 Myers RB, Grizzle WE: Biomarker expression in prostatic intraepithelial neoplasia. Eur Urol 1996;30:153–166.

17 Grubbs C, Eto I, Juliana M, Hardin J, Whitaker L: Effect of retinyl acetate and 4-hydroxyphenylretinamide on initiation of chemically-induced mammary tumors. Anticancer Res 1990;10:661–666.

18 Synchron LX Systems Chemistry Information Manual, Beckman Instruments, Fullerton, Calif., 1997.

19 Montironi R, Galluzzi CM, Diamanti L, Giannulis I, Pisani E, Scarpelli M: Prostatic intraepithelial neoplasia. Expression and localization of proliferating cell nuclear antigen in epithelial, endothelial and stromal nuclei. Virchows Arch A 1993;422:185–192.

20 McNeal JE, Haillot O, Yemoto C: Cell proliferation in dysplasia of the prostate: Analysis by PCNA immunostaining. Prostate 1995;27:258–268.

21 Bonkhoff H, Stein U, Remberger K: The proliferative function of basal cells in the normal and hyperplastic human prostate. Prostate 1994;24:114–118.

22 Myers RB, Kudlow JE, Grizzle WE: Expression of transforming growth factor alpha, epidermal growth factor and the epidermal growth factor receptor in benign prostatic hyperplasia and adenocarcinoma of the prostate. Mod Pathol 1993;6:733–737.

23 Harper ME, Goddard E, Glyne-Jones E, Wilson DW, Price-Thomas M, Peeling WB, Friffiths K: An immunocytochemical analysis of TGF-α expression in benign and malignant prostatic tumors. Prostate 1993;23:9–23.

24 Scher HI, Sarkis A, Reuter V, Cohen D, Netto G, Petrylak D, Lianes P, Fuks Z, Mendelsohn J, Cordon-Cardo C: Changing pattern of expression of the epidermal growth factor receptor and transforming growth factor-α in the progression of prostatic neoplasms. Clin Cancer Res 1995;1:545–550.

25 Myers RB, Lampejo O, Herrera GA, Srivastava S, Oelschlager D, Brown DA, Waterbor JW, Grizzle WE: TGF-α expression is a relatively late event in the progression of prostatic adenocarcinoma. J Urol Pathol 1995;3:195–203.

26 Maygarden SJ, Strom S, Ware JL: Localization of epidermal growth factor receptor by immunohistochemical methods in human prostatic carcinoma, prostatic intraepithelial neoplasia, and benign hyperplasia. Arch Pathol Lab Med 1992;166:269–273.

27 Ibrahim GK, Kems BM, MacDonald JA, Ibrahim SN, Kinney RB, Humphrey PA, Robertson CN: Differential immunoreactivity of epidermal growth factor receptor in benign, dysplastic and malignant prostatic tissues. J Urol 1993;149:170–173.

28 Maygarden SJ, Novotny DB, Moul JW, Bae VL, Ware JL: Evaluation of cathepsin D and epidermal growth factor receptor in prostate carcinoma. Mod Pathol 1994;7:930–936.

29 Mellon K, Thompson S, Charton RG, Marsh C, Robinson M, Lane DP, Harris AL, Wilson-Horne CH, Neal DE: p53, c-erbB-2 and the epidermal growth factor receptor in the benign and malignant prostate. J Urol 1992;147:496–499.

30 Veltri RW, Partin AW, Epstein JE, Marley GM, Miller GM, Singer DS, Patton KP, Criley SR, Coffey DS: Quantitative nuclear morphometry, markovian texture descriptors and DNA content captured on a CAS-200 image analysis system, combined with PCNA and HER-2-neu immunohistochemistry. J Cell Biochem Suppl 1994;19:249–253.

31 Kuhn EJ, Kurnot RA, Sesterhenn IA, Chang EH, Moul JW: Expression of the c-erbB-2 (HER-2/neu) oncoprotein in human prostatic adenocarcinoma. J Urol 1993;150:1427–1433.

32 Ware JL, Maygarden SJ, Koontz WW, Strom SC: Immunohistochemical detection of c-erbB-2 protein in human benign and neoplastic prostate. Hum Pathol 1991;22:254–258.

33 Sadasivan R, Morgan R, Jennings S, Austenfeld M, Van Veldhuizen P, Stephens R, Noble M: Overexpression of HER-2/neu may be an indicator of poor prognosis in prostate cancer. J Urol 1993;150:126–131.

34 Giri DK, Wadhwa SN, Upadhaya SN, Talwar GP: Expression of neu/HER-2 oncoprotein ($p185^{neu}$) in prostate tumors: An immunohistochemical study. Prostate 1994;23:329–336.

35 Myers RB, Srivastava S, Oelschlager DK, Grizzle WE: Expression of $p160^{erbB-3}$ and $p185^{erbB-2}$ in prostatic intraepithelial neoplasia and prostatic adenocarcinoma. J Natl Cancer Inst 1994;86:1140–1145.

36 Visakorpi T, Kallioniemi OP, Heikkinen A, Koivula T, Iosala J: Small subgroup of aggressive, highly proliferative prostatic carcinomas defined by p53 accumulation. J Natl Cancer Inst 1992;84:883–887.

37 Bookstein R, MacGrogan D, Hilsenbeck SG, Sharkey F, Allred DG: p53 is mutated in a subset of advanced-stage prostate cancers. Cancer Res 1993;53:3369–3373.

38 Henke RP, Kruger E, Ayhan N, Hubner D, Hammcrer P, Huland H: Immunohistochemical detection of p53 protein in human prostatic cancer. J Urol 1994;152:1297–1301.

39 Myers RB, Oelschlager D, Srivastava S, Grizzle WE: Accumulation of the p53 protein occurs more frequently in metastatic than in localized prostatic adenocarcinomas. Prostate 1994;25:243–248.

40 Navone NM, Troncoso P, Pisters LL, Goodrow TL, Palmer JL, Nichols WW, Von Eschenbach AC, Conti CJ: p53 protein accumulation and gene mutation in the progression of human prostate carcinoma. J Natl Cancer Inst 1993;85:1657–1669.

41 Hughes JH, Cohen MB, Robinson RA: p53 immunoreactivity in primary and metastatic prostatic adenocarcinoma. Mod Pathol 1995;8:462–466.

42 Heidenberg HB, Sesterhenn IA, Gaddipati JP, Weghorst CM, Buzard GS, Moul JW, Srivastava S: Alteration of the tumor suppressor gene p53 in a high fraction of hormone refractory prostate cancer. J Urol 1995;154:414–421.

43 Myers RB, Meredith RF, Schlom J, LoBuglio AF, Bueschen AJ, Wheeler RH, Stockard CR, Grizzle WE: Tumor-associated glycoprotein-72 is highly expressed in prostatic adenocarcinomas. J Urol 1994;152:243–246.

44 Myers RB, Schlom J, Srivastava S, Grizzle WE: Expression of tumor-associated glycoprotein-72 in prostatic intraepithelial neoplasia and prostatic adenocarcinoma. Mod Pathol 1995;8:260–265.

45 Brenner PC, Rettig WJ, Sanz-Moncasi MP, Reuter V, Aprikian A, Old LJ, Fair WR, Garin-Chesa P: TAG-72 expression in primary, metastatic and hormonally treated prostate cancer as defined by monoclonal antibody CC49. J Urol 1995;153:1575–1579.

46 Mazur MT, Schultz JJ: Prostatic adenocarcinoma: Evaluation of immunoreactivity to monoclonal antibody B72.3. Am J Clin Pathol 1990;93:466–471.

47 Shurbaji MS, Kuhajda FP, Pasternack GR, Thurmond TS: Expression of oncogenic antigen 519 (OA-519) in prostate cancer is a potential prognostic indicator. Am J Clin Pathol 1992;97:686–691.

48 Epstein JI, Carmichael M, Partin AW: OA-519 (fatty acid synthase) as an independent predictor of pathologic stage in adenocarcinoma of the prostate. Urology 1995;45:81–86.

49 Myers RB, Srivastivea S, Grizzle WE: Lewis Y antigen as detected by the monoclonal antibody BR96 is expressed srongly in prostatic adenocarcinoma. J Urol 1995;153:1572–1574.

50 Myers RB, Lieberman R, Kelloff GJ, Grizzle WE: Effects of chemopreventive agents on the growth of prostatic adenocarcinoma cell lines in vitro. Proc Am Assoc Cancer Res 1998;39:193.

51 Hsieh TC, Ng C, Wu JM: The synthetic retinoid N-(-hydroxyphenyl)retinamide (4-HPR) exerts antiproliferative and apoptosis inducing effects in H. androgen-independent human prostatic JCA-1 cells. Biochem Mol Biol Int 1995;37:499–506.

52 Igawa M, Tanabe T, Chodak GW, Rukstalis DB: N-(4-hydroxyphenyl)retinamide induces cell cycle specific growth inhibition in PC3 cells. Prostate 1994;24:299–305.

Molecular Targets for Chemoprevention of Prostate Cancer

European Urology

Eur Urol 1999;35:439–442

Factors Controlling the Expression of 5α-Reductase in Human Prostate: A Possible New Approach for the Treatment of Prostate Cancer

Fouad K. Habib Margaret Ross Colin W. Bayne

Prostate Research Group, Department of Oncology, University of Edinburgh, Western General Hospital, Edinburgh, UK

Key Words

5 alpha-reductase isoenzymes · Paracrine control · CaP · BPH · mRNA expression

Abstract

The functional activity of the 5α-reductase isoenzyme in the human prostate is gradually depleted as the gland undergoes transformation from the normal to the metastatic state. There are two isoforms of this enzyme expressed in the prostate and recent studies have demonstrated that the type II isoenzyme is the one most affected by the onset of neoplasia. To elucidate the mechanism(s) responsible for the down-regulation of the isoenzyme activity, we re-examined the nature of the interaction between stroma and epithelial cells in the human prostate. We noted that the control of the isoenzyme expression in the epithelial cells was regulated by a paracrine factor specific to the prostate fibroblast. In the absence of this factor the human prostate loses its capacity to express the 5α-reductase type II isoenzyme – a characteristic manifested simultaneously with the loss of differentiation in the tissues. This finding presents a totally new concept to the control of 5α-reductase in the human prostate and offers a possibility for an interesting and alternative approach to the management of prostate cancer.

Introduction

Research on the prostate and other male accessory sexual organs is producing new insights into the regulatory mechanisms responsible for the normal and abnormal growth of the prostate. This chapter will review the physico-chemical characteristics of testosterone 5α-reductase and attempt to identify the mechanism(s) regulating 5α-reductase gene expression in the human prostate. In rat, prostate dihydrotestosterone (DHT) induces expression of its own steroid 5α-reductase which is secondary to enhancement of 5α-reductase messenger RNA levels [1]. This in turn increases DHT synthesis thereby triggering a positive developmental cascade resulting in a feed-forward control of prostatic growth. Until recently it was thought that a similar mechanism might regulate the 5α-reductase activity in the human prostate but studies from this group have now demonstrated that the mRNA expression of this enzyme is under paracrine control with factors specifically associated with the prostate regulating the enzyme activity.

KARGER

Fax + 41 61 306 12 34
E-Mail karger@karger.ch
www.karger.com

0302–2838/99/0356–0439$17.50/0

Accessible online at:
http://BioMedNet.com/karger

Dr. Fouad K. Habib
Prostate Research Group, Department of Oncology
University of Edinburgh, Western General Hospital
Edinburgh EH4 2XU (UK)
Tel. +44 131 537 1568, Fax +44 131 343 6529, E-Mail fkh@srv0.med.ed.ac.uk

Table 1. Summary of clinical and biochemical parameters for CaP patients receiving endocrine therapy

Patient	Treatment	Gleason score	5α-Reductase activity[1]	Response
1	Cyproterone	4+3	54.1	Good
2	Stilboestrol	5+4	2.1	Good
3	Stilboestrol	3+2	33.1	Good
4	Cyproterone	3+3	32.5	Good
5	Cyproterone	2+3	66.2	Good
6	SCO	3+4	4.5	Partial response then
7	Cyproterone	3+2	14.5	progression
8	Cyproterone	5+4	2.5	Poor
9	Dinoerstrol	5+4	2.5	Poor
10	Cyproterone	4+3	6.1	Poor
11	Cyproterone	4+5	7.4	Poor
12	SCO	3+2	34.0	Stable
13	SCO	3+4	29.5	Stable
14	SCO	1+2	38.5	Stable

[1] 5α-Reductase activity in pmol/mg protein/30 min.

5α-Reductase in Benign Prostatic Hyperplasia and Prostate Cancer

In an earlier study incorporating 39 prostate cancer (CaP) patients with tumours at different stages of differentiation, an analysis of prostate tissue testosterone 5α-reductase activity was carried out [2]. The measurements were compared to values obtained from an age-matched group of patients with benign prostatic hyperplasia (BPH). The data demonstrated significant differences in the enzyme activity for both tissue types with the mean values of the CaP group being markedly depleted when compared to the hyperplastic specimens ($p < 0.005$). Furthermore, following the classification of the tumours according to their histological grade, we noted that there was a diminished propensity by testosterone to metabolize to its 5α-reduced metabolites as the tumour progressively became less differentiated. In those studies the Gleason grading system was employed as an index of the degree of differentiation.

Attempts were also made to relate the 5α-reductase activity to tumour bulk using the TNM system but the findings suggested that the staging of the disease bears no relationship to the capacity of the tissue to metabolize testosterone. The 5α-reductase activity of the gland was therefore perceived as being purely a function of tumour differentiation and as such it may be that the measurement of enzyme activities in tumours could be used as a further confirmatory evidence for the histopathological grading of CaP.

Is the 5α-Reductase a Marker for Hormone Sensitivity

In view of the reported association between the 5α-reductase activity and the differentiation of the tumour, we explored the possibility that the androgen-metabolizing enzyme might be more closely involved with the mechanism(s) controlling the hormone sensitivity of the gland: It is conceivable that specimens with a reduced or absent enzyme activity might become androgen insensitive and would therefore not respond to endocrine manipulation. This hypothesis was put to the test in a retrospective study involving 35 patients with CaP who had been receiving endocrine therapy at the Western General Hospital in Edinburgh over the previous 52 months. Prostate tissues removed from those patients, prior to the treatment, were analyzed for a number of biochemical parameters, histologically assessed and graded. Clinical response to endocrine therapy and relapse were assessed by urologists who were unaware of the results of the 5α-reductase assay.

Interestingly when 5α-reductase activity was correlated to the response to endocrine therapy, the results revealed a close association between the two parameters: Patients with a low enzyme activity were poor responders whereas those exhibiting high androgen metabolic activity showed, on the whole, good response (table 1). Clearly this preliminary study needs to be expanded further to confirm the initial findings and a larger population will have to be entered. Additionally the criteria for segregation of patients might benefit from some refining and survival patterns will have to be considered in any future study. Nonetheless, the present investigation underlines the importance of 5α-reductase not only as a biochemical marker for tumour differentiation but also as a potential prognostic aid in the management of CaP.

Distribution of 5α-Reductase Isoenzymes

The observations described above are providing new evidence to support the existence of a biological basis for the endocrine treatment of CaP. However, this needs to be established on a firm and sound scientific footing to produce significant improvement in patient response. Furthermore, there is the added problem of identifying the molecular events leading to the loss of 5α-reductase activity as the tumour becomes less differentiated. New developments on the cloning and sequencing fronts revealed the presence of two separate genes encoding two steroid 5α-reductase isoenzymes with 50% sequence homology designated type I and type II [3, 4]. The type I enzyme (5αR-I), which maps chromosome 5, has a neutral basic pH optimum and is expressed in large amounts in peripheral tissues such as skin and liver. The type II enzyme (5αR-II) on the other hand, is located on chromosome 2, has an acidic pH optimum and is predominantly associated with the prostate. Unlike type I, 5α-reductase type II is mutated in male pseudohermaphroditism [5] and may therefore be central to the normal development of the prostate. Until recently it was believed that the type II isoenzyme was the only one associated with the prostate, but recent work from this laboratory has conclusively demonstrated mRNA encoding activity for both the 5αR-I and 5αR-II isoenzymes in human prostate tissue [6]. Employing RT-PCR with specific primers to the type I and type II isoenzymes it has been possible to identify mRNA transcripts for both isoenzymes in most tissues analysed. This data was subsequently confirmed by in situ hybridization establishing the distribution of the isoenzymes in both the epithelial as well as in the stroma fibroblast components of the prostate. The isoenzymes are functionally active with the 5αR-II exhibiting approximately 3 times as much activity as that measured for the 5αR-I. However, the activity of 5αR-I and 5αR-II in fibroblast was variable and patchy with expression present in some areas and absent in others.

The findings on the tissue were supported by supplementary experiments on primary cultures which demonstrated that both the fibroblast and epithelial cells maintained a capacity to express both isoenzymes in vitro [7]. In the case of the fibroblast this capacity was maintained following sequential passaging of the cells up to passage 6 following which the cells no longer expressed either isoenzyme. The loss of expression, once cells are passaged, is in many ways reminiscent of our observations on the loss of 5αR-I and 5αR-II in prostate cancer metastases [paper submitted for publication]. Even though prostate-specific antigen (PSA) and androgen receptors were present in osteoblastic and lymph node metastasis [8], there was no 5αR-I and 5αR-II mRNA expression in cells which had escaped outwith the prostate capsule. The cultured epithelial cells and the metastasizing prostate tumours are essentially cells which have been removed from their natural prostate environment and in the process have lost some of their physico-chemical characteristics. The supplementation of primary grown cell media with DHT failed to restore the 5α-reductase activity to the cells, demonstrating that the down-regulation of 5α-reductase was not in any way linked to androgen starvation but is obviously a by-product of a more fundamental process as of yet unidentified.

Stromal-Epithelial Interactions and Prostate Homeostasis

Preliminary experiments have demonstrated that the restoration of the 5α-reductase activity in the epithelial cells was only possible if these cells were propagated in the proximity of the fibroblast stroma component. To test these observations further we developed a new co-culture model in which the stroma-fibroblast and epithelial characteristics of the in vivo prostate gland were maintained [9]. In this system the two growing populations of stroma-fibroblast and epithelial cells were separated by a microporous membrane to allow communication by means of diffusible factors but without physical contact between the different cell types. This new model exhibited many of the phenotypic characteristics of the prostate including the capacity to express 5α-reductase isoenzymes and androgen receptors by both the stroma and epithelial cells, to respond to androgens and for the epithelial cells to secrete PSA. In addition, morphological studies employing electron microscopy demonstrated that the cells grown in co-culture exhibited round nuclei, tonofibrils and microvilli in epithelial cells and elongated nuclei, large amounts of Golgi apparatus and cilia in the fibroblasts, all indicative of the differentiated state. This system highlights the importance of stroma/epithelial cross-talk towards preserving the phenotypic characteristics of the human prostate.

Paracrine Control of 5α-Reductase in the Epithelial Cells

A significant feature of the co-culture model described in this report is the capacity of both the fibroblast and epithelial cells to express 5α-reductase. This is distinctive from earlier models where 5α-reductase activity was either absent or depleted and no previous systems ever expressed both isoenzymes simultaneously. The properties of the 5α-reductase activity in the co-culture model resemble those which had previously been detected in the human tissue. We have no reason to believe that these are any different, furthermore the model highlights the need for interaction between the stroma and epithelium to induce 5α-reductase mRNA expression. However, we were not too sure whether the induction of the isoenzyme activity in the epithelia is specific to prostate fibroblast or whether the induction could be prompted by fibroblast derived from other sources. To this end, prostate epithelial cells were co-cultured with a variety of fibroblast cells from a number of tissues including breast, skin and testes. Interestingly whilst prostate fibroblast induced 5αR-II expression in the epithelial cells of the co-cultured system, none of the other fibroblast cells triggered this activity suggesting that the effect is specific to the prostate. Additionally since the co-culture model does not permit any contact between the fibroblast and epithelial cells, we believe that the regulatory action is mediated by a soluble factor secreted by the stroma/fibroblast component but which is acting in a paracrine fashion on the epithelial cells. Recent efforts have demonstrated that this factor is a protein of molecular weight in the region of 10 kD. We have, as of yet, not identified the nature of this protein though we know that it is not one of the common growth factors found in the human prostate. We are also in the process of cloning and sequencing the gene and with the help of gene banks identify the exact nature of this putative factor.

Conclusions

The identification of a fibroblastic stroma-derived putative factor triggering the expression of 5αR-II in epithelial cells of the human prostate is a rather exciting development. This opens the way towards understanding some of the mechanism(s) which may be responsible for controlling prostate growth, differentiation and the oncogenic process in the gland. Additionally, the information gleaned from this work might eventually help in the design of new drugs or even gene therapy for the treatment of CaP.

References

1 George FW, Russell DW, Wolfson JD: Feed-forward control of prostate growth: Dihydrotestosterone induces expression of prostate growth: Dihydrotestosterone induces expression of its own biosynthetic enzyme, steroid 5α-reductase. Proc Natl Acad Sci USA 1991;88:8044–8047.

2 Habib FK, Busuttil A, Robinson RA, Chisholm GD: 5α-Reductase activity in human prostate cancer is related to the histological differentiation of the tumour. Clin Endocrinol 1985;23:431–438.

3 Anderson S, Russell DW: Structural and biochemical properties of cloned and expressed human rat steroid 5α-reductases. Proc Natl Acad Sci USA 1990;87:3640–3644.

4 Jenkins EP, Andersson S, Imperato-McGinley J, Wilson JD, Russell DW: Genetic and pharmacological evidence for more than one human steroid 5α-reductase. J Clin Invest 1992;89:293–300.

5 Anderson S, Berman DM, Jenkins EP, Russell DW: Deletion of steroid 5α-reductase 2 gene in male pseudohermaphroditism. Nature 1991;354:159–161.

6 Habib FK, Ross M, Bayne CW, Grigor K, Buck AC, Chapman K: The localisation and expression of 5α-reductase type I and type II mRNA in human hyperplasmid prostate and in prostate primary cultures. J Endocrinol 1998;156:509–517.

7 Bayne CW, Donnelly F, Chapman K, Bollina P, Habib FK: A novel co-culture model for benign prostatic hyperplasia expressing both isoforms of 5α-reductase. J Clin Endocrinol Metab 1998;83:206–213.

8 Hobisch A, Culig Z, Radmayr C, Bartsch G, Klocker H, Hittmair A: Distant metastases from prostatic carcinoma express androgen receptor protein. Cancer Res 1995;55:3068–3072.

9 Bayne CW, Ross M, Donnelly F, Chapman K, Buck C, Bollina P, Habib FK: Selective interactions between prostate fibroblast and epithelial cells in co-culture maintain the BPH phenotype. Urol Int 1998;773:1–7.

Molecular Targets for Chemoprevention of Prostate Cancer

European Urology

Eur Urol 1999;35:443–455

Certain Aspects of Molecular Endocrinology That Relate to the Influence of Dietary Factors on the Pathogenesis of Prostate Cancer

K. Griffiths[a] M.S. Morton[a] L. Denis[b]

[a]Tenovus Cancer Research Centre, University of Wales College of Medicine, Cardiff, UK and
[b]Oncology Centre, Antwerp, Belgium

Key Words
Isoflavonoids · Lignans · Chemoprevention · Intracellular signalling

Abstract
Isoflavonoids, flavonoids and lignans are natural oestrogenic compounds derived from soya, tea, fruits and vegetables and they have been proposed as chemopreventive agents in Asian men, in whom the incidence of prostate cancer is much lower than in men from the West. In addition to their weak oestrogenic activity, oestrogen antagonistic activity has also been described for some of these compounds. Furthermore, the lignan, enterolactone and the soya-derived isoflavone genistein are inhibitors of several steroid metabolising enzymes, such as aromatase, 5α-reductase and 17β-hydroxysteroid dehydrogenase. Genistein is a potent inhibitor of tyrosine kinases and along with flavonoids such as kaempferol and apigenin is also an inhibitor of topoisomerases I and II, enzymes which are crucial to cellular proliferation. Genistein is also an inhibitor of angiogenesis and many experimental in vivo and in vitro models, including those for prostate cancer, are growth inhibited by isoflavonoids, flavonoids and lignans. It is estimated that the traditionally eating Japanese male consumes approximately 20 mg of isoflavones per day, whereas for Western men, the daily consumption would be less than 1 mg/day. This is reflected in a high mean plasma concentration of genistein (180 ng/ml, n = 72) in Japanese men, compared to a level of <10 ng/ml for Western males.

Introduction

In a symposium on the 'Biology of the Prostate and Related Tissues', at the National Cancer Institute in Washington in 1962, Professor Charles Huggins, in his opening remarks [1], talked of the fable of the three blind men who, for the first time, had encountered an elephant. In examining the different parts of the great beast, one was impressed by the tusks, reminiscent of a walrus and another thought the hide was tough like a turtle. A third was taken by the snake-like trunk. The magnificence of the complete entity was not easy to envisage. In like manner, Professor Huggins emphasized ... 'the importance of assembling the bits and pieces of prostatic problems in a unitary concept'. He emphasized the value of interdisciplinary discussion, the importance of bringing advances in science to the bedside and highlighted certain problems recognized at that time (fig. 1), *one of which was the geo-*

KARGER

Fax + 41 61 306 12 34
E-Mail karger@karger.ch
www.karger.com

0302–2838/99/0356–0443$17.50/0

Accessible online at:
http://BioMedNet.com/karger

K. Griffiths, DSc
Tenovus Cancer Research Center, University of Wales College of Medicine
Tenovus Building, Health Park
Cardiff, CF4 4XX (UK)
Tel. +44 1222 74 2579, Fax +44 1222 75 2642

graphical differences in prostatic cancer incidence. Such problems still exercise the minds of today's investigators, but certain bits and pieces are coming together and this text relates to possible reasons for the high prevalence of prostate cancer in the developed countries of the USA and Northern Europe relative to that in the countries of Asia.

It would now be accepted that our knowledge and understanding of the endocrine, biochemical and molecular processes implicated in the pathogenesis of prostatic disease is rapidly growing. Although long recognized that symptomatic clinical benign prostate hyperplasia (BPH) associated with bladder outlet obstruction is not a premalignant condition that leads to the development of prostatic cancer, current attitudes [2] are directed to the possibility that genetic instability associated with epithelial cell hyperplasia of microscopic BPH may develop into transition zone cancer. Prostatic enlargement associated with bladder outlet obstruction is generally considered the consequence of dysfunctional growth regulatory processes [3, 4] within the gland, resulting from an androgen-oestrogen imbalance at mid-life, the resultant oestrogenic stimulus promoting the development of the benign stromal adenoma.

It is also clear from our understanding of the natural history of BPH [4–6] that similar risk factors are associated with the pathogenesis of both BPH and prostatic cancer. Particularly important is the age factor [7], both clinical conditions generally presenting in men beyond 50 years of age and also the fact that neither disease presents in men castrated early in life, suggesting that functional testes, but presumably androgens, are implicated in disease aetiology. Moreover, both conditions clinically respond to androgen ablative therapy. Ethnicity and family history are other risk factors that are also recognized as exercising some influence on prostate cancer and the aetiology of the disease. Also well accepted is that early phases in the pathogenesis of cancer can be identified a number of years prior to the disease being clinically evident (fig. 2). Certain premalignant lesions, prostatic intraepithelial neoplasia (PIN), are recognized as an early stage in the multistep process of carcinogenesis [8], although the evidence that atypical adenomatous hyperplasia (AAH) is such a premalignant lesion remains equivocal [9]. As with cancer of the breast, it may well be that some part of the commonality [10] of cancers of breast and prostate relates to initiation at the time of adolescence, or puberty, when younger people are 'inflicted' with marked hormonal changes that resulted in periods of rapid growth of the breasts and prostate. It is noteworthy, also, that certain 'bothersome' symptoms are now being recognized in men in their 40s [11, 12] and 'histological BPH', epithelial cell hyperplasia and nodular hyperplasia, can be seen in the prostate glands of men in their early 20s [13, 14]. Moreover, these classical studies of Coffey's group emphasized the increasing prevalence of these foci of epithelial hyperplasia with increasing age, *in men from various parts of the world, both East and West.*

The molecular biology associated with these early stages in the development of prostatic disease is of particular interest and was the essential basis of the discussions of a committee of the recent International Consultation on BPH [4]. Its report highlighted the complexity of the processes concerned in the regulation of prostate growth, but a consensus viewpoint was that on the basis of a better understanding of these processes, greater emphasis should now be directed to intervention initiatives possibly related to dietary factors, that could lead to the prevention of prostatic cancer and BPH. Some of these dietary concepts are now considered in relation to molecular endocrinology implicated in the growth regulatory processes of the prostate gland.

Extrinsic and Intrinsic Factors: Steroid Hormones and Growth Regulatory Factors

The prostate is androgen dependent and a source of testosterone is necessary for the growth and function of the gland [15], although it is 5α-dihydrotestosterone (DHT), that as a DHT-androgen receptor (AR) complex, associates with specific hormone response elements (HREs) on the genome [16, 17] to modulate, in association with other transcription factors (TFs), the expression of androgen-responsive genes (fig. 3). DHT is essential for prostate growth [18] and exercises an important role in the regulation of gene activity.

Androgens, however, as well as oestrogens, glucocorticoids and any other 'endocrine related agents' that might for example be made available through the diet or even the environment, are often now referred to as *extrinsic factors* in the regulation of prostate growth [19, 20]. Their biological effects on the gland are seen to be mediated by various peptide growth regulatory factors. *These intrinsic factors*, which are produced by the gland, influence prostatic growth by promoting inter- and intracellular signalling between and within cell populations, through paracrine, autocrine and intracrine effects (fig. 4). It is the biological actions of these intrinsic factors such as *epidermal growth factor (EGF), keratinocyte growth factor (KGF), insulin-like growth factors (IGF-I and -II) and the fibro-*

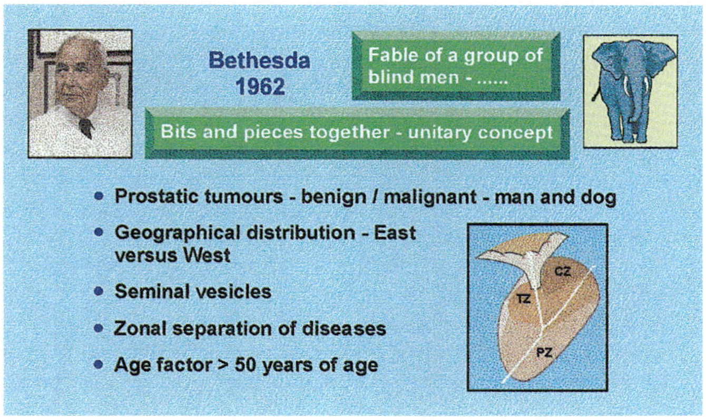

1

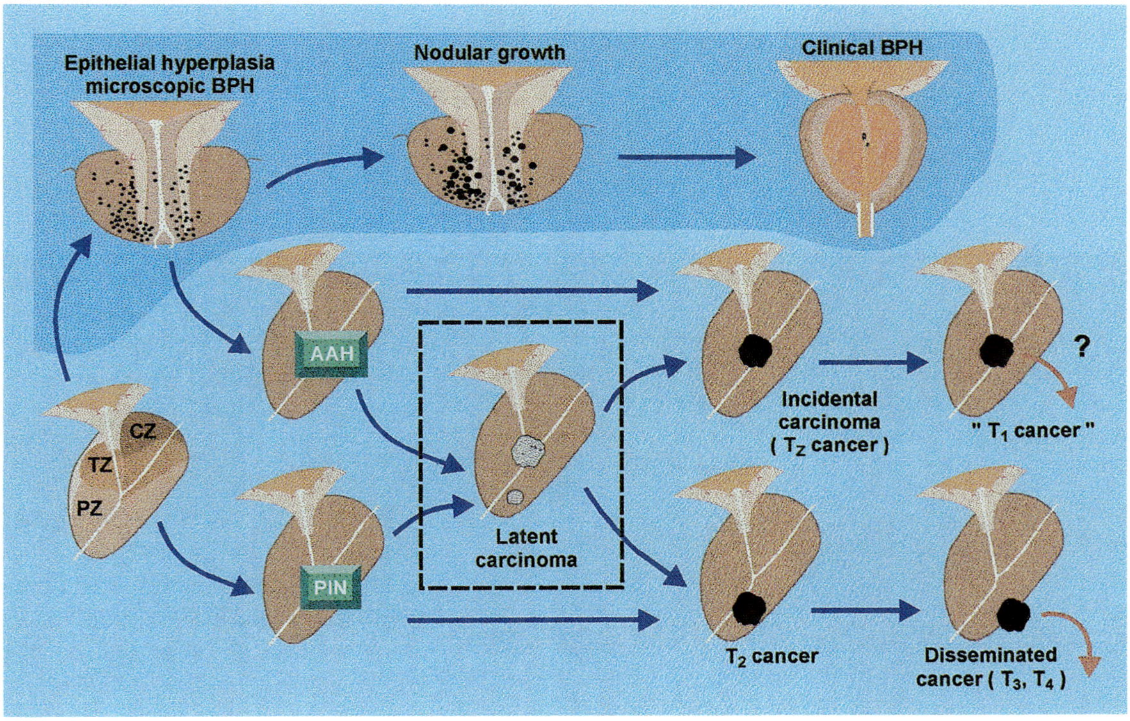

2

Fig. 1. Topics highlighted by Prof. C. Huggins in 1962 that he considered worthy of more investigation.

Fig. 2. The natural history of prostatic disease.

blast growth factors (FGFs), that promote the mitogenic effect and which directly stimulate cell proliferation under the modulating influence of the steroid hormones. The interrelationship, or *crosstalk*, between the signalling pathways influenced by DHT and those regulated by growth stimulatory factors is pivotal to growth regulation in the prostate.

Equally important in growth regulation is the intimate relationship between the stromal and epithelial compartments of the prostate, an interaction recognized many years ago by Franks et al. [21], who reported that the stromal elements influence epithelial cell proliferation. The more recent studies of Cunha et al. [22] have further emphasized the importance of this relationship. Essentially, DHT-mediated effects on the stromal compartment produce growth stimulatory factors, which induce signal transduction pathways within the epithelial cells that promote growth and differentiation (fig. 5).

Interest at present centres on KGF, one of the FGF family (FGF-7) and seen as a particularly important growth-promoting factor within the prostate [23–26]. KGF, produced by the fibroblasts within the stroma, elicits a paracrine mitogenic effect through an FGF receptor (FGF-R) protein located on the epithelial cell membrane. This receptor, FGF-R2-exonIIIb, a splice variant of the FGF-R2 (bek) gene, *specifically recognized KGF* [27].

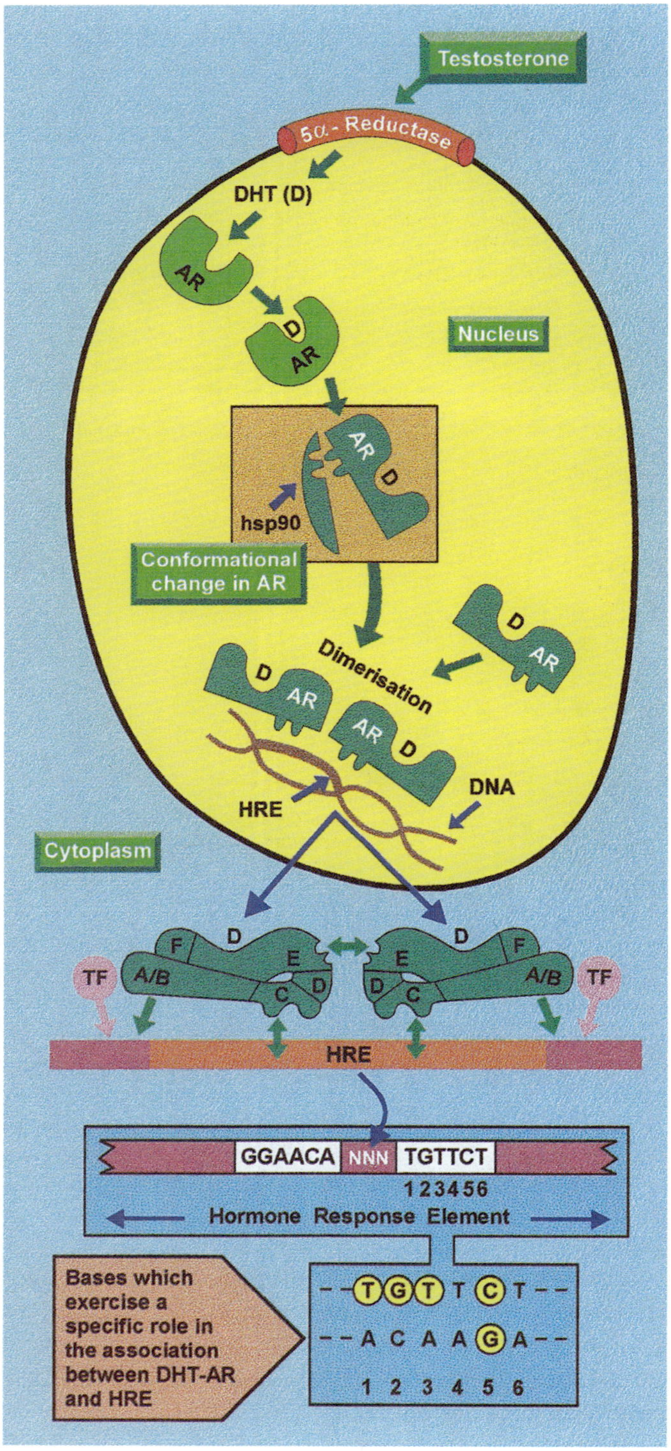

Fig. 3. Formation of the dihydrotestosterone-androgen receptor complex. DHT (D) = Dihydrotestosterone; AR = androgen receptor; HRE = hormone response element; TF = transcription factors.

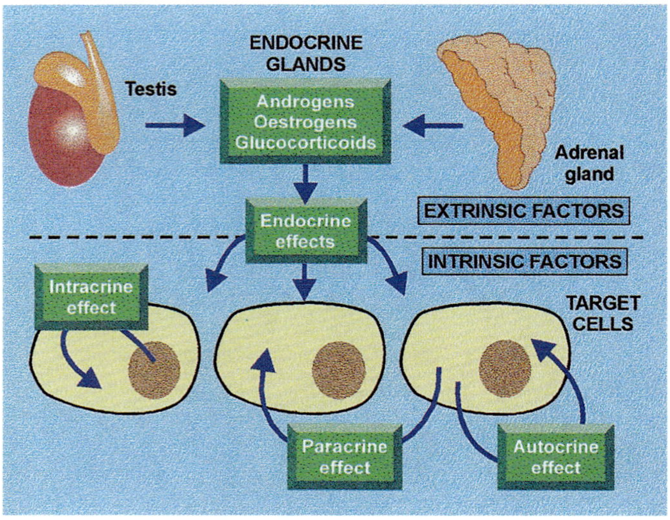

Fig. 4. Extrinsic and intrinsic growth regulatory factors.

Transforming growth factor (TGF)-β, originating in the smooth muscle-like cells of the stroma, inhibits this mitogenic action of KGF on epithelial cell proliferation.

KGF has no effect on the stromal cells, whereas FGF-2 promotes an autocrine mitogenic action, mediated by the receptor FGF-R1, on the stromal elements [28], but it has no effect on epithelial cells. FGF-R1, encoded by the FGF-R1 (flg) gene, is normally localized only in stromal tissue.

The FGF family (FGF-1 to FGF-10) would appear to have a major role in the regulation of prostate growth. The FGFs, as well as other growth stimulatory factors like EGF, associate with high affinity *receptors on the cell membrane, which have a tyrosine-specific protein kinase (TK) as part of the internal domain.* The FGFRs are encoded by four distinct genes, but alternative splicing generates various isoforms which consequently enhances the complexity of ligand-receptor interactions. FGF-8 mRNA was reported to be overexpressed in 71% of 31 human prostate cancers studied [29], has been identified in the androgen independent Du-145 prostate cancer cells [30] and could well be concerned in cancer progression. A change in FGF-R2 expression, FGF-R2exonIIIb to FGF-R2exonIIIc, has been identified [31] in the Dunning prostate tumour of the rat as it progresses to androgen independence. The different FGFs therefore associate with the FGF-Rs with varying affinities, although the precise part these interactions play in the growth regulatory processes, both normal as well as dysfunctional, remains to be determined.

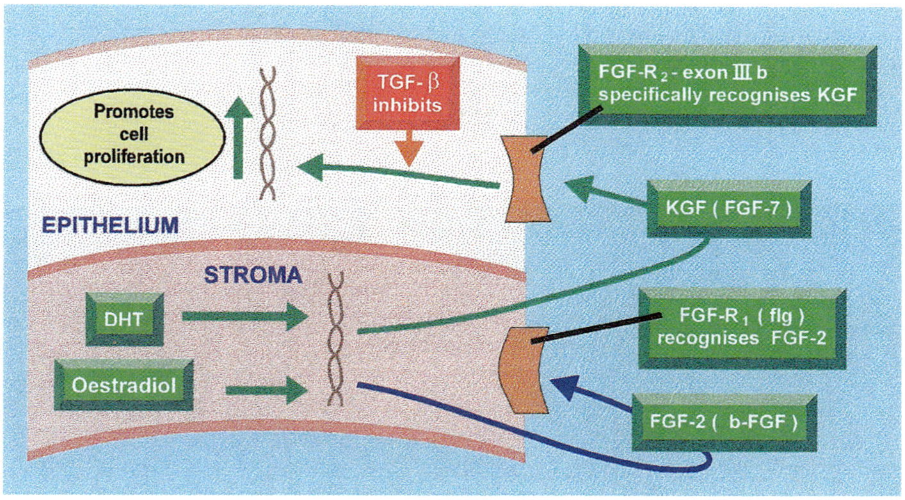

Fig. 5. Relationship between stromal and epithelial compartments of the prostate gland. DHT = Dihydrotestosterone; TGF = transforming growth factor; FGF = fibroblast growth factors; KGF = ketatinocyte growth factor.

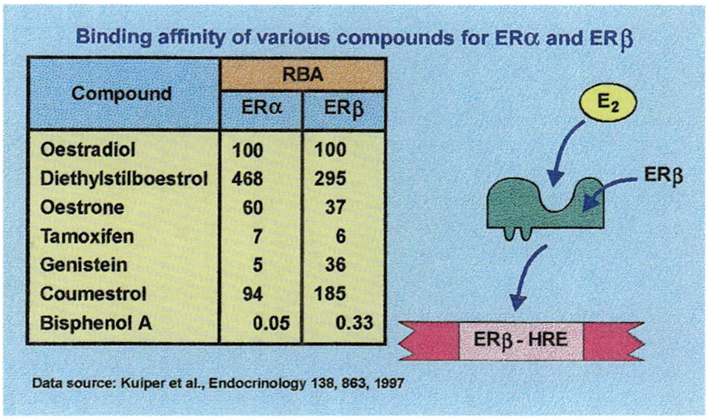

Compound	RBA	
	ERα	ERβ
Oestradiol	100	100
Diethylstilboestrol	468	295
Oestrone	60	37
Tamoxifen	7	6
Genistein	5	36
Coumestrol	94	185
Bisphenol A	0.05	0.33

Fig. 6. The 'new' oestrogen receptor, ERβ.

Oestrogens and the Prostate

Stromal hyperplasia is induced by oestrogens and in relation to this, it has been seen to be relevant that the 'classical' oestrogen receptor-α (ERα) is predominantly localized in the smooth muscle cells of the stroma of the human prostate [32]. This would suggest that oestradiol, as well as DHT, may be synergistically implicated in the production of FGF-2 by stromal cells (fig. 5). Oestrogens are clearly implicated in the growth regulatory mechanisms of the prostate [4], although a precise role remains to be established. Nonetheless, exciting have been recent reports [33, 34] of a complementary DNA clone that encodes a new, distinct oestrogen receptor, referred to as oestrogen receptor β (ERβ). *Especially of interest is that the human and rat ERβ clones were identified within cDNA libraries from human testis and rat prostate.* The ERβ also has a high affinity for oestradiol. The ERα, however, predominates in the female reproductive system, whereas ERβ would appear to be the principal oestrogen receptor component of the prostate, with cell-specific localization to the secretory epithelial cells of the gland [33] and research interest is now directed to the biological role of ERβ relative to that of ERα. Their roles may be quite distinct, complementary or antagonistic and in relation to this, it is reported [35] that certain other oestrogenic compounds preferentially bind to the ERβ (fig. 6).

Although similar amino acid sequences are recognized in both DNA and oestrogen-binding domains of these receptor proteins, suggesting that they would associate with the same recognition sites on the genome, the oestrogen response elements (fig. 7), the N-terminal A/B region and related TAF-1 activation functions are, however, different. Crosstalk (fig. 8) between signalling pathways involving steroid receptor function and those promoted by growth stimulatory factors [4], the synergistic functional interaction between the ERs and other cell specific co-activators and -repressors in juxtaposition on the genome of the prostate cells, could be different for the ERβ relative to ERα [36–40]. The nucleotide recognition se-

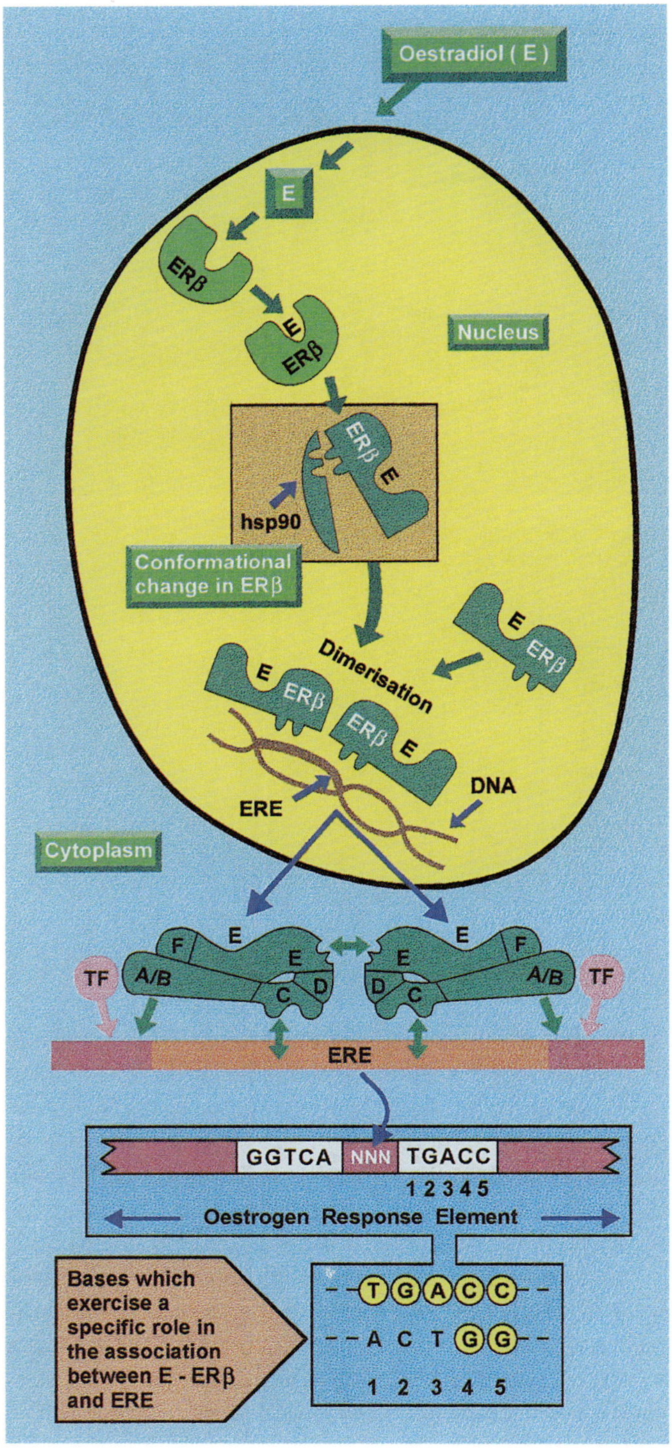

Fig. 7. Diagrammatic illustration of the intracellular processes relating to oestrogen action.

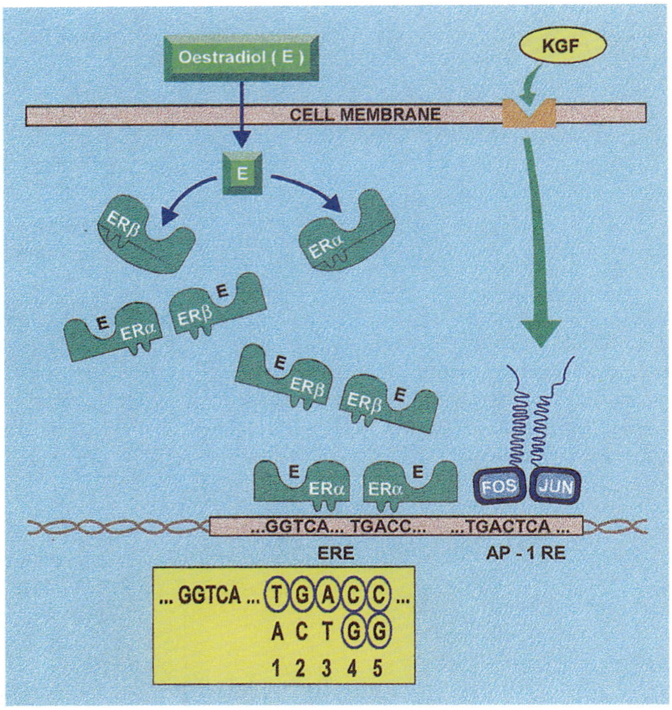

Fig. 8. Potential interrelationship between the estrogen binding domain of the receptor proteins and the genome. E = Estradiol; ER = estrogen receptor; KGF = keratinocyte growth factor.

quences could, for example, specifically interact with a ERα/ERβ heterodimer and it is now necessary to further investigate these molecular events. Such work will revitalize interest in the precise biological role of oestrogens within the human prostate gland, an interest which has already been particularly evoked by the recent studies of Rosner and co-workers [41], with regard to the mitogenic effect of sex hormone-binding globulin (SHBG) on the stromal tissue of the human prostate and of Chang and co-workers [42], with direct attention to the association of oestradiol with the ALA70 co-activator, which, as part of a tripartite unit (fig. 9), enhances the androgenic influence of DHT on gene transcription.

Inter- and Intracellular Signalling Pathways

The sophistication of the inter- and intracellular signalling pathways, between and within cells and the intrinsic growth regulatory factors that influence these pathways, is becoming increasingly more apparent. The cell-cell interactions between glandular epithelial cells and the muscle cells and fibroblasts of the stromal compartment

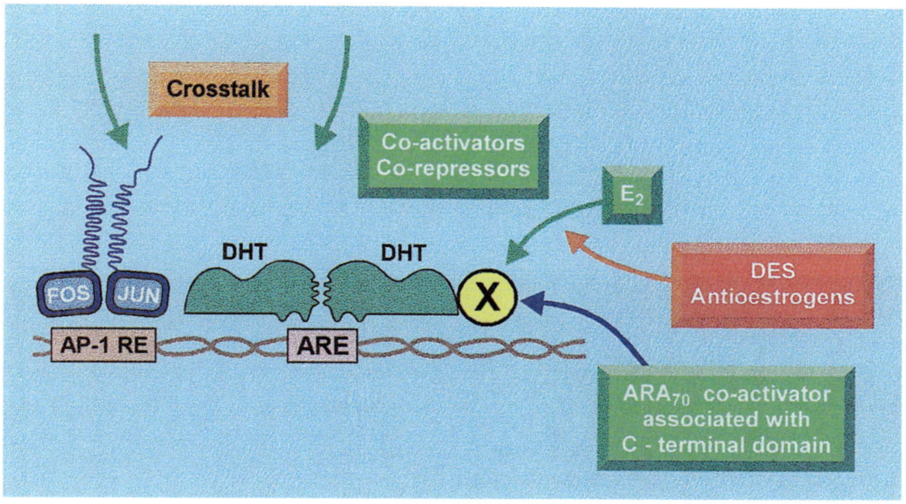

Fig. 9. Diagrammatic illustration of a co-activator X, influenced by oestradiol and part of the mechanism associated with androgen receptor action.

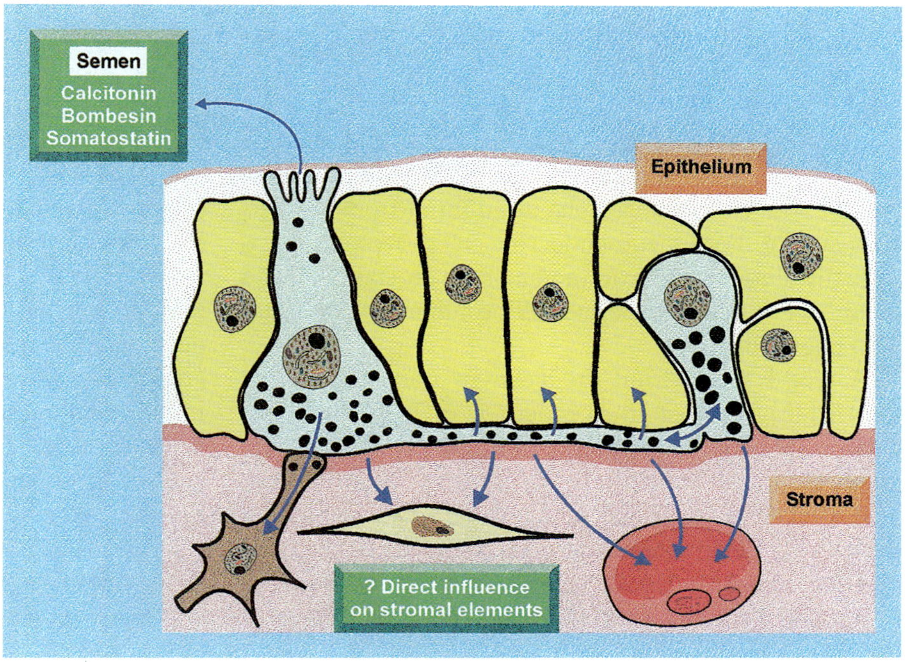

Fig. 10. Neuroendocrine cells, illustrating possible simple links to nerve and muscle cells.

have been briefly described. The prostatic neuroendocrine cells, located within the epithelial compartment, are rarely mentioned. These cells are basally-orientated (fig. 10) and morphologically are either of the *'open type'*, with apical processes extending to the lumen, or the *'closed type'*, both having long dendritic processes extending under and weaving between adjacent epithelial cells [43]. There is speculation regarding their role, but it generally would be considered to encompass the regulation of cell growth and differentiation as well as neuroendocrine, endocrine and exocrine secretion [44, 45]. They are specialized, differentiated cells that contain and secrete: (a) the biogenic amine, serotonin; (b) bombesin/gastrin-releasing peptide; (c) the chromogranin family of polypeptides; (d) the calcitonin family of peptides; (e) somatostatin; (f) parathyroid hormone-related protein (PHTrP); (g) thyroid-stimulating hormone (TSH)-like peptide, and (h) human chorionic gonadotropin (HCG)-like peptide.

Although the high levels of calcitonin, bombesin and somatostatin in semen suggest that these peptides are directly secreted by the neuroendocrine cells, little is known about the intercellular autocrine and paracrine local regulatory mechanisms by which the neuroendocrine cells interrelate with the neighbouring cells. This may involve interaction between neuroendocrine cells, factors produced by the stromal compartment, extrinsic,

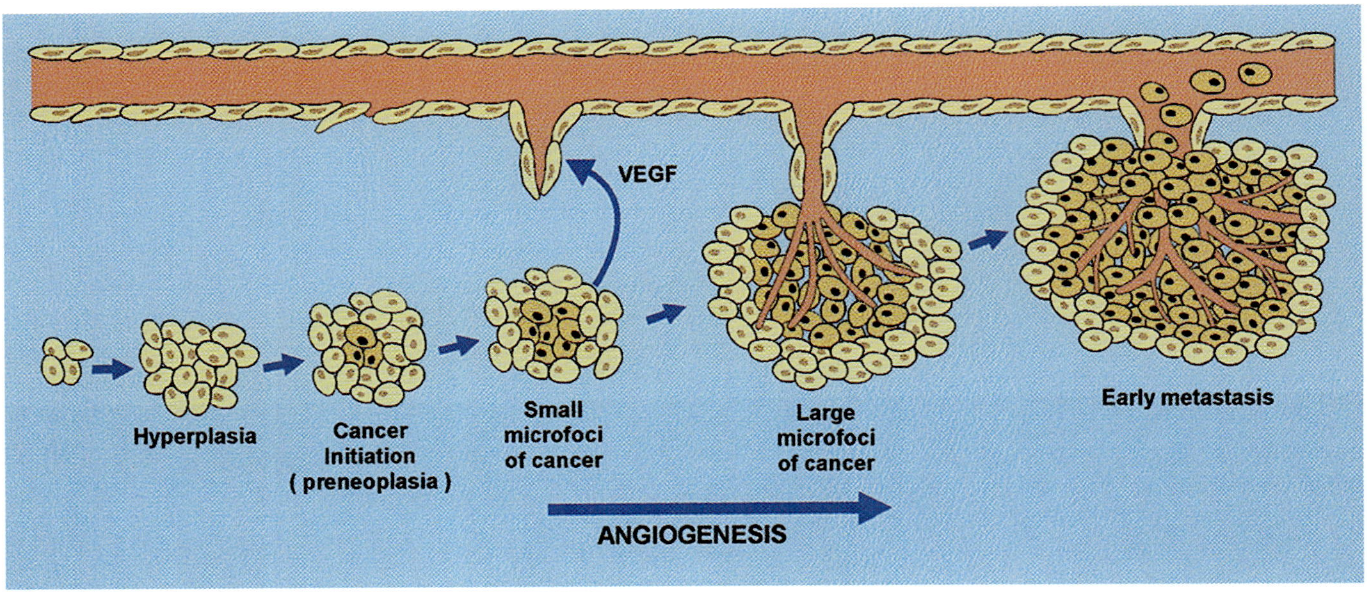

Fig. 11. Angiogenesis.

blood-borne endocrine agents, or an input from the nervous system. Focal neuroendocrine cell differentiation is virtually ubiquitous in carcinoma of the prostate [43] and the extent of neuroendocrine cell proliferation correlates with poor prognosis.

A recent report from the Tenovus Cancer Research Centre [46] relating to the production of TGF-α and vascular endothelial growth factor (VEGF) by neuroendocrine cells of the human prostate is of particular interest. TGF-α expression, which mediates its biological action through the EGF receptor, is generally associated with the proliferation of human prostatic cancer cells and VEGF is now recognized as a powerful promoter of angiogenesis (fig. 11). It is well accepted that once a tumour attains a volume of approximately 2 mm, an improved new blood supply is required for continued growth [47–49]. The production of VEGF by the neuroendocrine cells of the tumour and its activation of signalling pathways within the sprouting endothelial cells may well be a factor associated with the promotion of angiogenesis and cancer progression [50, 51].

The Complex Interrelationship between the Intrinsic Factors

The integrated response of the various populations of cells within the prostate to signalling language, reading sense from the many messages induced by the wide range of growth regulatory factors, as well as those initiated by the extrinsic endocrine factors that impact on the gland, is very clearly a finely-tuned and complex interactive system. As our understanding of these singalling pathways develops, the information that accumulates provides a greater insight into the potential consequences of their impairment and their relationship to the pathogenesis of prostate disease. Cells which respond to external stimuli such as those induced by KGF or FGF-2 depend on the presence of cell membrane-localized receptor proteins (fig. 12). The signalling pathways, sometimes referred to as the phosphorylation cascade, are complex and interest centres on the mechanisms by which these various kinases are controlled. As stated earlier, fundamental to the hormone responsiveness of the prostate gland is the interrelationship between the signalling pathways which induce biological responses through steroid receptors and those activated through the binding of the peptide growth regulatory factors to the transmembrane cell receptors. It would now appear that the mitogenic effect of DHT on prostate epithelial cells is mediated by peptide growth stimulatory factors, probably KGF (KGF-7), produced by the fibroblasts of the stromal compartment of the gland.

The association of the growth factor with the external domain of membrane receptor initiates the signalling processes related to mitogenesis. Through a *tyrosine-specific protein kinase (TK)* situated on the intracellular domain of the receptor, the binding of the peptide triggers a cascade of intracellular signalling events (fig. 12) that ultimately

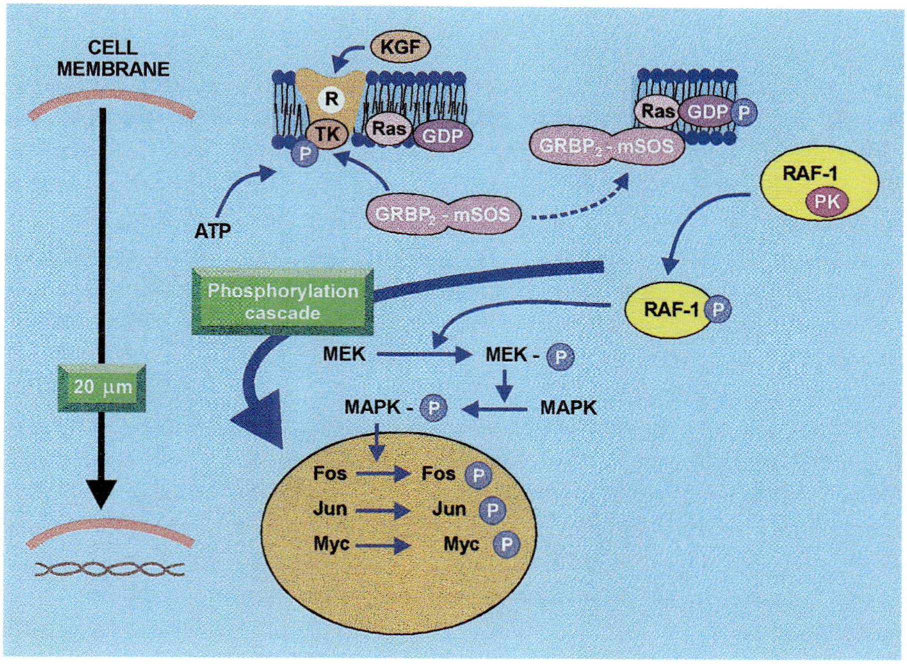

Fig. 12. Some complex aspects of signal transduction pathways.

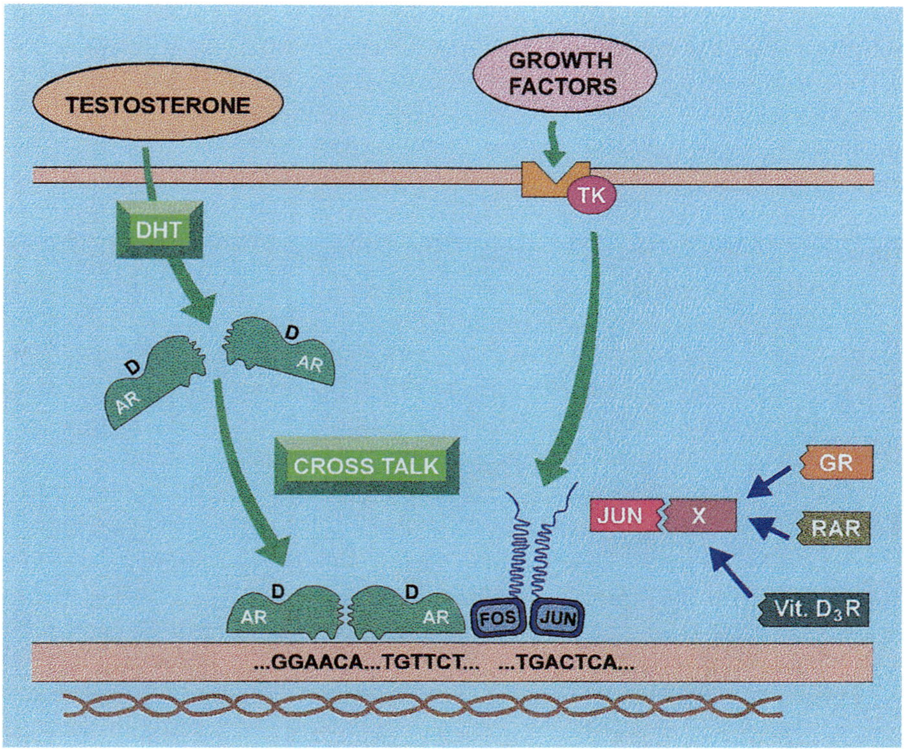

Fig. 13. Function interaction of crosstalk between signalling pathways. DHT (D) = Dihydrotestosterone; AR = androgen receptor; TK = tyrosine kinase; GR = glucocorticoid receptor; RAR = retinoic acid receptor; Vit.D_3R = vitamin D_3 receptor.

lead to the activation of proto-oncogenes and gene transcription [52, 53]. Such signals would activate the *c-myc, c-fos and c-jun proto-oncogenes*, all encoding proteins that are involved in normal growth regulatory processes within the prostate gland and which are referred to as *transcription factors (TFs)*. As well as encoding for transcription factors, proto-oncogenes would also encode growth regulatory factors and their corresponding membrane receptor proteins, as well as for the many and various components of the signal transduction pathways (fig. 12).

The Fos and Jun proteins, either as Fos/Jun heterodimers, or as Jun/Jun homodimers, are components of the AP-1 transcription factor that specifically associates with the AP-1 recognition sequences on the genome (fig. 8) characterized by the -TGACTCA- nucleotide sequence [54, 55]. The interaction between the two proteins on the genome represents a specific interaction between the 'leucine zipper' structural domains of the proteins [56]. The spatial disposition of the HREs, or androgen response elements alongside AP-1 recognition sites in juxtaposition along the promoter region of an androgen-responsive gene (fig. 8) would therefore lead to functional interaction, or synergism [57, 58], the interaction referred to as crosstalk between signalling pathways. It would be considered [59, 60] that the association of the steroid receptor complex to the genome would change the spatial orientation of the DNA such that the DNA strands 'bend', thereby offering easier accessibility to the transcription factors for their recognition sites.

Little is known about the concentrations of DHT-AR necessary to support growth factor signalling, nor of the sensitivity of these processes which may be greater than hitherto believed. An even greater sensitivity may be conferred on cancer cells [61]. AR expression is maintained in most androgen-resistant cancers of the prostate [62] and the presence of the AR itself may offer a growth advantage even in the presence of extremely low concentrations of androgen present in patients with prostate cancer on maximal androgenic blockade.

The complexity of these interrelationships is further emphasized in figure 13, which illustrates how other receptor proteins can probably interact with the TFs, to influence gene transcription [63, 64]. The illustration simply depicts the potential protein-protein interaction of the retinoic acid receptor (RAR), the glucocorticoid receptor (GR) and the 1,25-dihydroxyvitamin D_3 (1,25-diOHvitD_3) receptor (VDR) with the Fos/Jun heterodimer complex that could thereby influence transcription activity [58].

Some Early Phases of Cancer Development

Impairment of the growth regulatory balance can lead to cellular hyperplasia with consequent genetic instability and subversion of the normal processes of growth restraint. Furthermore, proto-oncogenes that become dysfunctional through point mutations, deletions, amplification, or other changes that alter the structure or influence the expression of these growth regulatory genes, can induce carcinogenesis.

From a study of the ductal budding and branching patterns in the developing prostate, Timms et al. [65] and Cunha and co-workers [66] re-emphasize the concept that the regional organization of the prostatic complex is determined by the regional heterogeneity of mesenchymal induction, with particular specific mesenchymal effects induced along a budding axis. The influence of stromal heterogeneity on prostatic growth and differentiation, *effects which are 'imprinted' on the gland during fetal life by the action of the various steroid hormones, in utero, including effects induced by oestrogens, is fundamentally important and relates to subsequent predisposition of various regions of the prostate to disease.*

This concept of imprinting and predisposition to disease is particularly important with regard to the role of oestrogens on the developing fetal prostate [67]. Timms and co-workers [68] reported that a *physiological*, 50% increase in the oestradiol concentration within the male mouse fetus, produced from a maternal silastic implant, subsequently resulted in the development of an enlarged adult prostate gland, with a 6-fold increase in AR levels relative to controls. A 5-fold increase in the total serum oestradiol levels resulted in a smaller adult prostate gland.

The results suggest that oestrogens can modulate the action of androgens by 'in utero', enhancing the sensitivity of the prostate to androgen and, moreover, *the effect is sustained throughout life*, probably forming the basis of growth regulatory dysfunction and disease in later years. It is of interest that the male mouse fetus, exposed to these physiological, small increases in oestradiol levels, showed an immediate significant increase in the number of prostatic glands throughout the dorsal urogenital sinus, including the dorsocranial region, a region considered homologous to the areas of the human prostate in which BPH originates. *It is certainly important to better understand the role of oestradiol in the prostate gland.*

Again, of particular interest, is that the biological action of oestrogens on vasculature is associated with the production of nitric oxide (NO), now seen as an important physiological regulator of endocrine systems, and implicated in the proliferation of smooth muscle cells. Moreover, in relation to intracellular signalling, the presence of a specific plasma membrane-located receptor to intracellular signalling, the presence of a specific plasma membrane-located receptor for an oestradiol-SHBG complex, that was found [69] in the stromal elements of the human prostate, provides another pathway by which oestradiol may influence prostatic growth. The oestradiol-SHBG complex can induce intracellular signalling by promoting an 8-fold elevation in cAMP levels, that in the absence of androgens can induce PSA expression.

Furthermore, studies with the rat insulinoma RINm5F cell line [70] suggest that the induction of NO-synthase and NO generation may influence apoptosis. The role of oestrogens in relation to apoptosis in the prostate gland is, as yet, still to be precisely determined. It has also been suggested [71] that the reaction between NO and superoxide that gives rise to the toxic peroxynitrite, may be implicated in the process of apoptosis, by which phagocytes engulf and destroy foreign proteins, with 'apoptotic genes' encoding free radical scavengers.

Diet and Prostate Disease: The Concept of Prevention

The relationship of diet to prostate disease has been the subject of a recent major review [72] and is discussed in an earlier section of this text (page 377). From the marked differences in the incidence of both prostate and breast cancer between the East and the West, it was not difficult to direct attention to fat and animal products which can provide up to 40% of the total caloric intake in some North American people, as possible *causative factors*. Recently [72], however, an alternative concept has emerged to suggest that *constituents of the Asian diet may restrain the processes of carcinogenesis*. The studies of migrating people from Japan and China, through Hawaii, to mainland USA, indicate that the migrants, in one or two generations, show a mortality rate for prostate cancer that comes close to that of the indigenous American people, thereby highlighting a possible influence of dietary factors [73, 74].

Interest now centres on certain *isoflavonoids, flavonoids and lignans*, products of vegetables, fruit, whole grains and soya, that are metabolized by the gut microflora to give rise to compounds such as enterolactone, daidzein and genistein, weak plant oestrogens, referred to generally as the phyto-oestrogens. As weak oestrogens, such compounds could act as 'natural tamoxifen-like' factors that could, like tamoxifen, also a weak oestrogen agonist, restrain the early processes associated with breast carcinogenesis by their *antagonistic antioestrogenic effect*.

The presence in plants of nonsteroidal substances with oestrogenic activity has been recognized for some time and many hundreds of plants manifest some degree of oestrogenic activity [75]. Soya bean and red clover are members of the leguminosae family which is a major source of isoflavonoids and soya is consumed daily in large amounts in a number of forms in China and Japan and in Asia generally. Many foods of plant origin contain varying amounts of isoflavonoids, flavonoids and lignans and it is not unreasonable to assume that at least some of these polyphenolic phyto-oestrogens could exercise an influence on oestrogen-sensitive growth regulatory processes of the prostate gland. The lignans are widely distributed in nature and precursors are found in many cereals, grains, fruits and vegetables, but the richest source is linseed (flaxseed) and other oilseeds such as sesame.

The flavonoids are closely related in structure to the isoflavonoids, the former having a 2-phenylchroman nucleus and the latter a 3-phenylchroman nucleus [75] and recently several commonly occurring plant flavonoids have been shown to possess weak oestrogenic activity [75]. Unlike isoflavonoids, the flavonoids are ubiquitous in nature, and are found in high concentration in many fruits, vegetables and crop species. In particular, apigenin and kaempferol, both of which are oestrogenic, are regarded as two of the major flavonoids because of their common occurrence among plants, and their significant concentrations when they are present. Apigenin, for example, is found in the leaves, seeds and fruits of flowering plants, with up to 7% of dry weight in leafy vegetables. Tea leaves are an excellent source of apigenin.

The levels of isoflavonoids are high in the urine and plasma of the Japanese and Chinese whose traditional foodstuffs contain large amounts of soya in the form of bean curd (tofu), soya bean milk, miso and tempeh. The concentration of lignans is high in the urine of vegetarians [76] whose diet contains whole grain cereals, vegetables and fruits. The concentrations of flavonoids in plasma and urine of different populations have yet to be determined and is an obvious programme for future research. However, as tea, fruit and vegetables are the principal source of flavonoids, it is probable that Asians with their high consumption of tea, and vegetarians, have significant circulating levels of these compounds.

Essentially, in relation to these growth regulatory processes and prostatic carcinogenesis, the other characteristics [72, 77, 78] of the phyto-oestrogens – i.e., 5α-reductase inhibition, tyrosine kinase inhibition, aromatase enzyme inhibition, angiogenesis inhibition, DNA topoisomerase inhibition, tumourigenesis inhibition and antioxidant activity – already discussed earlier, it is not too difficult to envisage the growth-restraining influence that such dietary factors could exercise on the development of prostatic disease.

References

1 Huggins CH: Introduction; in Vollmer EP, Kauffmann G (eds): Biology of the Prostate and Related Tissues. Nat Cancer Inst Monogr 12. Bethesda, NIH, 1963, pp xi–xii.

2 Bostwick DG: Origins of prostatic carcinoma. Cancer 1996;78:230–236.

3 Griffiths K, Coffey D, Cockett ATK, Di Sant'Agnese A, Ichikawa T, Krieg M, Lee C, McKeehan W, Schalken J, Sciarra F, Steiner G, Sugimura Y, Yamanaka H: The regulation of prostatic growth; in Cockett ATK, Khoury S, Aso Y, Chatelain C, Denis L, Griffiths K, Murphy G (eds): The 3rd International Consultation on Benign Prostatic Hyperplasia. Paris, SCI, 1996, pp 73–115.

4 Griffiths K, Cockett ATK, Coffey DS, Krieg M, Lee C, McKeehan W, Neal DE, Partin A, Di Sant'Agnese A, Schalken J: Regulation of prostate growth; in Denis L (eds): 4th International Consultation on BPH. Paris, SCI, 1998, pp 83–128.

5 Girman C, Panser L, Chute C et al: Natural history of prostatism: Urinary flow rates in a community-based study. J Urol 1993;887–892.

6 Guess HA: Epidemiology and natural history of benign prostatic hyperplasia. Urol Clin North Am 1995;22:247–261.

7 Franks LM: Benign nodular hyperplasia of the prostate: A review. Ann R Coll Surg England 1954;14:92–106.

8 Bostwick DG, Pacelli A, Lopez-Beltran A: Molecular biology of prostatic intraepithelial neoplasia. Prostate 1996;29:117–134.

9 Harper ME, Glynne-Jones E, Goddard L, Mathews P, Nicholson RI: Expression of androgen receptor and growth factors in premalignant lesions of the prostate. J Pathol 1998;186:169–177.

10 Lopez-Otin C, Diamandis EP: Breast and prostate cancer: An analysis of common epidemiological, genetic and biochemical features. Endocr Rev 1998;19:365–396.

11 Barry MJ, Boyle P, Fourcroy J, Garraway M, Gu FL, Harrison NW, Jacobsen SJ, O'Leary MP, Oishi K, Senge T, Tsukamoto T, Guess HA: Epidemiology and natural history of BPH; in Cockett ATK, Khoury S, Aso Y, Chatelain C, Denis L, Griffiths K, Murphy G (eds): The 3rd International Consultation on Benign Prostatic Hyperplasia. Paris, SCI, 1996, pp 21–36.

12 Garraway WM, Collins GN, Lee RJ: High prevalence of benign prostatic hypertrophy in the community. Lancet 1991;338:469–471.

13 Berry SJ, Coffey DS, Walsh PC, Ewing LL: The development of human benign prostatic hyperplasia with age. J Urol 1984;132:474–479.

14 Isaacs JT, Coffey DS: Etiology and disease process of benign prostatic hyperplasia. Prostate 1989;(suppl 2):33–50.

15 Bruchovsky N, Lesser B, Van Doorn E, Craven S: Hormonal effects on cell proliferation in rat prostate. Vitam Horm 1975;33:61–102.

16 Truss M, Beato M: Steroid hormone receptors: Interaction with deoxyribonucleic acid and transcription factors. Endocr Rev 1993;14: 459–479.

17 Gronemeyer H: Transcription activation by estrogen and progesterone receptors. Annu Rev Genet 1991;25:89–123.

18 Imperato-McGinley J, Guerro L, Gautier T, Peterson RE: Steroid 5α-reductase deficiency in man: An inherited form of male pseudohermaphroditism. Science 1974;186:1213–1215.

19 Griffiths K, Akaza H, Eaton CL, El Etreby M, Habib F, Lee C, Partin AW, Coffey DS, Sciarra F, Steiner G, Tenniswood MP: Regulation of prostate growth; in Cockett ATK, Khoury S, Aso Y, Chatelain C, Denis L, Griffiths K, Murphy G (eds): The 2nd International Consultation on Benign Prostatic Hyperplasia. Paris, SCI, 1993, pp 49–75.

20 Lee C, Kozlowski JM, Grayhack JT: Intrinsic and extrinsic factors controlling benign prostatic growth. Prostate 1997;31:131–138.

21 Franks LM, Riddle PN, Carbonell AW, Gey GO: A comparative study of the ultrastructure and lack of growth capacity of adult human prostate epithelium mechanically separated from its stroma. J Pathol 1970;100:113–119.

22 Cunha GR, Chung LWK, Shannon JM, Taguchi O, Fujii H: Hormone-induced morphogenesis and growth: Role of mesenchymal-epithelial interactions. Recent Prog Horm Res 1983; 39:559–595.

23 Yan G, Fukabori Y, Nikoloropolous S, Wang F, McKeehan WL: Heparin-binding keratinocyte growth factor is a candidate stromal to epithelial cell andromedin. Mol Endocrinol 1992; 6:2123–2128.

24 Peehl DM, Wong ST, Rubin JS: KGF and EGF differentially regulate the phenotype of prostatic epithelial cells. Growth Regul 1996;6:22–31.

25 Sugimura Y, Foster BA, Hom YK, Lipschutz JH, Rubin JS, Finch PW, Aaronson SA, Hayashi N, Kawamura J, Cunha GR: Keratinocyte growth factor can replace testosterone in the ductal branching morphogenesis of the rat ventral prostate. Int J Dev Biol 1996;40:941–951.

26 Culig Z, Hobixch A, Cronauer MV, Radmayr C, Trapman J, Hittmair A, Bartsch G, Klocker H: Androgen receptor activation in prostatic tumour cell lines by insulin-like growth factor I, keratinocyte growth factor and epidermal growth factor. Cancer Res 1994;54:5474–5478.

27 Miki T, Bottaro DP, Fleming TP, Smith CL, Burgess WH, Chan AML, Aarinson SA: Determination of ligand-binding specificity by alternate splicing: Two distinct growth factor receptors encoded by a single gene. Proc Natl Acad Sci USA 1992;89:246–250.

28 Sherwood ER, Fong CJ, Lee C, Kozlowski JM: Basic fibroblast growth factor: A potential mediator of stromal growth in the human prostate. Endocrinology 1992;130:2955–2963.

29 Leung HY, Dickson C, Robson CN, Neal DE: Overexpression of fibroblast growth factor-8 in human prostate cancer. Oncogene 1996;12: 1833–1835.

30 Schmitt JF, Hearn MT, Risbridger GP: Expression of fibroblast growth factor-8 in adult rat tissues and human prostate carcinoma cells. J Steroid Biochem Mol Biol 1996;57:173–178.

31 Yan G, Fukabori Y, McBride G, Nikolarapolous S, McKeehan WL: Exon switching and activation of stromal and embryonic fibroblast growth factor (FGF)-FGF receptor genes in prostate epithelial cells accompany stromal independence and malignancy. Mol Cell Biol 1993;13:4513–4522.

32 Krieg M, Bartsch W, Thomsen M, Voigt KD: Androgens and estrogens: Their interaction with stroma and epithelium of human benign prostatic hyperplasia and normal prostate. J Steroid Biochem 1983;19:155–161.

33 Kuiper GGJM, Enmark E, Pelto-Huikko M, Nilsson S, Gustafsson JA: Cloning of a novel estrogen receptor expressed in rat prostate and ovary. Proc Natl Acad Sci USA 1996;93:5925–5930.

34 Mosselman S, Polman J, Dijkema R: ERβ: Identification and characterisation of a novel human estrogen receptor. FEBS Lett 1996;392: 49–53.

35 Kuiper GGJM, Carlsson B, Grandien J, Enmark E, Haggblad J, Nilsson S, Gustafsson JA: Comparison of the ligand binding specificity and transcript tissue distribution of estrogen receptors α and β. Endocrinology 1997;138: 863–870.

36 Berry M, Metzger D, Chambon P: Role of the two activating domains of oestrogen receptor in the cell-type and promoter-context dependent agonistic activity of the anti-oestrogen 4-hydroxytamoxifen. EMBO J 1990;9:2811–2818.

37 Tzukerman MT, Esty A, Santiso-Mere D, Danielian P, Parker MG, Stein RB, Pike JW, McDonnell DP: Human estrogen receptor transactivational capacity is determined by both cellular and promoter-content and mediated by two functionally distinct intramolecular regions. Mol Endocrinol 1994;8:21–30.

38 Kraus WL, McInerny EM, Katzenellenbogen BS: Ligand-dependent, transcriptionally productive association of the amino- and carboxy-terminal regions of a steroid hormone nuclear receptor. Proc Natl Acad Sci USA 1995; 92:12314–12318.

39 Montano MM, Muller V, Trobaugh A, Katzenellenbogen BS: The carboxy-terminal F domain of the human estrogen receptor: Role in the transcriptional activity of the receptor and the effectiveness of antiestrogens as estrogen antagonists. Mol Endocrinol 1995;9:814–825.

40 Katzenellenbogen JA, O'Malley BW, Katzenellenbogen BS: Tripartite steroid hormone receptor pharmacology: Interaction with multiple effector sites as a base for the cell- and promoter-specific action of these hormones. Mol Endocrinol 1996;10:119–131.

41 Nakhla AM, Khan MS, Romas NP, Rosner W: Estradiol causes the rapid accumulation of cAMP in human prostate. Proc Natl Acad Sci USA 1994;91:5402–5405.

42 Yeh S, Miyamoto H, Shima H, Chang C: From estrogen to androgen receptor: A new pathway for sex hormones in prostate. Proc Natl Acad Sci USA 1998;10:5527–5532.
43 Di Sant Agnese P: Neuroendocrine differentiation in carcinoma of the prostate. Diagnostic, prognostic and therapeutic implications. Cancer 1992;70:254–268.
44 Larsson LI: On the possible existence of multiple endocrine, paracrine and neuroendocrine messengers in secretory cell systems. Invest Cell Pathol 1980;3:73–85.
45 Bishop A, Polak J: Gut endocrine and neural peptides. Endocr Pathol 1990;1:24.
46 Harper ME, Glynne-Jones E, Goddard L, Thurston VJ, Griffiths K: Vascular endothelial growth factor expression in prostatic tumours and its relationship to neuroendocrine cells. Br J Cancer 1996;74:910–916.
47 Folkman J: What is the evidence that tumors are angiogenesis dependent? J Natl Cancer Inst 1990;82:4–6.
48 Folkman J, Klagsbrun M: Angiogenic factors. Science 1987;235:442–447.
49 Weidner N, Carroll PR, Flax J, Blumenfeld W, Folkman J: Tumor angiogenesis correlates with metastasis in invasive prostate carcinoma. Am J Pathol 1993;143:401–409.
50 Cockett ATK, Di Sant Agnese PA, Gopinath P, Schoen SR, Abrahamsson PA: Relationship of neuroendocrine cells of prostate and serotonin to benign prostatic hyperplasia. Urology 1993; 42:512–519.
51 Cockett ATK, Di Sant Agnese PA, Gopinath P, Schoen S, Abrahamsson PA: Relationship of neuroendocrine cells of prostate and serotonin to benign prostatic hyperplasia. Adult Urol 1993;42:512–519.
52 Aaronson S: Growth factors and cancer. Science 1991;254:1146–1153.
53 Weinberg RA: The action of oncogenes in the cytoplasm and nucleus. Science 1983;230:770–776.
54 Curran T, Bravo R, Muller R: Transient induction of c-fos and c-myc is an intermediate consequence of growth factor stimulation. Cancer Surv 1985;4:655–681.
55 Jones N: Transcriptional regulation by dimerisation: Two sides to an incestuous relationship. Cell 1990;61:9–11.
56 Landschultz WH, Johnson PF, McKnight SL: The leucine zipper: A hypothetical structure common to a new class of DNA binding proteins. Science 1986;240:1759–1764.
57 Schule R, Muller M, Kaltschmidt C, Rentawitz R: Many transcription factors interact synergistically with steroid receptors. Science 1988; 242:1418–1420.
58 Shemshedini L, Knauthe R, Sassone-Corsi P, Pornon A, Gronemeyer H: Cell-specific inhibitory and stimulatory effects of fos and jun on transcription activation by nuclear receptors. EMBO J 1991;10:3839–3849.
59 Sabbah M, Le Recousse S, Redeuilh G, Beaulieu EE: Estrogen receptor-induced binding of the xenopus vitellogenin A2 gene hormone response element. Biochem Biophys Res Commun 1992;185:944–952.
60 Nardulli AM, Shapiro DJ: Binding of the estrogen receptor DNA-binding domain to the estrogen response element induces DNA binding. Mol Cell Biol 1992;12:2037–2042.
61 Griffiths K, Morton MS, Nicholson RI: Androgens, androgen receptors, antiandrogens and the treatment of prostate cancer. Eur Urol 1997;32(suppl 3):24–40.
62 Chodak GW, Krane DM, Puy LA, Takeda H, Johnson K, Chang C: Nuclear localization of androgen receptor in heterogeneous samples of normal, hyperplastic and neoplastic human prostate. J Urol 1992;147:798–803.
63 Beato M, Herrlich P, Schutz G: Steroid hormone receptors: Many actors in search of a plot. Cell 1995;83:851–857.
64 Mangelsdorf DJ, Evans RM: The RXR heterodimers and orphan receptors. Cell 1995;83: 841–850.
65 Timms BG, Mohs TJ, Didio LJA: Ductal budding and branching patterns in the developing prostate. J Urol 1994;151:1427–1432.
66 Sugimura Y, Norman JT, Cunha GR, Shannon JM: Regional differences in the inductive activity of the mesenchyme of the embryonic mouse urogenital sinus. Prostate 1985;7:253–260.
67 Santti R, Newbold RR, Makela S, Pylkkanen L, McLachlan JA: Developmental estrogenization and prostatic neoplasia. Prostate 1994;24:67–78.
68 Vom Saal FS, Timms BG, Montano MM, Palanza P, Thayer KA, Nagel SC, Dhar MD, Ganjam VK, Parmigiani S, Welshons WV: Prostate enlargement in mice due to fetal exposure to a low dose of estradiol or diethylstilbestrol, and opposite effects at high doses. Proc Natl Acad Sci USA 1997;94:2056–2061.
69 Ding VHD, Moller DE, Feeney WP, Didolkar V, Nakhla AM, Rhodes L, Rosner W, Smith R: Sex hormone-binding globulin mediates prostate androgen receptor action via a novel signaling pathway. Endocrinology 1998;139:213–218.
70 Suarez-Pinzon WL, Strynadka K, Schulz R, Rabinovitch A: Mechanisms of cytokine-induced destruction of rat insulinoma cells: The role of nitric oxide. Endocrinology 1994;134: 1006–1010.
71 Sarafian TA, Bredesen DE: Is apoptosis mediated by reactive oxygen species? Free Radic Res 1994;20:1–6.
72 Griffiths K, Adlercreutz H, Boyle P, Denis L, Nicholson RI, Morton M: Nutrition and Cancer. Oxford, Isis Medical Media, 1996.
73 Haenzel W, Kurihara M: Studies of Japanese migrants. I. Mortality from cancer and other diseases among Japanese in the United States. J Natl Cancer Inst 1968;40:43–68.
74 Shimizu H, Ropp RK, Bernstein L, Yatani R, Henderson BE, Mack TH: Cancers of the breast and prostate among Japanese and white immigrants in Los Angeles County. Br J Cancer 1991:63:963–966.
75 Miksicek RJ: Commonly occurring plant flavonoids have estrogenic activity. Mol Pharmacol 1993;44:37–43.
76 Adlercreutz H, Fotsis T, Bannwart C, Wahala K, Makela T, Brunow G, Hase T: Determination of urinary lignans and phytoestrogen metabolites, potential antiestrogens and anticarcinogens, in urine of women on various habitual diets. J Steroid Biochem 1986;25:791–797.
77 Morton MS, Griffiths K, Blacklock N: The preventive role of diet in prostatic disease. Br J Urol 1996;77:481–493.
78 Griffiths K, Denis L, Turkes A, Morton MS: Possible relationship between dietary factors and pathogenesis of prostate cancer. Int J Urol 1998;5:195–213.

Preclinical Models for Drug Discovery

European Urology

Eur Urol 1999;35:456–458

High-Grade Prostatic Intraepithelial Neoplasia in Dogs

David J. Waters

Cancer Biology Laboratory, School of Veterinary Medicine, Purdue University, West Lafayette, Ind., USA

Key Words

Prostate · Cancer · Carcinogenesis · Chemoprevention · Premalignant nature · Animal models

Abstract

The dog is the only nonhuman species in which high-grade intraepithelial neoplasia (HGPIN) and invasive carcinoma spontaneously occur. Our work was the first to describe HGPIN in the dog prostate. Canine HGPIN bears remarkable morphologic similarity to its human counterpart. There is also striking similarity between canine and human HGPIN with respect to basal layer disruption, proliferative index, and microvessel density. For each of these parameters, HGPIN is intermediate between benign epithelium and invasive carcinoma, strengthening the hypothesis that HGPIN is an intermediate step on the road to prostate cancer. In another study, we showed that HGPIN is present in the majority (55%) of elderly sexually intact pet dogs without clinical evidence of prostate cancer. These data suggest that the early events of prostate carcinogenesis may occur with high frequency within the prostates of pet dogs sharing the same environment as humans. We are currently conducting a large-scale autopsy-epidemiological study to further characterize the epidemiology of HGPIN and invasive carcinoma in pet dogs. We are also testing the potential utility of pet dogs for the rapid, cost-effective in vivo screening of chemopreventive agents by using the prevalence and extent of HGPIN in the dog prostate as a surrogate endpoint biomarker.

The dog is the only nonhuman species in which spontaneous prostate cancer occurs frequently [1]. Our group has been investigating the prostate cancers that arise spontaneously in pet dogs. Clinically apparent prostate cancer in pet dogs exhibits aggressive biological behavior, with metastasis to regional lymph nodes or lungs frequently present at the time of diagnosis [2, 3]. Similar to its human counterpart, canine prostate carcinoma frequently metastasizes to the skeleton. Several aspects of canine prostate carcinoma that support its relevance as a model for human prostate cancer are summarized in table 1 [2].

In 1997, our group was the first to describe high-grade prostatic intraepithelial neoplasia (HGPIN) in the dog prostate and demonstrate its close association with invasive carcinoma [4]. In addition, our data suggest that the early events in prostate carcinogenesis occur with high frequency in the prostates of elderly sexually intact pet dogs [5]. This paper will summarize our previously published data on HGPIN in dogs and discuss the potential implications of these findings.

HGPIN is the most likely precursor of many human prostate cancers [6, 7]. Morphologic findings, including basal layer disruption [8], increased proliferative capacity [9], and increased microvessel density [10], suggest that HGPIN is an intermediate stage in the progression from benign epithelium to carcinoma. Foci of HGPIN are present in 85% of men with prostate cancer [11], and the presence of HGPIN on biopsy is a significant risk factor for subsequent carcinoma [12, 13]. The recent identification of specific and consistent molecular changes in

KARGER

Fax +41 61 306 12 34
E-Mail karger@karger.ch
www.karger.com

0302–2838/99/0356–0456$17.50/0

Accessible online at:
http://BioMedNet.com/karger

David J. Waters, DVM, PhD
Purdue University, Cancer Biology Laboratory
1296 Lynn Hall
West Lafayette, IN 47907 (USA)
Tel. +1 765 494 9271, Fax +1 765 496 1108

Table 1. Relevance of spontaneous canine prostate cancer to human prostate cancer [modified from 2]

Aging stronly influences prevalence of HGPIN and spontaneous prostate cancer development
At autopsy, frequent existence of premalignant or malignant changes in elderly
HGPIN is apparently an intermediate step between benign epithelium and invasive carcinoma
Cancers are high-grade carcinomas that exhibit morphologic and phenotypic heterogeneity
End-stage, lethal cancers are apparently androgen-independent
Skeletal distribution and osteoblastic nature of bone metastases mimics human prostate cancer

HGPIN adds further support to the premalignant nature of this lesion [14]. Significant changes in the expression of oncogenes, growth factors and growth factor receptors occur during the apparent transition from benign epithelium to HGPIN, suggesting that HGPIN represents an important threshold for carcinogenesis.

To investigate the association between HGPIN and canine prostate cancer, we evaluated the prostates of pet dogs with spontaneous prostate carcinoma [4]. The prevalence of HGPIN was determined in formalin-fixed prostates from 29 dogs with spontaneous prostate carcinoma. Using immunoperoxidase technique, we compared basal layer integrity (high-molecular-weight keratin 34 β-E12), proliferative index (MIB-1), and microvessel density (factor VIII-related antigen) in 14 prostates which contained benign epithelium, HGPIN, and invasive carcinoma in the same tissue section.

Canine HGPIN showed cytologic features identical to the human counterpart, including cell crowding, loss of polarity, and nuclear and nucleolar enlargement. Our results indicated that HGPIN, the most likely precursor of human prostate cancer, is present in the majority (66%) of prostates of pet dogs with prostate carcinoma. This measure of the prevalence of HGPIN in canine prostates with carcinoma likely underestimates the true prevalence because exhaustive step-sectioning of the specimens was not undertaken. These findings are similar to the 85% prevalence of HGPIN reported in men with prostate carcinoma [11].

The immunophenotype of canine HGPIN was compared to carcinoma and benign epithelium. Immunohistochemistry showed that the basal layer is partially disrupted in HGPIN, whereas it is absent in prostate cancer. The proliferative index and microvessel density of canine HGPIN are intermediate between benign epithelium and carcinoma. The results are similar to those reported for human HGPIN and prostate cancer [9, 10] and indicate that HGPIN is part of a morphologic continuum in the progression of prostate cancer.

Although clinically apparent prostate carcinoma occurs sporadically in pet dogs, we hypothesized that early events in the carcinogenesis process may be occurring with much higher frequency. To test this hypothesis, we determined the prevalence of HGPIN in totally-embedded prostates of 35 dogs without clinical evidence of prostatic disease [5]. In this autopsy study, we evaluated three groups of dogs so that we could determine if the prevalence of HGPIN was influenced by age or testicular androgens: (1) 11 sexually intact dogs 7–17 years old (elderly sexually intact); (2) 13 sexually intact dogs 1–4 years old (young sexually intact), and (3) 11 dogs 7–17 years old that had been surgically castrated (elderly castrated). The prevalence of HGPIN was determined by systematic evaluation of hematoxylin and eosin and high-molecular-weight keratin 34 β-E12 stained tissue sections from formalin-fixed, paraffin-embedded prostates that had been serially sectioned at 4-mm intervals.

Our results indicated that the prevalence of canine HGPIN, like human HGPIN, is apparently influenced by age [15–17] and testicular androgens [18]. There was a high prevalence (55%) of HGPIN in the prostates of elderly sexually intact pet dogs. In contrast, foci of HGPIN were found in only 11% of the prostates of young sexually intact dogs and elderly castrated dogs. These data suggest that early events in prostate carcinogenesis may be occurring in elderly pet dogs at a frequency higher than previously recognized.

We have also studied the prevalence of HGPIN in the prostates of military working dogs [19]. Similar to our data from pet dogs [4], HGPIN was found in 72% of dogs with prostate carcinoma. In contrast to pet dogs, HGPIN was found in only 3% of single random histologic sections from the prostates of elderly military working dogs without clinical evidence of prostate cancer. In comparison to pet dogs, this represents more than 5-fold reduction in the percentage of tissue sections in which foci of HGPIN were identified. These data raise intriguing questions regarding the influence of genetic and environmental factors (e.g. diet) on the prevalence of HGPIN in dogs.

Recently, an International Workshop on Animal Models of Prostate Cancer was convened to discuss the strengths and limitations of existing animal models [20]. At that workshop, a consensus was reached that spontaneous prostate carcinoma in pet dogs represents an exciting and potentially valuable animal model [2]. Although ongoing work is beginning to characterize spontaneous prostate cancer in pet dogs, several important pieces of data are lacking. Determining the age-specific incidence of HGPIN and clinically latent prostate carcinoma in pet dogs was considered to be a priority for investigation [2]. This could be achieved by conducting an autopsy-epidemiological study similar to the human autopsy studies of Sakr et al. [16] and Billis [21]. A 3-year autopsy-epidemiological study in pet dogs has been recently funded in order to pursue this goal. It was also considered a high priority that further studies investigate the strength of association between HGPIN and invasive carcinoma in pet dogs. It was recommended that the relationship between invasive carcinoma and its putative precursor should be scrutinized using temporal (time interval between the two lesions), topographical (anatomic proximity, zonality, multifocality), genetic, and phenotypic analyses [2].

Among the human population, prevention rather than treatment may be the best approach to reduce the morbidity and mortality associated with prostate cancer. Animal models of HGPIN and invasive carcinoma are needed to evaluate the in vivo efficacy of chemopreventive agents. Widespread screening of chemopreventive agents using human subjects is impractical due to difficulties in selecting target populations, the expense of long-term clinical trials, and the infeasibility of using cancer diagnosis as an endpoint. In vivo screening of promising chemopreventive agents using the dog model of spontaneous prostate carcinogenesis represents a novel approach to the prevention of prostate cancer. In particular, the use of pet dogs that share the same environment as humans will allow for the simultaneous investigation of risk factors and biomarkers for prostate carcinogenesis in an outbred population. An interventional study using pet dogs has been designed to test the utility of pet dogs as a rapid, cost-effective model for the in vivo screening of promising chemopreventive agents. Ultimately, our plan is to utilize the dog as a preclinical model to pursue innovative strategies in prostate cancer prevention and treatment.

References

1 Rivenson A, Silverman J: The prostatic carcinoma in laboratory animals: A bibliographic survey from 1900 to 1977. Invest Urol 1979; 16:468–472.
2 Waters DJ, Sakr WA, Hayden DW, Lang CM, McKinney L, Murphy GP, Radinsky R, Ramoner R, Richardson RC, Tindall D: Workgroup 4: Spontaneous prostate carcinoma in dogs and nonhuman primates. Prostate 1998; 36:64–67.
3 Leav I, Ling GV: Adenocarcinoma of the canine prostate. Cancer 1960;22:1329–1345.
4 Waters DJ, Hayden DW, Bell FW, Klausner JS, Qian J, Bostwick DG: Prostatic intraepithelial neoplasia in dogs with spontaneous prostate cancer. Prostate 1997;30:92–97.
5 Waters DJ, Bostwick DG: Prostatic intraepithelial neoplasia occurs spontaneously in the canine prostate. J Urol 1997;157:713–716.
6 Graham SD Jr, Bostwick DF, Hoisaeter A, Abrahamsson P, Algaba F, di Sant'Agnese A, Mostofi F, Napallkov A: Report of the committee on staging and pathology. Cancer 1992; 70(suppl):359–361.
7 Bostwick DG: High grade prostatic intraepithelial neoplasia. Cancer 1995;75:1823–1836.
8 Bostwick DG, Brawer MK: Prostatic intra-epithelial neoplasia and early invasion in prostate cancer. Cancer 1987;59:788–794.
9 Montironi R, Galluz CM, Diamanti L, Giannulis I, Pisani E, Scarpelli M: Prostatic intraepithelial neoplasia: Expression and location of proliferating cell nuclear antigen in epithelial, endothelial and stromal nuclei. Virchows Archiv A 1993;422:185–192.
10 Montironi R, Galluzzi CM, Diamanti L, Taborro R, Scarpelli M, Pisani E: Prostatic intraepithelial neoplasia: Qualitative and quantitative analyses of the blood capillary architecture on thin tissue sections. Pathol Res Pract 1993; 189:542–548.
11 McNeal JE, Bostwick DG: Intraductal dysplasia: A premalignant lesion of the prostate. Hum Pathol 1986;17:64–71.
12 Brawer MK, Bigler SA, Sohlberg OE, Nagle RB, Lange PH: Significance of prostatic intraepithelial neoplasia on prostate needle biopsy. Urology 1991;38:103–107.
13 Davidson D, Bostwick DG, Qian J, Wollan P, Oesterling JE, Rudders RA et al: Prostatic intraepithelial neoplasia is a risk factor for adenocarcinoma: Predictive accuracy in needle biopsies. J Urol 1995;154:1295–1299.
14 Bostwick DG, Pacelli A, Lopez-Beltran A: Molecular biology of prostatic intraepithelial neoplasia. Prostate 1996;29:117.
15 Sakr WA, Haas GP, Cassin BJ et al: The frequency of carcinoma and intraepithelial neoplasia of the prostate in young male patients. J Urol 1993;150:379–385.
16 Sakr WA, Grignon DJ, Crissman JD, Heilbrun LK, Cassin BJ, Pontes JJE, Haas GP: High grade prostatic intraepithelial neoplasia and prostatic adenocarcinoma between the ages of 20–69: An autopsy study of 249 cases. In Vivo 1994;8:439–444.
17 Sakr WA, Haas GP, Cassin BJ et al: The frequency of carcinoma and intraepithelial neoplasia of the prostate in young male patients. J Urol 1993;150:379–385.
18 Qian J, Wollan P, Bostwick DG: The extent and multicentricity of high grade prostatic intraepithelial neoplasia in clinically localized prostatic adenocarcinoma. Hum Pathol 1997; 28:143–148.
19 Aquilina JW, McKinney L, Pacelli A, Richman LK, Waters DJ, Thompson I, Burghardt WF Jr, Bostowick DG: High grade prostatic intraepithelial neoplasia in military working dogs with and without prostate cancer. Prostate 1998;36: 189–193.
20 Waters DJ, Bostwick DG, Murphy GP: Conference summary: First international workshop on animal models of prostate cancer. Prostate 1998;36:46–48.
21 Billis A: Latent carcinoma and atypical lesions of prostate: An autopsy study. Urology 1986; 28:324–329.

Preclinical Models for Drug Discovery

European Urology

Eur Urol 1999;35:459–463

Use of Animal Models in Defining Efficacy of Chemoprevention Agents against Prostate Cancer

Maarten C. Bosland

Departments of Environmental Medicine and Urology, New York University School of Medicine, New York, N.Y., USA

Key Words

Prostate cancer · Chemoprevention · Animal models · Efficacy testing · Predictive value

Abstract

Animal models are crucial in preclinical efficacy testing of chemoprevention agents. The most feasible, realistic, and potentially effective target for prostate cancer chemoprevention is progression from prostatic intraepithelial neoplasia (PIN) to histologic cancer and from histologic to clinically manifest cancer. There are transgenic mouse models for prostate cancer and models for PIN, but these have not yet been fully developed and evaluated for chemoprevention studies. Human prostate cancer xenografts in mice and transplantable Dunning rat prostate carcinomas can be used to assess tumor growth inhibition. Several Dunning tumors metastasize, enabling detection of inhibition of metastases. Detection of inhibitory effects on de novo prostate cancer development requires induction of a high cancer incidence and similarity of induced tumors to human prostate carcinomas. Transgenic mice with oncogenes expressed in a prostate-specific fashion, combined chronic treatment of NBL rats with estradiol-17β and testosterone, and sequential treatment of rats with carcinogens such as *N*-methyl-*N*-nitrosourea (MNU) and chronic testosterone treatment all lead to a high incidence of prostatic adenocarcinomas. PIN occurs mostly in the former two models, and metastases are frequent in some transgenic models and the MNU-testosterone rat model. The latter model has been applied to chemoprevention agent efficacy testing. In 8 control groups, the carcinoma incidence was 77% in all accessory sex glands combined, 51% for small tumors confined to dorsolateral/anterior prostate, and 25% for large tumors of uncertain origin in the prostate area. This model was predictive of the lack of antiprostate cancer efficacy of *N*-(4-hydroxyphenyl)all-*trans*-retinamide in humans. Thus, rats given MNU and chronic testosterone represent a relevant and reliable model for efficacy testing of chemoprevention agents. In conclusion, there are now adequate animal models for prostate cancer proven to be suitable for preclinical chemoprevention studies.

Animal models are a crucial element in the development of cancer chemoprevention agents. The core objective of using animal models in this process is preclinical efficacy testing of candidate chemoprevention substances in in vivo models of cancer development to guide in the selection of agents for clinical trials. There are adequate animal models for many major human cancers, but such models for prostate cancer have long been lacking. In recent years, several animal models have been developed,

KARGER

Fax + 41 61 306 12 34
E-Mail karger@karger.ch
www.karger.com

0302–2838/99/0356–0459$17.50/0

Accessible online at:
http://BioMedNet.com/karger

Dr. Maarten C. Bosland
Department of Environmental Medicine, New York University School of Medicine
550 First Avenue, New York, NY 10016 (USA)
Tel. +1 212 951 5428, Fax +1 212 951 5424
E-Mail maarten.bosland@med.nyu.edu

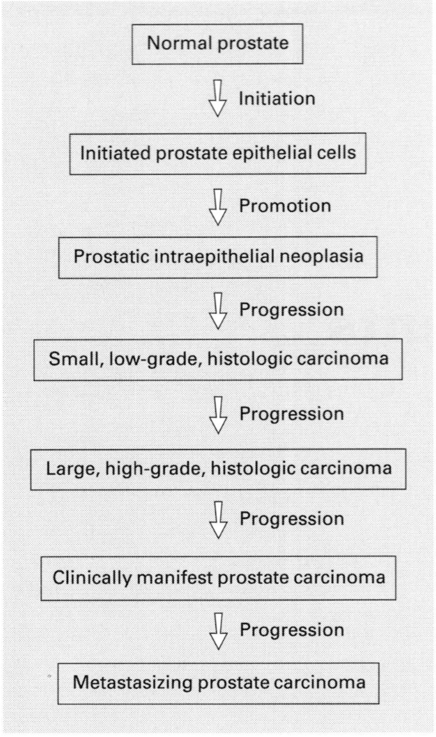

Fig. 1. Schematic representation of the putative multistep process of human prostate carcinogenesis. Although this figure suggests one single pathway of prostate cancer development, there are likely to be many pathways which may not each involve every stage depicted here and there are likely to be a variety of multistep molecular mechanisms involved.

characterized, and evaluated that allow detection of chemoinhibitory effects in various stages of prostate cancer development [1–4]. Critical issues in using prostate cancer animal models for chemoprevention studies are: (a) the relevance of the model for human prostate cancer; (b) the adequacy of the model for cancer chemoprevention studies; (c) the relevance of the lesion(s) occurring in the model for human lesions that are targets for chemoprevention, and (d) the predictive value of the results of model studies with specific agents for prostate cancer chemoprevention efficacy in humans.

Relevance and Adequacy

Requirements of an ideal adequate animal model of prostate cancer for chemoprevention experiments have been discussed previously [1]. In summary, the tumors developing in such a model must display a reasonable degree of similarity with human prostate cancer. Thus, they must be adenocarcinomas that are metastasizing, androgen-sensitive, and slowly growing. They should also originate in tissue that has homology to the human prostate; in mice and rats this is the dorsolateral or anterior prostate (not the ventral prostate lobe). In addition, the tumors should mimic the natural history and pathogenesis of human prostate cancer, and harbor similar molecular alterations and develop from similar precursor lesions such as prostatic intraepithelial neoplasia (PIN). The model should possess identifiable initiation, promotion, and progression stages that can be separately studied, and tumor incidence should be high, to allow detection of inhibition of carcinogenesis. However, tumor incidence should not be 100%, because overwhelmingly strong tumor-inducing stimuli may interfere with the model's sensitivity to identify cancer-inhibiting properties of candidate agents.

Target Lesions of Human Prostate Cancer

As traditionally defined, the concept of chemoprevention applies to interference with the development of cancer prior to the fully malignant state. With respect to prostate cancer, this implies interference with the development of PIN and with the progression of PIN to invasive cancer. However, not all prostate cancers develop from PIN and microscopic-size (or histologic) prostate cancer is very frequent, even at young age. There are several studies indicating that the prevalence of histologic prostate cancer may be as high as 35% in men between the ages of 30 and 40 [W.A. Sakr, this issue]. Histologic prostate cancer probably occurs in more than 50% of men of the age groups in which prostate cancer is usually detected clinically, apparently *regardless* of their risk for clinical prostate cancer; histologic prostate cancer is roughly equally frequent in male populations around the world that differ greatly in risk for clinically manifest prostate cancer [5; W.A. Sakr, this issue]. Clinical prostate cancer, however, is frequent only at old age, and risk in most Western countries is between 10 and 15%. Consequently, prostate cancer chemoprevention should not only target the development and progression of PIN, but also growth and progression of histologic prostate cancer. Locally extended prostate cancer is manageable, but prostate cancer metastases lead to death and their development should be an additional important target of chemoprevention. In other words, to be really effective, chemoprevention agents should inhibit several of the stages in the multistep process of prostate carcinogenesis summarized in figure 1, and they must be particularly active against the later steps in this process. Animal models that are adequate for prostate cancer chemoprevention studies must, therefore, comprise several, ideally all, of the various stages in prostate carcinogenesis depicted in figure 1.

Potential Models Relevant Target Lesions

There are to date no reliable and adequate animal models of PIN. PIN has only been reported to occur in the NBL rat model (NBL rats treated chronically with testosterone and estradiol-17β [6]), in one transgenic mouse model (the so-called TRAMP model [4, 7]), and spontaneously in aging dogs [D.J. Waters, this issue]. However, the PIN-like lesion in the NBL model is not the precursor of the prostate carcinomas found in this model [6], and the adequacy and feasibility of the transgenic mouse and dog models of PIN are uncertain at present. Histologic prostate cancer and clinical prostate cancer (symptom-producing and ultimately fatal) occurs in some transgenic mouse models and can be induced in the NBL rat model and in several rat prostate cancer induction models [2–4, 6, 8]. In addition, there is a growing number of human prostate cancer xenograft models and some rat transplantable tumors that provide models of prostate cancer growth and progression; good examples are the androgen-sensitive PC-82, PC-346, CWR-22, LAPC-4, and LuCaP-23 xenograft models [2, 8] and the Dunning rat R3327-H tumor [2, 3]. Prostate cancer metastases occur in some transgenic mouse models, most rat induction models, and some rat transplantable tumor systems, and when human prostate cancer cells are orthotopically injected into nude mice [2–4, 7, 8]. However, none of these models have been sufficiently evaluated with exception of some of the metastatic Dunning rat R-3327 models.

High Incidence Prostate Cancer Models Potentially Suited for Chemoprevention Studies

There are basically three different model approaches that lead to a high incidence of prostate cancer in experimental animals: (1) Prostate-targeted carcinogen treatment of rats followed by chronic androgen administration results in a 70–90% incidence of metastasizing adenocarcinomas in some rat strains, but no PIN is induced [8–13]. (2) Combined chronic treatment of NBL rats with testosterone and estradiol-17β induces a 65–100% incidence of PIN and nonmetastasizing adenocarcinoma [6, D.L. McCormick et al., unpubl. data]. (3) Prostate-targeted expression of SV40/T-antigen in mice achieved by transgenic techniques leads to a 100% incidence of metastasizing adenocarcinoma in some of these models and PIN in one model [4, 7]. Androgen sensitivity of the carcinomas induced in any of these models is uncertain, but very likely, because exogenous androgen treatment is required in the first two models [6, 8–13], and in some of the transgenic mouse models the expression of SV40/T-antigen is driven by androgen [4, 7]. Once the tumors in these models become very large and near fatal, they appear to have become androgen-independent. Thus, none of these models possesses all desired properties for an ideal prostate cancer animal model for preclinical chemoprevention studies. The very high (100%) prostate carcinoma incidence in the transgenic models may preclude adequate sensitivity to detect inhibitory activity of chemoprevention agents. The lack of progression to metastatic disease limits the significance of the NBL model. The only model systems that have been evaluated in chemoprevention experiments are induction models in rats treated with carcinogens and androgens [9, 10; D.L. McCormick and K.N.V Rao, this issue].

High Incidence Induction Rat Prostate Cancer Models

The induction of prostate cancer may to some extent be dependent on the rat strain used. Wistar rats, the HsdCpb:WU and the Lobund-Wistar strains, Fisher (F344) rats, and MRC (Wistar-derived?) rats have been used to induce prostate cancer by the following three different prostate-targeted carcinogen treatments: 10 repeat injections of 3,2′-dimethyl-4-aminobiphenyl (F344 rats) [11], or hormonal (androgenic) stimulation of prostatic cell proliferation followed by either 1–3 injections of *N*-nitrosobis(oxopropyl)amine (MRC rats) [12] or a single injection of *N*-methyl-*N*-nitrosourea (MNU) (WU and Lobund-Wistar rats) [8–10, 13]. In all three models chronic androgen administration (testosterone via slow-release Silastic implants) subsequent to carcinogen treatment is required to obtain a high incidence. Of these three models, only the MNU plus testosterone treatment of WU and Lobund-Wistar rats has been used for chemoprevention experiments in several laboratories [9; D.L. McCormick and K.N.V Rao, this issue]. The WU model reproducibly yields mostly adenocarcinomas of the dorsolateral and anterior prostate [8, 9], whereas the Lobund-

Table 1. Adenocarcinoma incidences of dorsolateral prostate, anterior prostate and seminal vesicles in eight repeat experiments in Wistar rats[a]

	% incidence (range)			
Number of studies	1	3	4	All 8
Number of animals	32	100	142	274
Study duration, months	15	14	13	13–15
Location and size of adenocarcinoma				
All accessory sex glands combined	84	76 (72–83)	75 (63–80)	77
Dorsolateral prostate region (large tumors[b])	53	35 (33–38)	10 (5–18)	25
Confined to dorsolateral/anterior prostate (histologic tumors[c])	44	49 (41–54)	53 (35–65)	51
Anterior prostate/seminal vesicle region (large tumors[b])	6	13 (6–9)	7 (3–11)	9
Confined to seminal vesicle only (no other tumors)	16	6 (0–6)	8 (3–20)	7

[a] In each experiment, HsdCpb:WU rats were given sequential treatment with cyproterone acetate, testosterone propionate, and MNU, followed by chronic testosterone administration [8, 9].
[b] The exact origin of these large tumors is not clear.
[c] Histologic tumors were 3 mm in diameter or smaller, most macroscopically evident tumors were at least 5 mm in diameter.

Wistar model results in more seminal vesicle tumors than prostate carcinomas [10].

To illustrate the consistency of the WU model, the incidences of accessory sex gland carcinomas in the control groups of eight separate chemoprevention experiments are presented in table 1. The overall incidence of accessory sex gland carcinomas was remarkably stable. As the study duration increased from 13 to 15 months, the number of large (>4 mm diameter) carcinomas of uncertain origin located in the dorsolateral prostate region increased while the number of small (<4 mm) tumors that clearly originated in the dorsolateral or anterior prostate decreased. The incidence of tumors located in the anterior prostate/seminal vesicle region (uncertain origin) or confined to the seminal vesicle was relatively low and was not substantially affected by study duration. These data clearly indicate that the vast majority of carcinomas in this model originate in the dorsolateral prostate and that modifying the duration of experiments allows to study growth and progression of prostate cancer. By starting intervention at different times after MNU injection and by separate analysis of small and large carcinomas one can define the stages of prostate cancer development and progression which are inhibited by agents [1, 8, 9; D.L. McCormick and K.N.V Rao, this issue]. Despite these strengths of this model, there are some problems associated with it and with the Lobund-Wistar model. Neither rat strain is generally available and there are several, poorly defined, breeding stocks of the Lobund-Wistar rat. The induction protocol of the WU model is somewhat complicated, time-consuming, and expensive. Further improvement of particularly the WU model is thus desirable. Preliminary results indicate that generally available strains (e.g., F344) may be suitable substitute for the WU rat strain [14].

Predictive Value of Preclinical Models

The predictive value of preclinical models of prostate cancer is to a large extent uncertain at present. There is only one example of a chemoprevention agent for which information about concordance of efficacy results across model systems is available, *N*-(4-hydroxyphenyl)all-*trans*-retinamide (4-HPR). 4-HPR lacks efficacy in both the WU and Lobund-Wistar models [9, 10], but in a mouse model of fetal urogenital sinus cells infected with v-*ras* and v-*myc* oncogenes which following implantation under renal capsule develop into cancer inhibition by 4-HPR was found [15]. 4-HPR also inhibited the growth of the transplantable Dunning R3327-Mat-LyLu rat prostatic carcinoma which is fast growing and metastatic [16]. This synthetic retinoid is the only compound for which there are some human data available at present. Pienta et al. [17] gave 4-HPR to men with elevated PSA (4–20 ng/ml) and negative biopsy. This study was stopped early because several men developed clinically detectable prostate cancer and no inhibitory effect of 4-HPR was evident. In a placebo-controlled study with 4-HPR administration to men during a 4- to 8-week period prior to radical prostatectomy no effect was found on histologic, morphometric, and other parameters [D. Urban et al., this issue]. Thus, both the WU and Lobund-Wistar models, but not the v-*ras*-v-*myc* mouse model or the Dunning rat model, were predictive for the observed (lack of) efficacy in human models.

Conclusions

The most feasible, realistic, and potentially effective target for prostate cancer chemoprevention is progression from PIN to histologic cancer and from histologic to clinically manifest cancer, including metastatic disease. There are several transgenic mouse models for prostate cancer and models for PIN and prostate cancer metastases, but these have not yet been fully developed and evaluated for use in chemoprevention studies. WU rats given MNU and chronic testosterone represent a relevant and reliable model for efficacy testing of chemoprevention agents in these stages of prostate cancer development. However, further refinement of this model is desirable in terms of a generally available rat strain and simplified induction treatment. Although the model of Lobund-Wistar rats given MNU and testosterone produces predominantly seminal vesicle tumors, it was equally predictive of the lack of antiprostate cancer efficacy of 4-HPR in humans as the WU rat model. In comparison with well-established animal models of major human cancer sites such as breast and colon cancer, there are now equally adequate animal models for prostate cancer that are proven to be suitable for preclinical chemoprevention studies.

Acknowledgments

This work was supported in part by PHS Grants CA46426, CA72290 and CA16087, and Contracts N01-CN-85097-08, N01-CN-85097-09, N01-CN-35566-02 and N01-CN-65120 from the National Cancer Institute. The author thank Drs. David L. McCormick and K.V.N. Rao for their continued collaboration and Larry Richards, Lori Horton and Joanne Schmoll for their expert technical assistance.

References

1 Bosland MC: Animal models for the study of prostate carcinogenesis. J Cell Biochem 1992;suppl 16H:89–98.
2 Bosland MC, Chung LWK, Greenberg NM, Ho SH, Isaacs JT, Lane K, Peehl DM, Thompson TC, van Steenbrugge GJ, van Weerden WM: Recent advances in the development of cell culture models for prostate cancer research. Urol Oncol 1996;2:99–128.
3 Lucia MS, Bostwick DG, Bosland M, Cockett ATK, Knapp DW, Leav I, Pollard M, Rinker-Schaeffer C, Shirai T, Watkins B: Rodent models of prostate cancer. Prostate 1998;36:49–55.
4 Green JE, Greenberg NM, Ashendel CL, Barrett JC, Boone C, Getzenberg RH, Henkin J, Matusik R, Janus TJ, Scher HI: Transgenic and reconstitution models of prostate cancer. Prostate 1998;36:59–63.
5 Bosland MC: The etiopathogenesis of prostate cancer with special reference to environmental factors. Adv Cancer Res 1988;51:1–106.
6 Bosland MC, Ford H, Horton L: Induction at high incidence of ductal prostate adenocarcinomas in NBL/Cr and Sprague-Dawley Hsd:SD rats treated with a combination of testosterone and estradiol-17β or diethylstilbestrol. Carcinogenesis 1995;16:1311–1317.
7 Greenberg NM: Transgenic models for prostate cancer research. Urol Oncol 1996;2:119–122.
8 Bosland MC: Chemical and hormonal induction of prostate cancer in animal models. Urol Oncol 1996;2:103–110.
9 McCormick DL, Rao KVN, Dooley L, Steele VE, Lubet RA, Kelloff GJ, Bosland MC: Influence of *N*-methyl-*N*-nitrosourea, testosterone, and *N*-(4-hydroxyphenyl)-all-*trans*-retinamide on prostate cancer induction in Wistar (WU) rats. Cancer Res 1998;58:3282–3288.
10 Lucia MS, Anzano MA, Slayter MV, Anver MR, Green DM, Shrader MW, Logsdon DL, Driver CL, Brown CC, Peer CW, Roberts AB, Sporn MB: Chemopreventive activity of tamoxifen, N-(4-hydroxyphenyl)retinamide, and the vitamin D analogue Ro24-5531 for androgen-promoted carcinomas of the rat seminal vesicle and prostate. Cancer Res 1995;55: 5621–5627.
11 Shirai T, Tamano S, Kato T, Iwasaki S, Takahashi S, Ito N: Induction of invasive carcinomas in the accessory sex organs other than the ventral prostate of rats given 3,2′-dimethyl-4-aminobiphenyl and testosterone propionate. Cancer Res 1991;51:1264–1269.
12 Pour PM, Stepan K: Induction of prostatic carcinomas and lower urinary tract neoplasms by combined treatment of intact and castrated rats with testosterone propionate and *N*-nitrosobis(2-oxopropyl)amine. Cancer Res 1987;47: 5699–5705.
13 Pollard M, Luckert PH: Production of autochthonous prostate cancer in Lobund-Wistar rats by treatments with *N*-nitroso-*N*-methylurea and testosterone. J Natl Cancer Inst 1986;77: 583–587.
14 Bosland MC, Horton L, Dennison J: Induction of prostatic adenocarcinomas by *N*-methyl-*N*-nitrosourea and testosterone in Lobund-Wistar rats and five other rat strains. Proc Am Assoc Cancer Res 1996;37:244.
15 Slawin K, Kadmon D, Park SH, Scardino PT, Anzano M, Sporn MB, Thompson TC: Dietary fenretinide, a synthetic retinoid, decreases the tumor incidence and the tumor mass of ras+myc-induced carcinomas in the mouse prostate reconstitution model system. Cancer Res 1993;53:4461–4463.
16 Pienta KJ, Nguyen NM, Lehr JE: Treatment of prostate cancer in the rat with the synthetic retinoid fenretinide. Cancer Res 1993;53:224–226.
17 Pienta KJ, Esper PS, Zwas F, Krzeminski R, Flaherty LE: Phase II chemoprevention trial of oral fenretinide in patients at risk for adenocarcinoma of the prostate. Am J Clin Oncol 1997; 20:36–39.

Preclinical Models for Drug Discovery

European Urology

Eur Urol 1999;35:464–467

Chemoprevention of Hormone-Dependent Prostate Cancer in the Wistar-Unilever Rat

David L. McCormick K.V.N. Rao

Experimental Toxicology and Carcinogenesis Division, IIT Research Institute, Chicago, Ill., USA

Key Words

Prostate cancer · Chemoprevention · Dehydroepiandrosterone · 9-*cis*-Retinoic acid · α-Difluoromethylornithine · *L*-Selenomethionine · *DL*-α-Tocopherol (vitamin E) · Liarozole fumarate · *N*-(4-Hydroxyphenyl)retinamide (fenretinide) · Oltipraz

Abstract

The high incidence and long latent period of prostate cancer make it an ideal target for chemoprevention. We have evaluated a series of agents for chemopreventive efficacy using a model in which hormone-dependent prostate cancers are induced in the Wistar-Unilever (WU) rat by sequential treatment with antiandrogen (cyproterone acetate), androgen (testosterone propionate), and direct-acting chemical carcinogen (*N*-methyl-*N*-nitrosourea), followed by chronic androgen stimulation (testosterone). This regimen reproducibly induces prostate cancers in high incidence, with no gross toxicity and a low incidence of neoplasia in the seminal vesicle and other non-target tissues. Dehydroepiandrosterone (DHEA) and 9-*cis*-retinoic acid (9-*cis*-RA) are the most active agents identified to date. DHEA inhibits prostate cancer induction both when chronic administration is begun prior to carcinogen exposure, and when administration is delayed until preneoplastic prostate lesions are present. 9-*cis*-RA is the most potent inhibitor of prostate carcinogenesis identified; a study to determine the efficacy of delayed administration of 9-*cis*-RA is in progress. Liarozole fumarate confers modest protection against prostate carcinogenesis, while *N*-(4-hydroxyphenyl)retinamide (fenretinide), α-difluoromethylornithine, oltipraz, *DL*-α-tocopherol acetate (vitamin E), and *L*-selenomethionine are inactive. Chemoprevention efficacy evaluations in the WU rat will support the identification of agents that merit study for prostate cancer chemoprevention in humans.

Introduction

Carcinoma of the prostate presents an excellent target for chemoprevention: the disease occurs in high incidence in Western populations [1], has a predictable natural history in terms of age of onset [2], and generally presents with an indolent clinical course that offers a relatively long time period for interventions directed at disease prevention or stabilization. The ubiquitous nature of prostatic intraepithelial neoplasia (PIN) and subclinical prostate cancer in otherwise healthy men [3, 4], when considered with the often long period of preneoplasia and in situ disease development in the prostate [4], suggests that inhibi-

KARGER

Fax + 41 61 306 12 34
E-Mail karger@karger.ch
www.karger.com

0302–2838/99/0356–0464$17.50/0

Accessible online at:
http://BioMedNet.com/karger

D.L. McCormick
IIT Research Institute, 10 West 35 Street
Chicago, IL 60616 (USA)
Tel. +1 312 567 4972, Fax +1 312 567 4466
E-Mail dmccormick@iitri.org

tion of tumor promotion or progression may result in significant decreases in morbidity and mortality associated with prostatic malignancy.

Since carcinoma of the prostate occurs primarily in older populations, any delay in the time course of neoplastic development achieved through pharmacologic intervention could result in a substantial reduction in cancer incidence. Furthermore, even a modest reduction in the slope of the tumor latency curve could delay the onset of prostate cancer in individuals at risk for the disease until much later in life. On this basis, development of effective drugs for prevention of prostate cancer may not only reduce disease incidence and associated morbidity, but may also result in a significant decrease in cancer mortality. To date, however, few drugs have been identified that confer significant protection against prostate cancer induction in relevant in vivo model systems.

Until recently, a significant limitation to drug discovery for prostate cancer chemoprevention was the lack of in vivo carcinogenesis models in which hormone-dependent prostate cancers are induced (a) in a time frame suitable for chemopreventive intervention, and (b) without significant neoplastic development in the seminal vesicle and other nontarget tissues. This limitation has been addressed through the development and validation of a model system in which male Wistar-Unilever (WU) rats are treated with a sequential regimen of antiandrogen, androgen, and chemical carcinogen, followed by chronic androgen stimulation [5–7]. This regimen induces hormone-dependent prostate adenocarcinomas in an anatomic site that is analogous to the primary location of prostate cancer in humans [5, 6]; induced cancers have a latency of 12–15 months. This report summarizes the results of a series of chemoprevention efficacy evaluations conducted using the WU rat prostate cancer model system, and identifies two agents whose anticarcinogenic efficacy suggests potential activity in human prostate cancer chemoprevention.

Materials and Methods

Experimental Animals. All studies are performed using male WU rats, obtained from American or European colonies maintained by Harlan/Sprague-Dawley. Rats are 7–8 weeks of age when received from the supplier, and are held in quarantine for a minimum of 1 week prior to the initiation of hormone pretreatment.

Hormone Pretreatment. Beginning 24 days prior to carcinogen administration, rats receive daily oral (gavage) administration of 50 mg cyproterone acetate per kg body weight for 21 consecutive days. One day after the final dose of cyproterone acetate, rats receive daily subcutaneous injections of 100 mg testosterone propionate per kg body weight for 3 days.

Carcinogen Administration and Androgen Promotion. Sixty hours after the first dose of testosterone propionate, rats receive a single intravenous injection of *N*-methyl-*N*-nitrosourea (MNU). We have conducted prostate cancer chemoprevention studies using MNU doses of 50 and 30 mg/kg body weight; use of the lower carcinogen dose improves animal survival and general health, reduces the incidence of neoplasms in nontarget tissues, and as a result, increases the incidence of prostate cancer. One to 2 weeks after carcinogen administration, rats receive subcutaneous implants of two silastic tubes containing 40 mg crystalline testosterone each. Silastic tubes are replaced at 6-month intervals throughout the studies.

Chemopreventive Agent Administration. In our standard protocol, chemopreventive agents are administered as dietary supplements, beginning 1 week prior to MNU administration. In follow-up studies to evaluate chemopreventive activity when drug administration is begun in the presence of preneoplastic prostate lesions, chemopreventive agents are administered beginning at 20 and 40 weeks after MNU administration. Administration of chemopreventive agents is continuous until termination of individual studies at approximately 13 months.

Necropsy, Histology, and Histopathology. At necropsy, all gross lesions are excised, and the accessory sex glands and urinary bladder are carefully removed en bloc from each rat and fixed in 10% neutral buffered formalin. After fixation, accessory sex glands are embedded in paraffin, and six step sections each are prepared at intervals of 200 μm from the dorsolateral prostate region and from the anterior prostate + seminal vesicle region. In addition, a single section is prepared from the ventral prostate of each animal. Tissues are stained with hematoxylin and eosin for histopathological evaluation. The approach used to classify accessory sex gland tumors in the rat has been described in detail [7, 8].

Results and Discussion

In order to maximize the probability of identifying active compounds, initial prostate cancer chemoprevention studies were focused on agents that demonstrate significant anticarcinogenic activity in other tissues. Subsequent studies have been designed to investigate mechanistic leads, to investigate the chemopreventive activity of agent combinations, and to determine whether chemopreventive activity is retained when agent administration is delayed until preneoplastic lesions are present in the prostate. The results of these studies are summarized in table 1.

We have identified two agents that confer significant protection against prostate cancer induction in the WU rat model system. The most potent inhibitor of prostate carcinogenesis identified to date is 9-*cis*-retinoic acid (9-*cis*-RA), the natural ligand for the retinoid 'X' nuclear receptor (RXR). Dietary administration of 9-*cis*-RA reduced cancer incidence in the dorsolateral and anterior

Table 1. Agents evaluated for efficacy in the prevention of prostate cancer in the WU rat

Agent	Dose levels mg/kg diet	Activity	Reference
9-*cis*-Retinoic acid	100 50	active active	9
9-*cis*-Retinoic acid (delayed administration)	100	in progress	–
Dehydroepiandrosterone (DHEA)	2,000 1,000	active active	10
Dehydroepiandrosterone (delayed administration)	2,000	active	11
Liarozole fumarate	160 120	marginal marginal	13
N-(4-Hydroxyphenyl)retinamide (4-HPR)	391	inactive	7
L-Selenomethionine	3.0 1.5	inactive inactive	9
DL-α-Tocopherol acetate (vitamin E)	4,000 2,000	inactive inactive	9
α-Difluoromethylornithine (DFMO)	2,000 1,000	inactive inactive	13
Oltipraz	250 125	inactive inactive	13

prostate of MNU-treated rats by more than two-thirds, and did not induce characteristic 'retinoid-like' toxicities upon chronic administration [9]. When considered with its ligand binding profile, the potent chemopreventive activity of 9-*cis*-RA may provide insight into mechanisms of retinoid chemoprevention in the prostate. 9-*cis*-RA is a pan-agonist that binds both to RXR and to the nuclear receptor for retinoic acid (RAR). By contrast, *N*-(4-hydroxyphenyl)-all-*trans*-retinamide (4-HPR; fenretinide), the hydroxyphenylamide analog of all-*trans*-retinoic acid, is inactive as a chemopreventive agent in the WU prostate cancer model system [7]. 4-HPR and metabolites do not bind to RXR, suggesting that RXR binding may be essential for retinoid chemopreventive activity in this target tissue.

The adrenal 17-ketosteroid, dehydroepiandrosterone (DHEA), also confers significant protection against prostate cancer induction in the WU model system [10]. DHEA appears to act primarily by suppressing the transition from carcinoma in situ to invasive (microscopic and macroscopic) prostate cancer. Supporting this hypothesis is the finding that DHEA retains essentially all of its chemopreventive activity when its administration is delayed until 20 or 40 weeks after carcinogen administration [11]. At these times, incipient neoplastic lesions are present in the prostate of WU rats; DHEA appears to prevent the progression of these lesions into invasive carcinoma.

In addition to its efficacy in prostate cancer chemoprevention [10, 11], DHEA is the most potent inhibitor of rat mammary carcinogenesis ever evaluated in our laboratory [12]. Its suppression of androgen-dependent as well as estrogen-dependent cancers suggests that DHEA action is not effected through a simple hormonal or antihormonal mechanism. Unfortunately, the toxicity of DHEA may make it unsuitable for chronic administration to humans. To identify an agent with a more desirable toxicity profile, a study to evaluate the activity of a fluorinated DHEA analog (fluasterone) as an inhibitor of prostate carcinogenesis is currently in progress.

Other agents have demonstrated at most modest efficacy in prostate cancer prevention in the WU model system. Dietary administration of liarozole fumarate, an imidazole derivative, resulted in a significant reduction in the number of macroscopic cancers induced by MNU + testosterone [13]; however, the compound had no effect on total cancer incidence. These data suggest that while liarozole may suppress the transition of carcinomas from microscopic to macroscopic size, the compound has little effect on other stages of neoplastic development in the prostate.

The retinoid, 4-HPR [7], and several other agents with a broad range of chemopreventive activity in animal models confer no protection against prostate cancer induction. No differences from the prostate cancer incidence observed in dietary control groups were seen in rats receiving chronic dietary exposure to maximum tolerated dose levels of: the ornithine decarboxylase inhibitor, α-difluoromethylornithine [13]; *DL*-α-tocopherol acetate (vitamin E) [14]; the natural organoselenium compound, *L*-selenomethionine [9]; or the inducer of phase II enzyme activity, oltipraz [13].

Acknowledgements

Research supported by contracts N01-CN-85097-08, N01-CN-85097-09, N01-CN-35566-02, and N01-CN-65120 from the US National Cancer Institute. The authors thank Drs. Maarten Bosland, Ronald Lubet, Vernon Steele and Gary Kelloff for their continued collaboration, and Teresa Bowman-Gram, Lawrence Dooley and Gloria Smith for excellent technical assistance.

References

1 Landis SH, Murray T, Bolden S, Wingo PA: Cancer statistics, 1998. CA Cancer J Clin 1998; 48:6–29.
2 Lalani el-N, Laniado ME, Abel PD: Molecular and cellular biology of prostate cancer. Cancer Metastasis Rev 1996;16:29–66.
3 Nelson PS, Gleason TP, Brawer MK: Chemoprevention for prostatic intraepithelial neoplasia. Eur Urol 1996;30:269–278.
4 Bostwick DG: Prospective origins of prostate carcinoma. Prostatic intraepithelial neoplasia and atypical adenomatous hyperplasia. Cancer 1996;78:330–336.
5 Bosland MC, Prinsen MK: Induction of dorsolateral prostate adenocarcinomas and other accessory sex gland lesions in male Wistar rats by a single administration of *N*-methyl-*N*-nitrosourea, 7,12-dimethylbenz(*a*)anthracene, and 3,2′-dimethyl-4-aminobiphenyl after sequential treatment with cyproterone acetate and testosterone propionate. Cancer Res 1990;50: 691–699.
6 Bosland MC, Prinsen MK, Dirksen TJM, Spit BJ: Characterization of adenocarcinomas of the dorsolateral prostate induced in Wistar rats by *N*-methyl-*N*-nitrosourea, 7,12-dimethylbenz(*a*)anthracene, and 3,2′-dimethyl-4-aminobiphenyl, following sequential treatment with cyproterone acetate and testosterone propionate. Cancer Res 1990;50:700–709.
7 McCormick DL, Rao KVN, Dooley L, Lubet RA, Steele VE, Kelloff GJ, Bosland MC: Influence of *N*-methyl-*N*-nitrosourea, testosterone, and *N*-(4-hydroxyphenyl)-all-*trans*-retinamide on prostate cancer induction in Wistar (WU) rats. Cancer Res 1998;58:3282–3288.
8 Bosland MC: Age-related lesions in the male accessory sex glands and penis of the rat; in Mohr U, et al (eds): Monographs on Pathology of the Aging Rat. Washington, ILSI Press, 1992, vol 1, pp 443–467.
9 McCormick DL, Rao KVN, Steele VE, Lubet RA, Kelloff GJ, Bosland MC: Chemoprevention of rat prostate carcinogenesis by 9-*cis*-retinoic acid. Cancer Res 1999;59:521–524.
10 McCormick DL, Rao KVN, Bosland MC, Steele VE, Lubet RA, Kelloff GJ: Inhibition of rat prostatic carcinogenesis by dietary dehydroepiandrosterone but not by N-(4-hydroxyphenyl)-all-*trans*-retinamide. Proc Am Assoc Cancer Res 1995;36:126.
11 Rao KVN, Bosland MC, Lubet RA, Steele VE, Kelloff GJ, McCormick DL: Inhibition of rat prostate carcinogenesis by delayed administration of dehydroepiandrosterone. Proc Am Assoc Cancer Res 1997;38:580.
12 McCormick DL, Rao KVN, Johnson WD, Bowman-Gram TA, Steele VE, Lubet RA, Kelloff GJ: Exceptional chemopreventive activity of low dose dehydroepiandrosterone in the rat mammary gland. Cancer Res 1996;56:1724–1726.
13 Rao KVN, McCormick DL, Bosland MC, Steele VE, Lubet RA, Kelloff GJ: Chemopreventive efficacy evaluation of liarozole fumarate, difluoromethylornithine, and oltipraz in the rat prostate. Proc Am Assoc Cancer Res 1996;37:273.
14 McCormick DL, Rao KVN, Lubet RA, Steele VE, Kelloff GJ, Bosland MC: Differential activity of 9-*cis*-retinoic acid, α-tocopherol, and selenomethionine as chemopreventive agents in the rat prostate. Proc Am Assoc Cancer Res 1997;38:261.

Surrogate Endpoint Biomarkers for Clinical Trials of Prostate Cancer Chemoprevention

European Urology

Eur Urol 1999;35:468–473

Subtle Morphological and Molecular Changes in Normal-Looking Epithelium in Prostates with Prostatic Intraepithelial Neoplasia or Cancer

Rodolfo Montironi[a] Peter W. Hamilton[b] Marina Scarpelli[a]
Deborah Thompson[c] Peter H. Bartels[c]

[a]Institute of Pathological Anatomy and Histopathology, School of Medicine, University of Ancona, Italy;
[b]Department of Pathology, The Queen's University of Belfast, N. Ireland; [c]Optical Sciences Center, University of Arizona, Tucson, Ariz., USA

Key Words

Prostate · Prostatic intraepithelial neoplasia · Invasive adenocarcinoma · Malignancy-associated changes · Enzyme-altered foci · Glutathione S-transferase · Telomerase · DNA adducts · Image analysis

Abstract

Background: Prostate cancer develops over an extended period of time. Until recently, the events initiating the process and the developments concomitant with the evolution towards invasive disease were largely unknown. ***Methods:*** Analytical and quantitative methods are applied to provide insights into certain individual molecular events and their effects on the complex multiple feedback system of cellular metabolism and regulation in prostate neoplasia. ***Results:*** Prostatic intraepithelial neoplasia (PIN) and prostate cancer (PCa) are associated with or possibly preceded by changes in the chromatin of secretory cell nuclei. The changes are detectable with a Bayesian belief network and quantifiable by computer image analysis in prostatic tissue that still appears histologically normal. In addition, normal-looking prostate epithelium shows some molecular changes similar to those present in the associated preneoplastic and neoplastic lesions. Such changes are also occasionally present in normal prostate glands without PIN and cancer. ***Conclusions:*** The subtle morphological and molecular changes of normal-looking epithelium might be seen as the onset of the development of prostatic neoplasia.

Introduction

One of the two main issues in prostate pathology is the identification of those prognostic factors that could predict the exact outcome in individual patients with prostate cancer. The goal is to tailor the therapeutic approach to the clinical, morphological and biological features of each patient. The other issue involves the early detection of PCa, preferably in the preinvasive phase, to treat the patient efficaciously. Therefore, understanding the morphology and biology of the preinvasive or precursor lesions has become increasingly important [1].

Precursors of PCa

Prostatic intraepithelial neoplasia is the most likely precursor of PCa, especially of peripheral zone carcinoma [2]. The progression from PIN to PCa is a complex process in which the kinetic organization of the normal epi-

KARGER

Fax + 41 61 306 12 34
E-Mail karger@karger.ch
www.karger.com

0302–2838/99/0356–0468$17.50/0

Accessible online at:
http://BioMedNet.com/karger

Prof. Rodolfo Montironi, FRC Path
Institute of Pathological Anatomy and Histopathology
University of Ancona School of Medicine, Nuovo Ospedale Regionale
Via Conca, I–60020 Torrette di Ancona (Italy)
Tel. +39 071 5964830, Fax +39 071 889985, E-Mail r.montironi@popcsi.unian.it

thelium is altered. This depends on several factors, including hormonal status and growth factor's milieu. Quantitative analysis was originally used to accurately compare PIN and PCa, thus contributing to the detection of the morphological changes which characterize the continuous spectrum seen in PIN and the similarities existing between high-grade PIN and PCa. Recently, more powerful quantitation techniques have become available, making feasible the detection of some subtle changes in the prostate gland structure and components (or lesions) [3]. Molecular pathology has allowed the detection of concomitant abnormal expression of oncogenes and enzymes and the identification of alterations at the chromosomal level [4].

The role of other precursors, such as atypical adenomatous hyperplasia (AAH), has been considered worthy of exploration. However, the data are insufficient to conclude that AAH is a premalignant lesion and its link to PCa has not yet been proved [5, 6]. Recently, subtle (or nonobvious and subvisual) morphological changes and the concomitant molecular alterations have been described in the normal-appearing tissue in prostates with PIN and/or PCa. These changes or alterations could be related to the development of prostatic neoplasia [3].

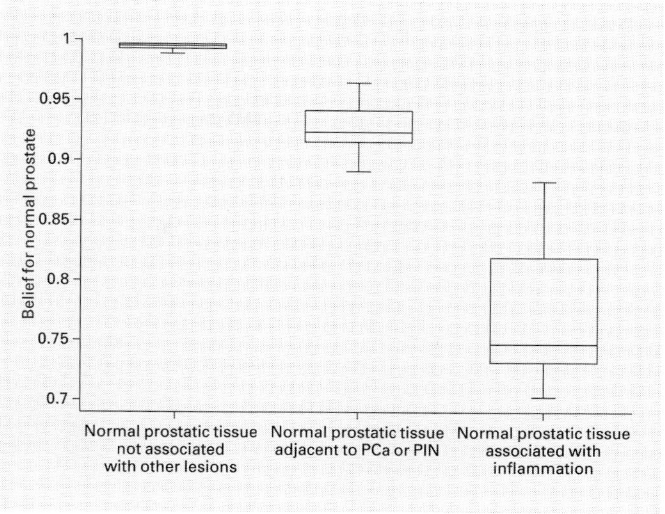

Fig. 1. Box-whisker plot of the three groups of normal prostatic tissue. It displays the mean and the range of the belief values for normal prostate. It shows an excellent separation of the cases of normal tissue adjacent to PCa or high-grade PIN from those associated with acute and/or chronic inflammation and not associated with other diseases [modified from 9].

Normal-Looking Epithelium in Prostates with PIN and/or Cancer

Subtle Morphological Changes

Diagnostic decision support systems (DDSSs) are applied to prostate histopathology to provide guidance in situations involving complex decision sequences. The decisive advantage of DDSSs is their ability to process symbolic information, e.g. linguistic or descriptive terms, words and concepts. DDSSs have been implemented as Bayesian belief networks (BBNs) in studies on the uncertainty assessment in the diagnosis and grading of prostate neoplasia, with particular reference to PIN [7, 8]. The results obtained have shown that the belief for the diagnostic alternatives reaches high values, often close to 1.0. Therefore, BBNs can provide a useful quantitative measure of certainty that characterizes individual cases according to the level of progression from PIN toward cancer.

Cases of normal-looking epithelium showing nonobvious morphological changes have been identified with a BBN-based analysis in a basic feasibility study [9]. The investigation included specimens of benign prostatic tissue subdivided as follows: (1) adjacent to PCa or high-grade PIN; (2) associated with acute and/or chronic inflammation, and (3) not associated with other diseases. For the cases evaluated in specimens with PCa or high-grade PIN, the belief values for normal prostate are intermediate between those for normal prostatic tissue associated with inflammation and those not associated. Subtle changes are detectable with the BBN at a certain distance from PCa or PIN. Therefore, the network can be used to identify with high certainty cases of benign prostate adjacent to PCa or PIN and distinguish them from those of benign prostatic tissue either associated or not with inflammation (fig. 1).

It is possible to use the subvisual morphological changes detected with a BBN as a tool in the management of patients with PIN or PCa. In particular, the possibility of identifying cases with subtle alterations may be applicable to specific clinical situations, such as the detection of malignancy in the prostate when only benign-appearing tissue is observed in a biopsy due to inadequate sampling [9].

Quantitative Analyses of Subvisual Morphological Changes

Bartels et al. [10–12] have documented the changes in the chromatin pattern in secretory cell nuclei from prostates with PIN and/or PCa. High-resolution images of

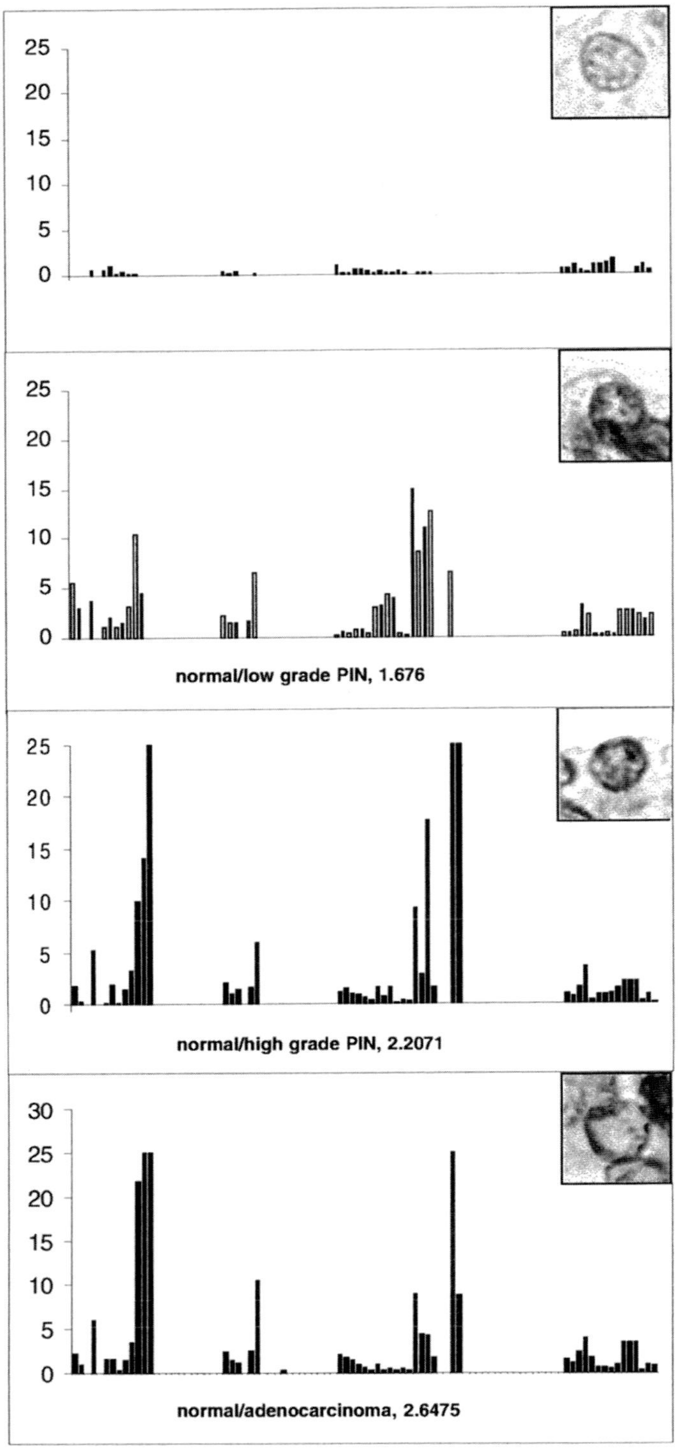

Fig. 2. Signature of individual nuclei from normal-appearing tissue of prostates harbouring low- and high-grade PIN and adenocarcinoma lesions [modified from 11].

nuclei have been recorded and a set of features descriptive of the chromatin texture and spatial distribution have been computed. From these data sets, features undergoing a monotonic trend of progression have been selected and plotted to reveal trends of lesion progression.

It has been shown that the nuclear chromatin in secretory cells in prostates with either PIN or PCa undergoes distinct changes in its texture and spatial distribution (fig. 2). Two trends of progressive change have been documented. The values of a number of features descriptive of the clumpiness of the chromatin increase from values found in normal prostate to those recorded for nuclei in the histologically normal-appearing tissue of prostates with PIN or PCa. There is a further increase in values for nuclei from low-grade PIN to high-grade PIN lesions. The second trend is a decrease in the values of the same features from those found in nuclei in high-grade PIN lesions still facing an intact basal cell layer, to those no longer facing a basal cell layer. This may be a possible first step in progression towards development of a malignant lesion. A further decrease occurs in nuclei from glands immediately adjacent to a malignant lesion, and in adenocarcinoma itself.

Sets of images have been recorded in the histologically normal-appearing tissue of prostates with high-grade PIN or PCa at a defined distances from the margin of lesions to explore the spatial extension of the subvisual morphological changes. The described changes appear to be detectable in the histologically normal-appearing tissue for distances of up to 10 mm from the margin of PIN or PCa (fig. 3) [11, 12]. Changes in the distribution and organization of the nuclear chromatin in cells of nontumour tissue in the vicinity of PCa have been documented also by Mairinger et al. [13] by means of high-resolution image analysis.

Molecular Changes

Recent studies have pointed out that the normal-looking prostate epithelium may show some molecular changes similar to those present in the associated preneoplastic and neoplastic lesions. Such changes are also occasionally present in normal prostate glands without PIN and cancer. Here are two examples of molecular changes, one concerning glutathione S-transferase (GST) and the other telomerase activity.

The most studied function of the GST enzymes is their role in cellular detoxification. GSTs may prevent carcinogenesis through inactivation of reactive electrophiles by conjugation to reduced glutathione. The immunohistochemical staining with anti-GST-π antibodies is primarily seen in the cytoplasm of the basal cell layer of the normal ducts and acini. Anti-GST-π antibodies fail to detect the enzyme in most prostatic adenocarcinomas. Additionally, it has been reported that the regulatory sequences near the gene GSTP1, which encodes the human p class GST, appear to be commonly hypermethylated during prostatic carcinogenesis [14, 15].

Two patterns are detectable in high-grade PIN lesions. One is represented by a type of GST-π staining very similar to that of the normal tissue. The other deviates from the normal in terms of extension and intensity because the gaps in the stained basal cell layer are wider and the cells themselves appear paler than in the normal. This indicates that the expression of GST-π deteriorates with the level of progression of PIN toward cancer. The same level of deterioration is not present in all the ducts and acini with high-grade PIN features. The normal-looking ducts and acini adjacent to either high-grade PIN or to PCa show the same dual pattern of staining, even though the second pattern with deterioration is less frequent and less severe than in high-grade PIN. Both distribution types are also recognizable in normal tissue from prostates without preneoplastic and neoplastic lesions, even though the latter is present in occasional cases [unpubl. data].

Telomerase activity is considered to be a useful diagnostic marker of prostate cancer [16]. Its expression is occasionally detected in benign prostatic tissue bordering prostate cancer and may result from either the presence of a primary undetected preneoplastic lesion or a secondary response of the benign elements to adjacent neoplastic lesions. The finding of telomerase activity in a certain proportion of biopsies from patients with benign prostatic hyperplasia (BPH) has been indicated as an early change in prostate carcinogenesis. It has been suggested that telomerase activity may be of use as a biomarker in patients diagnosed with BPH and who may subsequently develop prostate cancer [17].

These observations are related to the so-called 'enzyme-altered foci' as putative preneoplastic markers. According to Pretlow et al. [18] the most abundant of these lesions with molecular alterations show minimal or no morphological changes. Genetic abnormalities can occasionally be detected in normal prostate tissue [19].

Stromal Changes (Including Angiogenesis)

Substantial changes, including angiogenesis, occur in the stroma surrounding ducts and acini with PIN [20]. It has been shown that, going from normal prostate through PIN to PCa, an increasing proportion of capillaries become shorter, with open lumen, an undulated external contour and with a greater number of endothelial cells. The highest proportion of touching capillaries has been seen in normal prostate, while the lowest is in PCa, being intermediate in PIN. When the PIN samples have been divided into low-grade and high-grade, the feature values in the low-grade approach those in normal prostate, whereas in the high-grade they are close to invasive adenocarcinoma. The feature values in normal prostate samples from total prostatectomies performed because of a preoperative diagnosis of prostatic adenocarcinoma or PIN, have been reported to be close to those of low-grade PIN.

Siegal et al. [21] investigated the specific site of neovascularity within PCa and adjacent benign tissue. The highest microvessel density was found within the tumour and a stepwise increase in vessel density toward the centre of the neoplasm was observed. A less pronounced topographic gradient was evident within the benign region;

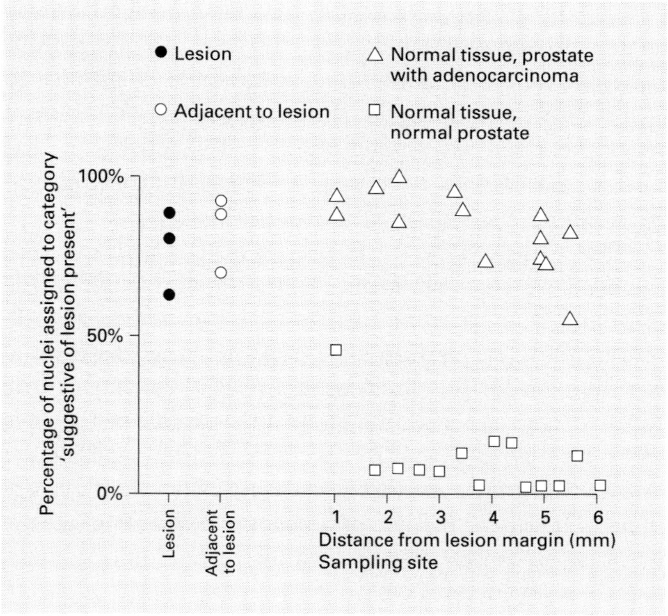

Fig. 3. Result of the classification of nuclei in normal-appearing tissue from prostates with adenocarcinoma, as compared to nuclei measured in normal prostates. In this study, samples of nuclei were recorded at different distances from the margin of the lesions, ranging from 1.1 to 6 mm. For each location in the histologically normal-appearing tissue regions of these prostates, the proportion of nuclei assigned to the category 'suggestive of lesion present' was determined. It is evident that all of the sites in the prostates with PCa, >50% of nuclei were assigned to the 'suggestive of lesion' category. In all the sites measured in normal prostates, only a small percentage of nuclei, < 10%, were thus assigned, with one exception [modified from 12].

benign tissue just outside the tumour was significantly more vascularized than that at a distance of 2.5 mm from the tumour. The apparent angiogenic field effect proved to have a limited radius in benign tissue, as tissue 5.0 mm from the edge has similar microvessel density to that 2.5 mm closer to the tumour edge. These findings are similar to those oberved by Montironi et al. [20].

These studies show the presence of qualitative and quantitative changes in the capillary architecture in the normal tissue adjacent to preneoplastic and neoplastic lesions [20–22]. Neovascularization may be an essential requirement for the development of PIN, such as is true for invasive adenocarcinoma, or it may be a consequence of factors arising in PIN or PCa. Understanding the events controlling angiogenesis could allow the development of new therapeutic approaches to prevent neoplastic progression as well as to induce the regression of cancers and their precursors.

Malignancy-Associated Cellular Markers

There is no agreement in the significance of the changes in the normal tissue adjacent to premalignant and malignant lesions [23]. They are hypothesized to represent either: (1) the surrounding tissue's response to signals given off by the premalignant or malignant lesion, or (2) a response in the surrounding tissue to the field effect of the agents that caused the initial lesion.

Evidence for the first hypothesis can be found in the results of a study of bronchial biopsies from patients with and without lung cancer by MacAulay et al. [24]. This investigation showed that changes in the distribution and organization of the nuclear chromatin, interpreted and defined as malignancy-associated change (MAC), were present in lung cancer patients and absent in healthy individuals. MACs were found in some precancerous lesions. The disappearance of MACs was noted in the subgroup of patients in which the lung with the tumour had been resected. The same authors produced similar changes in vitro using cultured epithelial cells. These experimental results support the hypothesis that the changes are due to some communication from already transformed cells to the normal cells in the vicinity. However, loss of heterozygosity (LOH) was detected in a set of bronchial biopsies with MACs [24]. Therefore, the possibility that MACs are related to genetic changes caused by some field affect was not excluded.

Evidence for the second hypothesis can be found in a study in which allelic loss was reported in normal lobules adjacent to breast cancer [25]. Cell populations that were unequivocally malignant or nonmalignant by histologic criteria were microdissected from tumour tissue for subsequent genetic analysis. Sixty-four percent of invasive tumours displayed LOH within the 3p22–25 region. Of these cases, 24% also showed loss of the same allele in benign lobules interspersed within the tumour tissue. Generally, the tumour cells displayed a more extensive region of loss than benign lobules. At the morphological level, the genetically altered lobules demonstrated no evidence of hyperplastic or neoplastic changes. According to Dairkee [25], these observations may reflect the existence of a 'predisposing field' within which a morphologically normal, yet aberrant, focal area becomes committed to malignant progression, leading eventually to invasive cancer.

The data collected in the literature point towards the possibility that also in the prostate the cases with malignancy-associated cellular markers may represent two distinct groups [23–29]. One represents the response to factors secreted by a premalignant or malignant lesion, and the other is related to the field effect of the agents that caused the initial lesion. Support to the existence of the latter group comes from the observation that some abnormalities usually seen in the preneoplastic and neoplastic lesions are occasionally detected in normal-appearing prostate tissue [19, 30]. The findings that some of the malignancy-associated cellular markers can be detected in prostates without cancer or PIN as well as at a distance from the preneoplastic and neoplastic lesions are seen as to favour the existence of the latter group.

The changes related to the field effect of the agents that caused the initial lesion might be seen as the onset of the development of prostatic neoplasia [12]. It might well be that under certain conditions the lesion can progress to a premalignant stage and may then, due to severe genetic instability, result in a clone that has the ability to invade. Data related to the formation of DNA adducts in normal tissue adjacent to cancer in humans support this hypothesis [31, 32]. According to Han et al. [33], the selective occurrence of a DNA adduct in the tissue of origin of carcinomas and preceding carcinoma development suggests a causal relation between adduct formation and PCa development in testosterone plus estradiol-17β-treated rats.

Conclusions

With the understanding and characterization of the sequence of events comes the ability to determine accurately the stage of progression neoplasia. All of the developmental stages in this evolutionary process are potential targets for chemoprevention. The identification of subtle morphological changes might represent the key to an effective search for chemopreventive strategies based on measurable, numerically defined criteria for success.

Acknowledgements

This research has been supported by a grant from the University of Ancona (R.M.) and, in part, by a grant from the NIH, National Cancer Institute, Bethesda, Md., R35 CA 53877 (P.H.B.). The content of this paper is solely the responsibility of the authors and does not necessarily represent the official views of the University of Ancona and the National Cancer Institute.

References

1 Bostwick DG: High grade prostatic intraepithelial neoplasia: The most likely precursor of prostate cancer. Cancer 1995;75:1823–1836.

2 Montironi R, Bostwick DG, Bonkhoff H, Cockett A, Helpap B, Troncoso P, Waters D: Workshop 1: Origins of Prostate Cancer. Cancer 1996;78:362–365.

3 Montironi R, Schulman CC: Precursors of prostatic cancer: Progression, regression and chemoprevention. Eur Urol 1996;30:133–137.

4 Bostwick DG, Pacelli A, Lopez-Beltran A: Molecular biology of prostatic intraepithelial neoplasia. Prostate 1996;29:117–134.

5 Parkinson MC: Pre-neoplastic lesions of the prostate. Histopathology 1995;27:301–311.

6 Montironi R, Thompson D, Bartels PH: Premalignant conditions of the prostate. Recent Adv Histopathol 1998;18, in press.

7 Bartels PH, Thompson D, Weber JE: Diagnostic and prognostic decision support systems. Pathologica 1995;87:221–236.

8 Montironi R, Bartels PH, Thompson D, Scarpelli M, Hamilton PW: Prostatic intraepithelial neoplasia. Performance of Bayesian belief network for diagnosis and grading. J Pathol 1995; 177:153–162.

9 Montironi R, Diamanti R, Pomante R, Thompson D, Bartels PH: Subtle changes in benign tissue adjacent to prostate neoplasia detected with a Bayesian belief network. J Pathol 1997;182:442–449.

10 Bartels PH, Montironi R, Thompson D, Vaught L, Hamilton PW: Statistical histometry of the basal cell/secretory cell bilayer in prostatic intraepithelial neoplasia. Analyt Quant Cytol Histol 1998;20:381–388.

11 Bartels PH, da Silva Vinicius D, Montironi R, Hamilton PW, Thompson D, Vaught L, Bartels HG: Chromatin texture signatures in nuclei from prostates lesions. Analyt Quant Cytol Histol 1998;20:407–416.

12 Bartels PH, Montironi R, Hamilton PW, Thompson D, Vaught L, Bartels HG: Nuclear chromatin texture in prostate. PIN and malignancy-associated changes. Analyt Quant Cytol Histol 1998;20:397–406.

13 Mairinger T, Mikuz G, Gschwendtner A: Malignancy-associated changes and prostatic cancer. Proceedings of the 12th International Congress on Diagnostic Quantitative Pathology, Vancouver, Canada, Oct 1–3, 1998, p 29A.

14 Lee WH, Morton RA, Epstein JI, Brooks JD, Campbell PA, Bova GS, Hsieh WS, Isaacs WB, Nelson WG: Cytidine methylation of regulatory sequences near the p-class glutathione S-transferase gene accompanies human prostatic carcinogenesis. Proc Natl Acad Sci USA 1994; 91:11733–11737.

15 Montironi R, Mazzucchelli R, Pomante R, Thompson D, Duval da Silva V, Vaught L, Bartels PH: Immunohistochemical expression of π-class glutathione S-transferase in the basal cell layer of benign prostate tissue following chronic treatment with finasteride. J Clin Pathol 1998, in press.

16 Kallabury BVS, Brien TP, Lowry CV, Muraca PJ, Fisher HAG, Kaufman RP, Toss JS: Telomerase activity in human benign prostate tissue and prostatic adenocarcinoma. Diagn Mol Pathol 1997;6:192–198.

17 Scates DK, Muir GH, Venitt S, Carmichael PL: Detection of telomerase activity in human prostate: A diagnostic marker for prostatic cancer? Br J Urol 1997;80:263–268.

18 Pretlow TG, Nagabhushan M, Pretlow TP: Prostatic intraepithelial neoplasia and other changes during promotion and progression. Pathol Res Pract 1995;191:842–849.

19 Sandberg AA: Chromosomal abnormalities in human prostate cancer: Their detection and pathological significance; in Foster CS, Bostwick DG (eds): Pathology of the Prostate. Major Problems in Pathology. Philadelphia, Saunders, 1998, vol 34, pp 400–427.

20 Montironi R, Magi-Galluzzi C, Diamanti L, Taborro R, Scarpelli M, Pisani E: Prostatic intraepithelial neoplasia. Qualitative and quantitative analyses of the blood capillary architecture on thin tissue sections. Pathol Res Pract 1993;189:542–548.

21 Siegal JA, Yu E, Brawer MK: Topography of neovascularity in human prostate carcinoma. Cancer 1995;75:2545–2551.

22 Montironi R, Diamanti L, Thompson D, Bartels HG, Bartels PH: Analysis of the capillary architecture in the precursor of prostate cancer: Recent findings and new concepts. Eur Urol 1996;30:191–200.

23 Nieburgs H: Malignancy-associated cellular markers; in Wied GL, Keebler CM, Koss LG, Patten SF, Rosenthal DL (eds): Compendium on Diagnostic Cytology, ed 7. Chicago, Tutorials of Cytology, 1992, pp 409–418.

24 MacAulay C, Payne P, Wilton D, Lam S, Palcic B: MAC: Some answers, more questions. Analyt Quant Cytol Histol 1996;19:78A.

25 Dairkee SH: Allelic loss in normal lobules adjacent to breast cancer. Cancer Detect Prev 1998; 22(supppl 1):135A.

26 Hutchinson ML, Isenstein LM, Martin JJ, Zahniser DJ: Measurement of subvisual changes in cervical squamous metaplastic cells for detecting abnormality. Analyt Quant Cytol Histol 1992;14:330–334.

27 Montag AG, Bartels PH, Lerma-Puertas E, Dytch HE, Leelakusolvong S, Bibbo M: Karyometric marker features in tissue adjacent to in situ cervical carcinomas. Analyt Quant Cytol Histol 1989;11:275–280.

28 Bibbo M, Michelassi F, Bartels PH, Dytch H, Bania C, Lerma E, Montag AG: Karyometric marker features in normal-appearing glands adjacent to human colonic adenocarcinoma. Cancer Res 1990;50:147–151.

29 Fleischhacker M, Lee S, Spira S, Takeuchi S, Koeffler P: DNA aneuploidy in morphologically normal colons from patients with colon cancer. Mod Pathol 1995;8:360–365.

30 Berner A, Danielsen HE, Nesland J, Reith A: Prognostic importance of DNA 'single' cell aneuploidy in normal, hyperplastic, intraepithelial/carcinomatous prostate. Analyt Quant Cytol Histol 1996;18:50A.

31 Li D, Zhang W, Sahin AA, Hittelman WN: DNA adducts in normal tissue adjacent to breast cancer. Cancer Detect Prev 1998; 22(suppl 1):134A.

32 De Waziers I: DNA adduct in normal tissue adjacent to colon cancer. Cancer Detect Prev 1998;22(suppl 1):134A.

33 Han X, Liehr JG, Bosland MC: Induction of a DNA adduct detectable by ^{32}P-postlabelling in the dorsolateral prostate of NBL/Cr rats treated with estradiol-17-beta and testosterone. Carcinogenesis 1995;16:951–954.

European Urology

Eur Urol 1999;35:474–478

Prostatic Intraepithelial Neoplasia: A Marker for High-Risk Groups and a Potential Target for Chemoprevention

Wael A. Sakr

Department of Pathology, Wayne State University and Karmanos Cancer, Institute, Detroit, Mich., USA

Key Words
Prostate cancer · Prostatic intraepithelial neoplasia · Epidemiology · Chemoprevention

Abstract
Both the incidence of, and the mortality due to, prostate cancer in the USA are higher in African-American men than in Caucasian men. This is particularly true in men less than 60 years of age. Our findings indicate that both the prevalence and the extensiveness of high-grade prostatic intraepithelial neoplasia (PIN) are higher in African-American men compared to Caucasians and that this discrepancy starts as early as the third decade of life. In an autopsy series comprising 650 men, extensive high-grade PIN with diffuse involvement of the prostate gland was evident in 25 (7%) of 364 African-American men less than 50 years of age compared to 4 (2%) of 208 Caucasian men in the same age group ($p = 0.002$). In a series of more than 1,200 men undergoing radical prostatectomy for clinically localized prostate cancer, extensive high-grade PIN was significantly and consistently higher in the African-American cohort than the Caucasian cohort. The difference was more evident in younger patients and those with smaller, organ-confined tumors. In a subset of 216 men (71 African-Americans and 138 Caucasians) with clinical stage T1C prostate cancer, extensive high-grade PIN was identified in 33% and 12% of the two groups respectively ($p = 0.001$). Moreover, in patients with organ-confined disease, both Gleason score and the extensiveness of high-grade PIN were significant predictors of biochemical recurrence. Our findings suggest an important role for high-grade PIN in the development of clinically significant, potentially aggressive prostate cancer in African-American men. In this epidemiologically identifiable high-risk group, there is a potential opportunity for chemoprevention strategies in younger men with high-grade PIN.

Introduction

The spectrum of neoplastic changes of the prostate gland is diverse and complex encompassing extremely prevalent preclinical 'histologic' carcinomas evident in postmortem examination and prostatic tissue samples removed for benign diagnoses, a complex array of atypical epithelial lesions with some presenting compelling arguments for a precursor status and finally, clinically manifest prostatic carcinoma which is in turn a heterogeneous disease with a wide range of biological potential and ability to progress. This pathobiologic heterogeneity is paralleled by an equally intriguing discrepancy in the geographic and ethnic variations of prostate cancer incidence and mortality among different populations and regions of the world. While these figures are higher in Caucasian men living in the Western hemisphere compared to those

KARGER

Fax + 41 61 306 12 34
E-Mail karger@karger.ch
www.karger.com

0302–2838/99/0356–0474$17.50/0

Accessible online at:
http://BioMedNet.com/karger

Wael A. Sakr, MD
Department of Pathology, Harper Hospital
3990 John R
Detroit, MI 48201 (USA)
Tel. +1 313 745 2525, Fax +1 313 745 9299

reported from the Far East and Eastern Europe, African-American men have the highest reported incidence and mortality rates due to prostate cancer in the world [1]. Detailed discussion of the potential reasons for these variations within the different population is beyond the scope of this limited report. Our objective rather, is to focus on one component of the multifaceted aspects of prostatic neoplasia, namely high-grade prostatic intraepithelial neoplasia (PIN), explore its potential contribution to these discrepancies and present an argument advocating a role for chemoprevention for this lesion for an ultimate goal of preventing the development of clinically evident, potentially life-threatening prostate cancer.

Why is high-grade PIN an important lesion in prostate carcinogenesis? The reasons for this are several, spanning the epidemiological, clinical and, increasingly so, the molecular aspects of prostate cancer. It has been shown that the prevalence of both high-grade PIN and prostatic carcinoma increase steadily with advancing age [2] and also that this lesion is more frequent in prostate glands that harbor carcinoma when compared to benign glands [3]. Morphologically, high-grade PIN and prostate cancer share several important features in terms of spatial distribution, architectural and cytologic characteristics. Both lesions are found mainly in the peripheral zone of the prostate gland [4, 5]. The basal cell layer normally present in benign prostatic ducts and acini is variably interrupted in high-grade PIN and is absent in adenocarcinoma [6]. The cytologic features of high-grade PIN cells, uniform nuclear enlargement and prominent nucleoli evident in most lining cells of the ducts harboring the lesion, are similar to those of carcinoma. Furthermore, areas of transition between high-grade PIN and cancer are frequent in the peripheral zone of the prostate. In these microscopic foci the ducts harboring high-grade PIN appear to give rise or to be in continuity with smaller, separate malignant acini of prostatic adenocarcinoma. This transition between high-grade PIN and areas of prostatic adenocarcinoma depicted morphologically has been used to suggest a 'progression' of prostatic neoplasia from a noninvasive into an invasive form with high-grade PIN representing the noninvasive phase [7].

The clinical implications of identifying high-grade PIN in prostate biopsies that have no evidence of cancer has gained increasing attention during the last several years. This is due to several studies indicating that this finding is an indicator for the presence of cancer in the gland. It has been shown that the probability of finding prostate cancer on subsequent biopsies in this setting is about 50% [8, 9].

The literature documenting the overlapping molecular/genetic characteristics between high-grade PIN and prostate cancer continues to expand. Numerous studies investigating parameters such as nuclear DNA ploidy, cellular proliferation and an extensive array of 'biomarkers' have been reported. The markers studied range from apoptotic index to expression of cell adhesion molecules, growth factors, oncogenes, tumor suppressor genes to specific chromosomal loci [10–15]. Most investigators found high-grade PIN to have an intermediate position with respect to many of these markers between benign and malignant prostatic epithelium [6]. Are there correlations between the variable incidence and mortality due to prostate cancer among different ethnic and geographic groups and the prevalence of high-grade PIN in these groups? If so, is there a role for preventive strategies in high-risk cohorts? We hope the following data and discussion contribute to answering this question.

Material and Methods

We reviewed studies that have reported on the epidemiology and prevalence of high-grade PIN in ethnic/geographic populations known to have different rates of prostate cancer incidence and mortality. Subsequently, the rationale and reports of studies exploring the potential applicability of different preventive strategies in men with higher prevalence of this lesion are summarized. A major proportion of the epidemiology of high-grade PIN in African-American and Caucasian men has been published by our group using the Wayne State University and the Karmanos Cancer Institute prostate database [4, 16]. There are additional studies reporting on similar aspects in other populations. These include data from Brazil and Japan by Billis [17] and Fujita et al. [18] respectively. The data from our institution are driven from two major sources, an ongoing autopsy study designed in collaboration with the Wayne County Medical Examiner Office and supported by the National Cancer Institute, and a large cohort of patients undergoing radical prostatectomy for clinically localized prostate cancer. The objective of the autopsy study is to determine the prevalence of prostate cancer and high-grade PIN in African-American and Caucasian men who died from trauma and accident and in whom antemortem history of prostate cancer is not established. More than 1,000 intact prostate glands have been procured with approximately 700 in which complete microscopic evaluation has been completed. The glands are procured from men of both races starting at 20 years of age whose death was estimated (according to Medical Examiners' report) to have occurred within the last 24 h. The confidentiality of the identity of the individuals is maintained throughout the study; the biostatistician on the project receives only the race and age information on the subjects whose specimen has been analyzed blindly. During the procurement process, the prostate gland with the seminal vesicles are removed en bloc and fixed in 10% neutral buffered formalin for 24–48 h. After trimming, the excess soft tissues are weighed and each prostate is completely sectioned at 2.5-mm intervals perpendicular to the posterior 'rectal' surface using a long disposable knife. The resulting slices are hand-processed, embedded in paraffin and later sectioned to produce 5-μm whole-mount sections that are stained with hematoxylin and eosin. After microscopic evaluation, the following parameters are documented for every gland: (1) The presence of prostate cancer and/or high-grade PIN determined according to criteria described by Bostwick and Montironi [19] and Gleason [20] respectively. Additionally the grade (Gleason score), volume and number of foci for cancers are recorded. (2) The zonal distribution of these lesions in the prostate gland according to the anatomy described by McNeal [21]. (3) The spatial relationship between high-grade PIN and cancer foci in the gland. (4) The number of foci and the extent of high-grade PIN in the prostate determined. Subsequently, according to the last parameters, high-grade PIN in every prostate harboring the lesion is classified as focal multifocal or extensive. These parameters are mapped on an individual specimen diagram and are correlated with the age and race of the subjects included in the study.

The surgical cohort of this study comprises over 1,600 patients with clinically localized prostate cancer who were treated by radical prostatectomy at one institution. The radical prostatectomy specimens are handled uniformly according to a previously published institutional protocol [22]. Briefly, after the gland is weighed, measured and inspected, it is sectioned fresh from apex to base at 3- to 4-mm intervals perpendicular to the posterior surface using a sharp disposable knife. Following gross inspection, small amounts of benign and malignant tissue samples with subsequent histologic confirmation are harvested from the 'inside' of the slices to avoid interference with the ability to evaluate the status of surgical margins and extraprostatic tissue. The rest of the glandular tissue is entirely submitted for histologic examination. This results in the documentation of the final Gleason score for the radical prostatectomy based on the index tumor when present. In glands without a distinct main tumor nodule, our approach is to estimate the relative proportions of grades in the entire gland and assign the final Gleason score accordingly. Reporting tumor extent and pathologic staging is based on the consensus of a recent conference [23]. This is a 'variation' of pTNM staging.

Results

High-grade PIN data from Japan: The study by Fujita et al. [18] reviewed 53 clinical stage T2 or T3 prostatic cancers of Japanese patients living in Osaka. The cases were subdivided into a preoperatively noncastrated group (34 cases) and a medically or surgically castrated group (19 cases) [18]. Overall the authors found high-grade PIN in 27 (50%) of the cases. The prevalence of the lesion was significantly lower in the castrated compared with the noncastrated groups (21% and 67.6% respectively). The overall prevalence of the high-grade PIN of 50% however is significantly lower than the rate of 80–90% reported in prostate glands harboring cancer from US men [24, 25].

High-grade PIN data from Brazil: These come from Billis [17] who reported a higher prevalence of high-grade PIN in Brazilian men from African descent compared to those from Caucasian origin.

High-grade PIN data from Wayne State University and Karmanos Cancer Institute: The autopsy component of our cohort had an overall racial composition of approximately 60% African-American and 40% Caucasians contrasting with a reverse proportion of the radical prostatectomy patients. With 650 prostate glands from men in the autopsy study analyzed, high-grade PIN was documented in 18, 31, 69, 78 and 86% of African-American men in the 4th, 5th, 6th, 7th and 8th decades respectively. These percentages were higher than those encountered in Caucasian men in the study in whom the prevalence of high-grade PIN for the corresponding age groups was 14, 21, 38, 50 and 63% respectively. Subsequently, high-grade PIN was quantitated into focal and extensive according to the degree of glandular involvement; the extensive form of the lesion was significantly more prevalent in the African-American cohort of the study particularly in men less than 50 years of age. In this subset, 25 (7%) of 364 African-American men harbored the extensive form of the lesion compared to 4 (2%) of 208 Caucasian men in the same age group ($p = 0.002$). The difference in age distribution appeared to follow a chronological pattern with high-grade PIN in African-American preceding that of Causasian males by approximately a decade. When the amount of high-grade PIN in the glands of patients treated by radical prostatectomy was subjected to similar semiquantitative analysis, similar trends of difference between the two race groups were also observed.

This was also true for the entire cohort of more than 1,600 patients but particularly in the subsets of African-American and Caucasian patients who were younger, and with a smaller and/or organ-confined prostate. In patients undergoing radical prostatectomy for clinical stage T1C disease (prostate cancer diagnosed based on an abnormal serum prostate-specific antigen value but without palpable abnormalities), the African-American cohort of this stage category had a consistently more diffuse involvement of the prostate by high-grade PIN when compared to Caucasian men within the same clinical stages. Extensive glandular involvement by the lesion was found in 24 of 71 (33%) African-Americans and 14 of 117 (12%) Caucasians with clinical stage T1C ($p = 0.001$). The same analysis was applied to patients with pathologic stage pT2 prostate cancer (pathologically organ-confined carcinoma with no extraprostatic extension or involvement of the surgical margins, seminal vesicles or regional lymph nodes). In this early disease category, extensive high-grade PIN was also significantly more prevalent in the African-American cohort (57 of 309, 18%) compared to Caucasian men (41 of 344, 12%) ($p = 0.003$). Furthermore, when we correlated biochemical recurrence data with the distribution of high-grade PIN in the gland, we found patients with organ-confined tumors who had extensive high-grade PIN with diffuse involvement of the prostate to experience higher rates of recurrence compared to those with focal or multifocal distribution of the lesion: 3 of 47 (6%) compared to 7 of 257 (3%) ($p = 0.05$).

Comments and Conclusions

Our data and those of others suggest at least an epidemiologic link between the prevalence of high-grade PIN and that of prostate cancer in different population segments. The limited data from Japan suggest a significantly lower prevalence of this lesion in Japanese men compared to Caucasian men in the USA, who in turn appear to have lower prevalence of this lesion than African-American men. It is of interest to notice that prostate cancer incidence and mortality in these three population groups have similar trends to those of high-grade PIN prevalence data. Moreover, Billis [17] reports more prevalent high-grade PIN in Brazilian men of African descent compared to Brazilian men of Caucasian origin. Considering that the author indicates a higher prostate cancer incidence and mortality in African-Brazilian men, the high-grade PIN prevalence data from his study is also consistent with the above trends.

These observations could be contrasted with data indicating a similar worldwide prevalence of the so-called 'latent' prostate cancer, a form of the disease discovered in the postmortem examination setting, usually representing small foci of cancer evident on microscopic examination. Unlike the lack of correlation between the prevalence of 'latent' small cancers and the clinical trends of prostate cancer, a more compelling correlation appears to be present between the latter and the prevalence of high-grade PIN.

If high-grade PIN could predict for the subsequent development of prostate cancer that is more likely to be clinically significant and potentially life-threatening, the lesion may be a good candidate for chemopreventive trials in men who have high-grade PIN but not prostate cancer. What are the appropriate nutritional/pharmaceutical agents for such trials? Some investigators have addressed these issues recently in both a conceptual and practical manner. Recent reports from the Chemoprevention Branch at the National Cancer Institute have advocated approaches aiming at developing drugs that will slow or stop the progression to invasive cancer of precancerous (preinvasive) lesions (intraepithelial neoplasia) [26]. The Chemoprevention Branch reports that over 40 short-term clinical trials are in progress, testing the effect of a variety of agents (antimutagens, antiproliferatives, antioxidants, anti-inflammatories and hormonally active agents) on precancerous lesions in the different major organ systems including the prostate. The effect(s) of these agents are to be evaluated by a panel of surrogate endpoint biomarkers (SEBs) that are based on the individual cellular morphological and functional changes universally used by pathologists to diagnose the lesion of intraepithelial neoplasia.

Similar studies were proposed by Bostwick [27]. This author and colleagues have strongly advocated the use of androgen ablation preventive therapy for patients with high-grade PIN in a comprehensive recent review [28]. A similar evaluation is proposed by Nelson et al. [29] who provided a literature review on chemoprevention of prostate cancer and concluded that synthetic retinoids, polyamine synthesis inhibitors, and antiandrogens are among the compounds shown to have in vitro or in vivo chemopreventive effects in prostate carcinogenesis. Other authors have proposed a similar molecular pathogenesis of prostate cancer and high-grade PIN. Brooks et al. [30] suggested that the loss of expression of the pi-class glutathione S-transferase enzyme GSTP1 is extremely common in prostate cancer. This phenomenon, associated with the hypermethylation of deoxycytidine residues in the 5′-regulatory CG island region of the GSTP1 gene, is a near-universal finding in human prostate cancer. These authors reported that unlike the abundant immunohistochemical expression of the enzyme polypeptide evident in normal prostatic epithelium, all foci of high-grade PIN and prostate cancer were completely devoid of GSTP1. These observations may provide additional mechanistically oriented approaches for chemoprevention trials.

In conclusion, there are compelling data that associate high-grade PIN with clinically significant, potentially more biologically aggressive prostate cancer. Of particular interest are the data indicating a more prevalent and extensive anatomic distribution of this lesion in population groups known to experience a higher incidence and mortality due to prostate cancer. Furthermore, there are multiple studies indicating the sensitivity of high-grade PIN to androgen ablation therapy and increasing number of reports showing similar molecular carcinogenesis between high-grade PIN and prostate cancer. Taken collectively, these data advocate the role of high-grade PIN as marker for high-risk groups and a suitable target for chemoprevention.

References

1 Merrill RM, Potosky AL, Feuer EJ: Changing trends in US prostate cancer incidence rates. J Natl Cancer Inst 1996;88:1683–1705.

2 Sakr WA, Haas GP, Cassin BJ, Pontes JE, Crissman JD: Frequency of prostatic intraepithelial neoplasia and invasive carcinoma in young males. J Urol 1993;150:379–385.

3 McNeal JE, Bostwick DG: Intraductal dysplasia: A premalignant lesion of the prostate. Hum Pathol 1986;17:64–71.

4 Sakr WA, Grignon DJ, Haas GP, Schomer KL, Heilbrun LK, Cassin BJ, Powell J, Montie JA, Pontes JE, Crissman JD: Epidemiology of high-grade prostatic intraepithelial neoplasia. Pathol Res Pract 1995;191:838–841.

5 Bostwick DG, Brawer MK: Prostatic intra-epithelial neoplasia and early invasion in prostate cancer. Cancer 1987;59:788–794.

6 Bostwick DG, Pacelli A, Lopez Beltran A: Ultrastucture of prostatic intraepithelial neoplasia. Prostate 1997;33:32–37.

7 McNeal JE, Villers A, Redwine EA, Freiha FS, Stamey TA: Microcarcinoma in the prostate: Its association with duct-acinar dysplasia. Hum Pathol 1991;22:644–652.

8 Raviv G, Janssen T, Zlotta AR, Descamps F, Verhest A, Schulman CC: Prostatic intraepithelial neoplasia: Influence of clinical and pathological data on the detection of prostate cancer. J Urol 1996;156:1050–1055.

9 Langer JE, Rovner ES, Coleman BG, Yin D, Arger PH, Malkowicz SB, Nisenbaum HL, Rowling SE, Tomaszewski JE, Wein AJ, Jacobs JE: Strategy for repeat biopsy of patients with prostatic intraepithelial neoplasia detected by prostate needle biopsy. J Urol 1996;155:228–231.

10 Haggman MJ, Macoska JA, Wojno KJ, Oesterling JE: The relationship between prostatic intraepithelial neoplasia and prostate cancer: Critical issues. J Urol 1997;158:12–22.

11 Erbersdobler A, Gurses N, Henke RP: Numerical chromosomal changes in high-grade prostatic intraepithelial neoplasia and concomitant invasive carcinoma. Pathol Res Pract 1996; 192:418–427.

12 Drachenberg CB, Ioffe OB, Papadimitriou JC: Progressive increase of apoptosis in prostatic intraepithelial neoplasia and carcinoma: Comparison between in situ end-labeling of fragmented DNA and detection by routine hematoxylin-eosin staining. Arch Pathol Lab Med 1997;121:54–58.

13 Stattin P, Damber JE, Karlberg L, Nordgren H, Bergh A: Bcl-2 immunoreactivity in prostate tumorigenesis in relation to prostatic intraepithelial neoplasia, grade, hormonal status, metastatic growth and survival. Urol Res 1996;24: 257–264.

14 Yang Y, Hao J, Liu X, Dalkin B, Nagle RB: Differential expression of cytokeratin mRNA and protein in normal prostate, prostatic intraepithelial neoplasia, and invasive carcinoma. Am J Pathol 1997;150:693–704.

15 Sakr WA, Macoska JA, Benson P, Grignon DJ, Wolman SR, Pontes JE, Crissman J: Allelic loss in locally metastatic, multisampled prostate cancer. Cancer Res 1994;54:3273–3277.

16 Sakr WA, Grignon DJ, Haas GP: Pathology of premalignant lesions and carcinoma of the prostate in African-American men Semin Urol Oncol 1998;16:214–220.

17 Billis A: Age and race distribution of high-grade prostatic intraepithelial neoplasia: An autopsy study in Brazil (South America). J Urol Pathol 1996;5:175–181.

18 Fujita MQ, Shin M, Yasunaga Y, Sekii K, Itatani H, Tsujimura T, Miki T, Okuyama A, Aozasa K: Incidence of prostatic intra-epithelial neoplasia in Osaka, Japan. Int J Cancer 1997;73:808–811.

19 Bostwick DG, Montironi R: Prostatic intraepithelial neoplasia and the origins of prostatic carcinoma. Pathol Res Pract 1995;191:828–832.

20 Gleason DF: Atypical hyperplasia, benign hyperplasia, and well-differentiated adenocarcinoma of the prostate. Am J Surg Pathol 1985;9 (suppl 1):53–67.

21 McNeal JE: Normal histology of the prostate. Am J Surg Pathol 1988;12:619–633.

22 Sakr WA, Grignon DJ, Visscher DW, Wolman SR, Crissman JD: Evaluating the radical prostatectomy specimen. I. A protocol for establishing prognostic parameters and harvesting fresh tissue samples. J Urol Pathol 1995;3/4: 377–384.

23 Sakr WA, Henson D, Mostofi FK, Blute ML, Wojno KD, Zinke CH, Budo M: Staging and reporting of prostate cancer. Sampling the radical prostatectomy specimen. Cancer 1996;78: 366–368.

24 McNeal JE, Bostwick DG: Intraductal dysplasia: A premalignant lesion of the prostate. Hum Pathol 1986;17:64–71.

25 Oyasu R, Bahnson RR, Nowels K, Garnett JE: Cytological atypia in the prostate gland: Frequency, distribution and possible relevance to carcinoma. J Urol 1986;135:959–962.

26 Boone CW, Kelloff GJ: Biomarker end-points in cancer chemoprevention trials. IARC Sci Publ 1997;142:273–280.

27 Bostwick DG: Target populations and strategies for chemoprevention trials of prostate cancer. J Cell Biochem Suppl 1994;19:191–196.

28 Aquilina JW, Lipsky JJ, Bostwick DG: Androgen deprivation as a strategy for prostate cancer chemoprevention. J Natl Cancer Inst 1997;89: 689–696.

29 Nelson PS, Gleason TP, Brawer MK: Chemoprevention for prostatic intraepithelial neoplasia. Eur Urol 1996;30:269–278.

30 Brooks JD, Weinstein M, Lin X, Sun Y, Pin SS, Bova GS, Epstein JI, Isaacs WB, Nelson WG: CG island methylation changes near the GSTP1 gene in prostatic intraepithelial neoplasia. Cancer Epidemiol Biomarkers Prev 1998; 7:531–536.

Surrogate Endpoint Biomarkers for Clinical Trials of Prostate Cancer Chemoprevention

European Urology

Eur Urol 1999;35:479–483

Genetic and Chromosomal Alterations in Prostatic Intraepithelial Neoplasia and Carcinoma Detected by Fluorescence in situ Hybridization

Junqi Qian Robert B. Jenkins David G. Bostwick

Department of Laboratory Medicine and Pathology, Mayo Clinic, Rochester, Minn., USA

Key Words

Prostatic intraepithelial neoplasia · Prostatic carcinoma · Metastasis · Fluorescence in situ hybridization · Chromosomal anomaly · Genetic alterations

Abstract

Objective: In this review, we discuss the utility of fluorescence in situ hybridization (FISH) in the determination of genetic and chromosomal alterations in prostate cancer specimens. We also discuss the genetic association between prostatic intraepithelial neoplasia (PIN) and adenocarcinoma as detected by FISH and other techniques. ***Methods and Results:*** FISH is a commonly used technique for the determination of gene and chromosome dosage. In tissue sections, FISH allows precise histopathologic correlation of multiple foci of normal epithelium, premalignant lesions, and carcinoma within a single specimen, including study of intratumoral heterogeneity. PIN and prostatic carcinoma foci have a similar proportion of genetic changes, but foci of carcinoma usually have more alterations. This supports the hypothesis that PIN is the most likely precursor of prostatic carcinoma. The most common genetic alterations in PIN and carcinoma are: (1) gain of chromosome 7, particularly 7q31; (2) loss of 8p and gain of 8q, and (3) loss of 10q, 16q and 18q. Inactivation of tumor suppressor genes and/or overexpression of oncogenes in these regions may be important for the initiation and progression of prostate cancer. ***Conclusions:*** FISH is a useful technique to determine genetic relationships between cancer and its precursors. PIN and prostatic carcinoma foci have a similar proportion of genetic alterations, suggesting that PIN is often a precursor of prostatic carcinoma. Genes on chromosomes 7, 8, 10, 16 and 18 may play an important role in both initiation and progression of prostatic carcinoma.

Introduction

High-grade prostatic intraepithelial neoplasia (PIN) represents the most likely precursor of prostatic adenocarcinoma, the most common malignancy in men in the United States [1–4]. High-grade PIN harbors substantial genetic changes, and these changes are similar to those in primary and metastatic carcinoma [3–8]. An understanding of the genetic events which accompany the progression of PIN to prostatic adenocarcinoma and the subsequent development of metastases would be useful for prevention, early detection, and treatment.

Fluorescence in situ hybridization (FISH) is a commonly used method for the determination of gene and chromosome dosage in human specimens. In this review, we discuss the advantages and disadvantages of FISH technique for detecting chromosomal anomalies and genetic changes in human tumor samples. We also discuss the genetic associations of PIN and adenocarcinoma as detected by FISH, and other techniques.

KARGER

Fax + 41 61 306 12 34
E-Mail karger@karger.ch
www.karger.com

0302–2838/99/0356–0479$17.50/0

Accessible online at:
http://BioMedNet.com/karger

Robert B. Jenkins, MD, PhD
Cytogenetic Laboratory, Mayo Clinic
200 First Street, S.W., Rochester, MN 55905 (USA)
Tel. +1 507 284 9617, Fax +1 507 284 0043
E-Mail jenkins.robert@mayo.edu

Table 1. Review of literature describing chromosomal anomalies in paired PIN and carcinoma specimens using FISH with chromosome centromere-specific probes

Group (first author)	Chromosome studied	Tissue material	PIN foci	Cancer foci	Chromosome anomalies in PIN		Chromosome anomalies in cancer	
					% foci with any anomaly	most common anomaly	% foci with any anomaly	most common anomaly
Macoska [3]	4, 7, 8, 10, Y[1]	5-µm paraffin sections	2	15	50	–10	80	+8, +7
Takahashi [5]	7, 8, 11, 12	Needle biopsy core Touch preparation	3	50	33	+7, +8	48	+7, +8
Alers [8]	1, 7, 8, 10, 15, Y	4-µm paraffin sections, with biotin-labeled probes	17	25	12	–Y	52	–Y, +8
Qian [6]	7, 8, 10, 12, Y	5-µm paraffin sections of whole-mount prostates	68	78	50	+8, +10	51	+7, +8
Erbersdobler [20]	7, 8, 10, 17, X	5-µm paraffin sections, with biotin-labeled probes	30	15	57	+8, +X	73	+7, +8
Jenkins [7]	7, 8, 10, 12, Y	5-µm paraffin sections of whole-mount prostates	48	84	62	+8, +10	61	+7, +8

– or + represent loss or gain of chromosome.

1 Chromosome Y DNA probe was specific for mid-distal Yq (Yq12) region.

The Utility of FISH in the Determination of Gene and Chromosome Alterations

FISH is a useful method for the detection of gene and chromosome anomalies in cell lines [9], touch preparations from fresh tissue [5], isolated nuclei from formalin-fixed, paraffin-embedded tissue [10], and routine histologic sections from paraffin blocks [11, 12]. When FISH is applied to histologic sections, tumor cells can be precisely evaluated, and the genetic heterogeneity of tumor foci can be assessed [6, 7]. Normal ranges of FISH signals can be determined by studying regions of apparently normal tissue [6, 7]. Furthermore, in tissue sections, FISH allows precise histopathologic correlation of multiple foci of normal epithelium, premalignant lesions, and carcinoma within a single specimen [6, 7]. This is a useful approach for understanding carcinogenesis, especially for the study of clonal origin of multifocal prostate cancer [6, 7]. FISH can easily distinguish chromosomal centromere gain and loss [5–11]. With appropriate probes, the copy number of specific chromosomal regions can also be determined [7]. However, interphase FISH studies of gene dosage in paraffin-embedded materials require relatively large probes that target one locus, or at most, a few loci at a time [7]. Also, the counting of FISH signals is labor-intensive.

Polymerase chain reaction (PCR), and comparative genomic hybridization (CGH) are also commonly used techniques for the determination of gene and chromosome dosage. When used together, FISH, PCR, and CGH analyses can sensitively identify and define gene and chromosomal anomalies in cancer specimens [13–19].

The Most Frequently Gained and Deleted Chromosomal Regions in PIN and Carcinoma

Tables 1 and 2 summarize results of in situ hybridization (ISH) analyses and PCR-based microsatellite analyses of paired PIN and carcinoma reported in the English language literature [3–8, 20–22].

Gain and Loss of Chromosome 7

Cytogenetic analyses have demonstrated that gain, deletion, and translocation of 7q22-q31 are common in prostate adenocarcinoma [23]. FISH studies have demonstrated that aneusomy of chromosome 7 is frequent in prostate cancer and associated with higher tumor grade, advanced pathologic stage, and early patient death from prostate cancer [5, 9–11]. Using PCR analysis of microsatellite markers, we and others have identified frequent imbalance of alleles mapped to 7q31 in prostate and other cancers [14, 16]. In prostate cancer, allelic imbalance of 7q31 is strongly correlated with tumor aggressiveness, progression, and cancer-specific death [3–5]. These findings suggest that genetic alterations of the 7 q-arm play an important role in the development of prostate cancer.

We have previously reported that the frequency of trisomy 7 was much higher in carcinoma than PIN [6]. Bost-

Table 2. Review of literature describing genetic changes in paired prostatic intraepithelial neoplasia and carcinoma specimens using PCR-based microsatellite analysis and/or FISH with region-specific I

Group (first author)	Tissue material	PIN foci	Cancer foci	Genetic changes in informative PIN foci, %							Genetic changes in informative cancer foci, %						
				7q	8p	8q	10q	12p	16q	18q	7q	8p	8q	10q	12p	16q	18q
Sakr [4]	PCR, paraffin-embedded tissue	9	29	–	29	–	25	0	20	–	–	29	–	18	0	42	–
Macoska [3]	FISH, PCR, frozen tissue	1	10	–	100	0	–	–	–	–	–	70	43	–	–	–	–
Emmert-Buck [21]	PCR, frozen tissue	54	32	–	63	–	–	–	–	–	–	91	–	–	–	–	–
Jenkins [7]	FISH, paraffin-embedded tissue	48	84	–	–	50	–	–	–	–	–	–	44	–	–	–	–
Bostwick [22]	PCR, paraffin-embedded tissue	84	95	17	41	30	–	–	–	19	30	50	33	–	–	–	52

– = Not studied.

wick et al. [22] observed that allelic imbalance at 7q31 was slightly more frequent in prostate cancer than PIN (30 vs 17%). This indicates that gain of chromosome 7 may play a role in the progression of precursor lesions to carcinoma.

We recently undertook a molecular cytogenetic study of 25 prostate specimens with FISH probes for the chromosome 7 centromere and for 5 loci mapped to 7q31 [24]. We found that alterations of chromosome 7, the 7 q-arm, and particularly, 7q31, are common in prostate cancer. Unexpectedly, overrepresentation (gain) of 7q31 was more common than deletion of 7q31 and was strongly correlated with tumor Gleason score [24]. We also found that the DNA probe for D7S522 spans the common fragile site FRA7G at 7q31. The coincidence of FRA7G with the region showing the greatest allelic imbalance suggests that the instability in this fragile site may be responsible for both the gains and losses of this region. Our observations have two possible implications. It is possible that overrepresentation of the 7 q-arm, of 7q31 and/or genes in these regions may be important for the development and/or progression of a significant proportion of prostate cancer. Conversely, it is also possible that prostate cancer progression is associated with increased chromosomal fragility, perhaps as a result of other genetic alterations [24].

Loss of 8p and Gain of 8q

The chromosome 8 p-arm is one of the most frequently deleted regions in prostate cancer [21, 25–27]. Band 8p22 has been the most intensively studied region [26, 27]. The rate of 8p22 loss ranged from 29 to 50% in PIN, 32 to 69% in primary tumors, and 65 to 100% in metastatic cancer [25–27]. Other frequently deleted 8p regions in prostate cancer include 8p21 and 8p12 [21]. Emmert-Buck et al. [21] found loss of 8p12–21 in 63% of PIN foci and 91% of cancer foci using microdissected frozen tissue. Bostwick et al. [22] detected loss of 8p12–21 in 37% of PIN foci and 46% of cancer foci. These findings suggest that more than one tumor suppressor gene may be located on 8p, and inactivation of these tumor suppressor genes may be important for the initiation of prostate cancer.

In addition to loss of the 8 p-arm, gain of the 8 q-arm has been reported in prostate cancer [7, 13, 18]. Bova et al. [26] found gain of 8q in 11% of primary tumors and 40% of lymph node metastases. Van Den Berg et al. [28] found amplification of 8q DNA sequences in 75% of cancers metastatic to lymph nodes. Similarly, Visakorpi et al. [18] found gain of 8q far more frequently in locally recurrent cancer than in the primary cancer. Cher et al. [13] also detected frequent gain of 8q in metastatic and androgen-independent prostate cancer. Using FISH, Qian et al. [6] observed that gain of chromosome 8 was the most frequent chromosomal anomaly in metastatic foci, and the frequency was much higher than in PIN and carcinoma. Jenkins et al. [7] identified c-myc gene amplification in 22% of metastatic foci, which was much more frequent than in primary cancer (9%), suggesting that the 8 q-arm may harbor a gene(s) whose amplification and overexpression may play a key role in the progression and evolution of prostatic carcinoma. This gene may be c-myc.

Interestingly, gain of the chromosome 8 centromere or the 8 q-arm occurs simultaneously with loss of portions of the 8 p-arm in PIN and carcinoma [7, 13, 18, 19]. One simple genetic mechanism that could explain these prior observations is the presence of multiple copies of isochromosome 8q in tumor cells [28].

Gain and Loss of Other Chromosomal Regions

There is a high frequency of allelic imbalance at 10p and 10q in prostate cancer [29]. The most commonly deleted region on the 10 q-arm includes bands 10q23–24, and allelic loss of this region may inactive the MXI-1 gene [30]. Recently, another candidate gene in this region has been cloned: PTEN [31]. Four of 4 prostate cancer cell lines have recently been shown to have mutations of this gene [31]. Trybus et al. [32] mapped the common region of 10p deletion to 10p11.2. Chromosome 16 also had frequent allelic imbalance in prostate cancer. Carter et al. [33] observed ~30% allelic imbalance at 16q in clinically localized prostate cancer. Cher et al. [15] found a high frequency of allelic imbalance at 16q23-q24. The most commonly deleted region is located at 16q24.1-q24.2, and this deletion was significantly associated with tumor progression [15]. The frequency of loss of 18q22.1 varied from 20 to 40% in prostate cancer [28]. Recently, Cunningham et al. [34] detected allelic imbalance at 21q22.2–22.3 in 23% of cases of prostate cancer and at 3p25–26 in 20%. Other regions demonstrating frequent allelic imbalance include 5q12–23, 6q, 13q and 17p31.1 [34]. Loss of 10q, 16q and 18q has also been reported in PIN [4, 22]. Bostwick et al. [22] found loss of 18q12.2–12.3 was higher in prostate cancer than PIN (52 vs 19%, p = 0.01), indicating that this region may harbor a gene whose inactivation may be important for the progression of PIN to carcinoma.

Pathogenetic Relationship between PIN and Carcinoma

Since 1992, a small number of molecular biologic studies in PIN has been reported [3–8, 20, 22]. In earlier studies, only a few of PIN foci were analyzed with a limited number of centromere-specific probes [3, 5]. We previously reported numerical chromosomal anomalies in multiple foci of PIN and carcinoma in 40 whole-mount radical prostatectomy specimens with centromere-specific probes to chromosomes 7, 8, 10, 12 and Y [6]. The overall frequency of numeric chromosomal anomalies in PIN and carcinoma foci was remarkably similar [6]. To further evaluate the genetic relationship between PIN, primary adenocarcinoma and lymph node metastases, we studied c-myc gene amplification and numerical chromosomal anomalies in multiple foci of PIN and carcinoma in 25 totally embedded whole-mount radical prostatectomy specimens and 23 matched lymph node metastases [7]. Generally, within each prostate, carcinoma foci contained more chromosomal anomalies and extra copies of c-myc than matched PIN foci. The overall frequency of extra c-myc copy number anomalies and numeric chromosomal anomalies in PIN and carcinoma foci were remarkably similar, suggesting that they share a similar underlying pathogenesis [7]. Together with the anatomic association of PIN with cancer that we and others have observed, these findings suggest that PIN is a precursor of carcinoma [6–8]. However, in some prostates, one or more foci of PIN contained more anomalies than the carcinoma foci [6, 7]. This indicates that either some PIN foci may have a divergent pathogenesis, that some PIN foci may morphologically progress to cancer more slowly than other PIN foci, or that foci of carcinoma may occasionally be derived from other precursor lesions such as atypical adenomatous hyperplasia [35].

The molecular basis for prostate cancer metastasis remains unclear [4, 6, 7, 13]. In a recent study, we carefully mapped and compared the genetic changes and chromosomal anomalies in all multiple primary cancer foci and matched lymph node metastases [7]. We found that all 23 metastatic foci showed multiple FISH anomalies. The frequency of c-myc gene amplification and chromosomal aneusomy and the average number of extra c-myc copies and abnormal chromosomes per nucleus were higher than that of the primary tumor, indicating that primary tumor cells with multiple genetic anomalies usually metastasize and/or that metastatic lesions are genetically unstable [7]. Interestingly, one or more primary tumors usually shared the same FISH alteration as the matched ipsilateral metastasis, suggesting that this tumor focus gave rise to the metastatic lesions [6, 7].

Conclusions

FISH is a useful technique to determine genetic relationships between cancer and its precursors. PIN and prostatic carcinoma foci have a similar proportion of genetic changes, but foci of carcinoma usually have more alterations. This supports the hypothesis that PIN is often a precursor of prostatic carcinoma. The most common genetic alterations in PIN and carcinoma are (1) gain of chromosome 7, particularly 7q31; (2) loss of 8p and gain of 8q, and (3) loss of 10q, 16q and 18q. Inactivation of tumor suppressor genes and/or overexpression of oncogenes at theses regions may be important for the initiation and progression of prostate cancer.

References

1 Bostwick DG, Brawer MK: Prostatic intra-epithelial neoplasia and early invasion in prostate cancer. Cancer 1987;59:788–794.

2 Bostwick DG, Amin MB, Dundore P, Marsh W, Schultz DS: Architectural patterns of high-grade prostatic intraepithelial neoplasia. Hum Pathol 1993;24:298–310.

3 Macoska JA, Micale MA, Sakr WA, Benson PD, Wolman SR: Extensive genetic alterations in prostate cancer revealed by dual PCR and FISH analysis. Genes Chromosom Cancer 1993;8:88–97.

4 Sakr WA, Macoska JA, Benson PD, Grignon DJ, Wolman SR, Pontes JE, Crissman JD: Allelic loss in locally metastatic, multisampled prostate cancer. Cancer Res 1994;54:3273–3279.

5 Takahashi S, Qian J, Brown JA, Alcaraz A, Bostwick DG, Lieber MM, Jenkins RB: Potential markers of prostate cancer aggressiveness detected by fluorescence in situ hybridization. Cancer Res 1994;54:3574–3579.

6 Qian J, Bostwick DG, Takahashi S, Borell TJ, Herath JF, Lieber MM, Jenkins RB: Chromosomal anomalies in prostatic intraepithelial neoplasia and carcinoma detected by fluorescence in situ hybridization. Cancer Res 1995;55:5408–5414.

7 Jenkins RB, Qian J, Lieber MM, Bostwick DG: Detection of c-myc oncogene amplification and chromosomal anomalies in metastatic prostatic carcinoma by fluorescence in situ hybridization. Cancer Res 1997;57:524–531.

8 Alers CA, Krijtenburg PJ, Vissers KJ, Bosman FT, van der Kwast TH, Dekken H: Interphase cytogenetics of prostatic adenocarcinoma and precursor lesions: Analysis of 25 radical prostatectomies and 17 adjacent prostatic intraepithelial neoplasias. Genes Chromosom Cancer 1995;12:241–250.

9 Bandyk MG, Zhao L, Troncoso P, et al: Trisomy 7: A potential cytogenetic marker of human prostate cancer progression. Genes Chromosom Cancer 1994;9:19–27.

10 Alcaraz A, Takahashi S, Brown JA, Herath JF, Bergstralh E, Larson-Keller J, Lieber MM, Jenkins RB: Aneuploidy and aneusomy of chromosome 7 detected by fluorescence in situ hybridization are markers of poor prognosis in prostate cancer. Cancer Res 1994;54:3998–4002.

11 Takahashi S, Alcaraz A, Brown JA, Borell TJ, Herath JF, Bergstralh EJ, Lieber MM, Jenkins RB: Aneusomies of chromosomes 8 and Y detected by fluorescence in situ hybridization are prognostic markers for pathologic stage C ($pT_3N_0M_0$) prostate carcinoma. Clin Cancer Res 1996;2:137–145.

12 Qian J, Bostwick DG, Takahashi S, Borell TJ, Brown JA, Lieber MM, Jenkins RB: Comparison of fluorescence in situ hybridization analysis of isolated nuclei and routine histological sections from paraffin-embedded prostatic adenocarcinoma specimens. Am J Pathol 1996;149:1193–1199.

13 Cher ML, Bova GS, Moore DH, Small EJ, Carroll PR, Pin SS, Epstein JI, Isaacs WB, Jensen RH: Genetic alterations in untreated metastases and androgen-independent prostate cancer detected by comparative genomic hybridization and allelotyping. Cancer Res 1996;56:3091–3102.

14 Zenklusen JC, Thompson JC, Troncoso P, Kagan J, Conti CJ: Loss of heterozygosity in human primary prostate carcinoma: A possible tumor suppressor gene at 7q31.1. Cancer Res 1994;54:6370–6373.

15 Cher ML, MacGrogan D, Bookstein R, Brown JA, Jenkins RB, Jensen RH: Comparative genomic hybridization, allelic imbalance, and fluorescence in situ hybridization on chromosome 8 in prostate cancer. Genes Chromosom Cancer 1994;11:153–162.

16 Takahashi S, Shan A, Ritland SR, Delacey K, Bostwick DG, Lieber MM, Thibodeau SN, Jenkins RB: Frequent loss of heterozygosity at 7q31.1 in primary prostate cancer is associated with tumor aggressiveness and progression. Cancer Res 1995;55:4114–4119.

17 Jenkins RB, Takahashi S, Delacey KA, Bergstralh E, Lieber MM: Prognostic significance of allelic imbalance of chromosome regions 7q, 8p, 16q, and 18q in stage T3N0M0 prostate cancer. Genes Chromosom Cancer 1998;21:131–134.

18 Visakorpi T, Kallioniemi AH, Syvanen AC, Hyytinen ER, Karhu R, Tammela T, Isola JJ, Kallioniemi OP: Genetic changes in primary and recurrent prostate cancer by comparative genomic hybridization. Cancer Res 1995;55:342–347.

19 Cher ML, MacGrogan D, Bookstein R, Brown JA, Jenkins RB, Jensen RH: Comparative genomic hybridization, allelic imbalance, and fluorescence in situ hybridization on chromosome 8 in prostate cancer. Genes Chromosom Cancer 1994;11:153–162.

20 Erbersdobler A, Gurses N, Henke RP: Numerical chromosomal changes in high-grade prostatic intraepithelial neoplasia and concomitant invasive carcinoma. Pathol Res Pract 1996;192:418–427.

21 Emmert-Buck MR, Vocke CD, Pozzatti RO, Duray PH, Jennings SB, Florence CD, Zhuang Z, Bostwick DG, Liotta LA, Linehan WM: Allelic loss on chromosome 8p12–21 in microdissected prostatic intraepithelial neoplasia. Cancer Res 1995;55:2959–2962.

22 Bostwick DG, Shan A, Qian J, Darson M, Maihle NJ, Jenkins RB, Cheng L: Independent origin of multiple foci of prostatic intraepithelial neoplasia. Cancer 1998;83:1995–2002.

23 Brothman AR, Peehl DM, McNeal JE: Frequency and pattern of karyotypic anomalies in human prostate cancer. Cancer Res 1990;50:3795–3803.

24 Jenkins RB, Qian J, Lee HK, Huang H, Hirasawa K, Bostwick DG, Proffitt J, Wilber K, Lieber MM, Liu W, Smith DI: A molecular cytogenetic analysis of 7q31 in prostate cancer. Cancer Res 1998;58:759–766.

25 Cheng L, Song SY, Pretlow TG, Abdul-Karim FW, Kung HJ, Dawson DV, Park WS, Moon YW, Tsai ML, Linehan WM, Emmert-Buck MR, Liotta LA, Zhuang Z: Evidence of independent origin of multiple tumors from patients with prostate cancer. J Natl Cancer Inst 1998;90:233–237.

26 Bova GS, Carter BS, Bussemakers MJG, Emi M, Fujiwara Y, Kyprianou N, Jacobs SC, Robinson JC, Epstein JI, Walsh PC, Isaacs WB: Homozygous deletion and frequent allelic loss of chromosome 8p22 loci in human prostate cancer. Cancer Res 1993;53:3869–3873.

27 Vocke CD, Pozzatti RO, Bostwick DG, Florence CD, Jennings SB, Strup SE, Duray PH, Liotta LA, Emmert-Buck MR, Linehan WM: Analysis of 99 microdissected prostate carcinoma reveals a high frequency of allelic loss on chromosome 8p12-21. Cancer Res 1996;56:2411–2416.

28 Van Den Berg C, Guan XY, Von Hoff D, Jenkins RB, Bitter M, Griffin C, Kallioniemi O, Visakorpi T, McGill J, Herath JF, Epstein JI, Scarosdy M, Meltzer P, Trent J: DNA sequence amplification in human prostate cancer identified by chromosome microdissection: Potential prognostic implications. Clin Cancer Res 1995;1:11–18.

29 Ittman M: Allelic loss on chromosome 10 in prostate adenocarcinoma. Cancer Res 1996;56:2143–2147.

30 Eagle L, Yin X, Brothman A, William BJ, Atkin N, Prochownik E: Mutation of the MXI 1 gene in prostate cancer. Nat Genet 1995;9:249–255.

31 Li J, Yen C, Liaw D, Podsypanina K, Bose S, Wang SI, Puc J, Miliaresis C, Rodgers L, McCombie R, Bigner SH, Giovanella BC, Ittmann M, Tycko B, Hibshoosh H, Wigler MH, Parsons R: PTEN, a putative protein tyrosine phosphatase gene mutated in human brain, breast, and prostate cancer. Science 1997;275:1943–1947.

32 Trybus TM, Burgess AC, Wojno KJ, Glover TW, Macoska JA: Distinct areas of allelic loss on chromosomal regions 10p and 10q in human prostate cancer. Cancer Res 1996;56:2263–2267.

33 Carter BS, Ewing CM, Ward WS, Treiger BF, Aalders TW, Schalken JA, Epstein JI, Isaacs WB: Allelic loss of chromosomes 16q and 10q in human prostate cancer. Proc Natl Acad Sci USA 1990;87:8751–8755.

34 Cunningham JM, Shan A, Wick MJ, McDonnell SK, Schaid DJ, Tester DJ, Qian J, Takahashi S, Jenkins RB, Bostwick DG, Thibodeau SN: Allelic imbalance and microsatellite instability in prostatic adenocarcinoma. Cancer Res 1996;56:4475–4482.

35 Cheng L, Shan A, Cheville JC, Qian J, Bostwick DG: Atypical adenomatous hyperplasia of the prostate: A premalignant lesion? Cancer Res 1998;58:389–391.

Surrogate Endpoint Biomarkers for Clinical Trials of Prostate Cancer Chemoprevention

European Urology

Eur Urol 1999;35:484–491

Tissue Architecture Analysis in Prostate Cancer and Its Precursors: An Innovative Approach to Computerized Histometry

Peter H. Bartels[a] Rodolfo Montironi[b] Vinicius Duval da Silva[c]
Peter W. Hamilton[d] Deborah Thompson[a] Linda Vaught[a]
Hubert G. Bartels[a]

[a]Optical Sciences Center, University of Arizona, Tucson, Ariz., USA; [b]Institute of Pathological Anatomy and Histopathology, University of Ancona, Torrette di Ancona, Italy; [c]Coordenação de Aperfeiçoamento de Pessoal de Nível Superior, Brasília, and Federal University of Rio Grande do Sul, Porto Alegre, Brazil, and [d]Department of Pathology, The Queen's University of Belfast, N. Ireland

Key Words

Prostatic intraepithelial neoplasia · Histometry · Karyometry · Progression index

Abstract

Aims: It is the aim of these studies to derive a numerically defined progression index for prostatic intraepithelial neoplasia (PIN) lesions. ***Methods:*** Histometric and karyometric features were automatically extracted from images of histopathologic sections by a machine vision system. ***Results:*** Both histometric and karyometric measures lend themselves to the defining of a progression index. Karyometric features were found to be more sensitive. They allow the detection of very early change. ***Conclusions:*** It is possible to measure progression of PIN lesions with precision. The methodology would lend itself for measurement of regression due to chemopreventive intervention.

Introduction

Micromorphometric analysis can provide numerically defined measures of lesion progression, or regression in response to chemopreventive intervention. Both histometric criteria [1] and karyometric features [2, 3] lend themselves to the derivation of a progression index. In the case of karyometric features, they can be shown to point to changes in nuclei from histologically normal appearing tissue of prostates harboring a lesion – changes which are visually not perceived. These provide the means for the detection of very early change. The nuclear chromatin texture may be used to define a 'nuclear chromatin texture signature' [4], which allows a very specific characterization of individual nuclei and of an individual lesion.

The extraction of such progression measures has become possible and feasible due to advances in the design of knowledge-guided systems, adapted here to control the image analysis based on automated machine vision [5, 6].

KARGER

Fax + 41 61 306 12 34
E-Mail karger@karger.ch
www.karger.com

0302–2838/99/0356–0484$17.50/0

Accessible online at:
http://BioMedNet.com/karger

Peter H. Bartels, PhD
Optical Sciences Center
University of Arizona
Tucson, AZ 85721 (USA)
Tel. +1 520 621 2032, Fax +1 520 621 6778

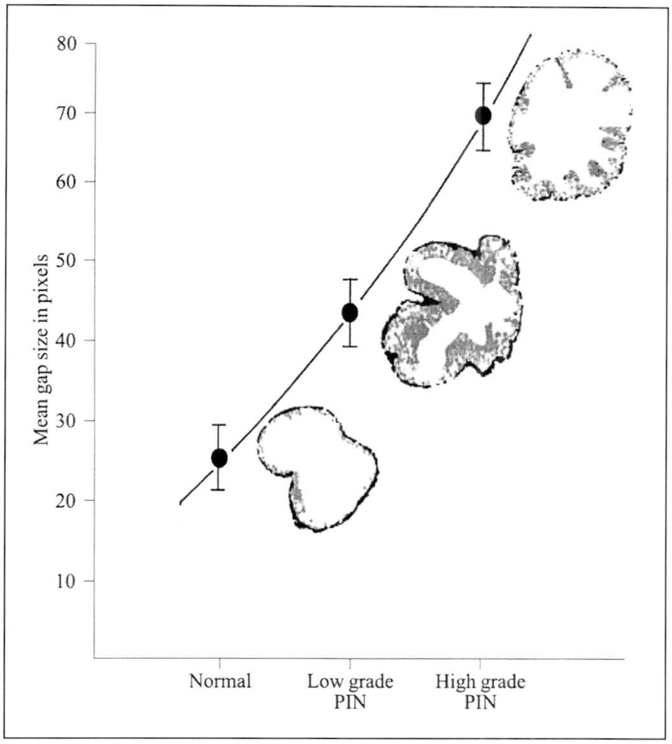

Fig. 1. Histometric measure of PIN lesion progression.

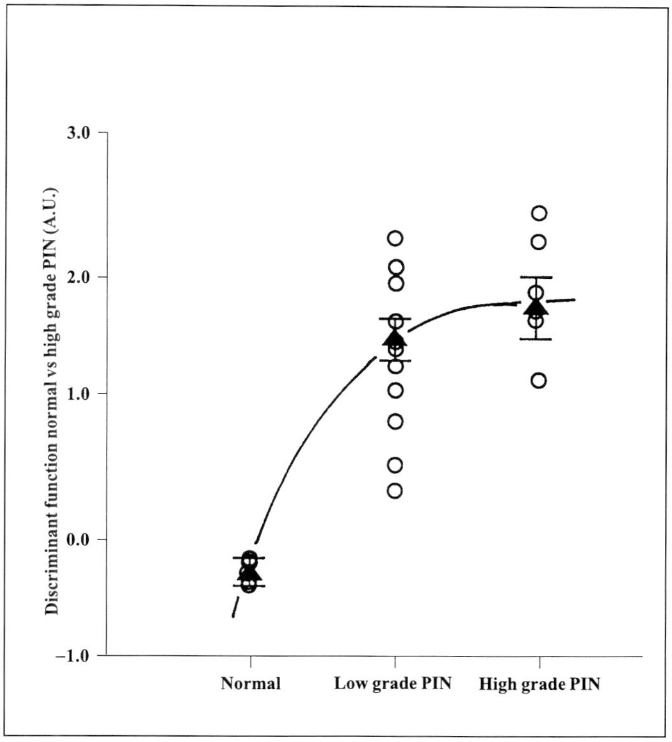

Fig. 2. Mean discriminant function score per case as a function of PIN lesion grade.

Histometry

The derivation of a histometric progression index is based on original work by Bostwick and Brawer [7] in 1987. These authors reported the disruption of the basal cell layer concomitant with the progression of prostatic intraepithelial neoplasia. The machine vision system was set up to generate a binary image showing only the basal cell layer, and to record such histometric variables as the number of gaps and gap sizes, in relation to gland perimeter. Several such histometric features show a monotonic trend as a function of lesion progression and could be used for a numeric assessment of lesion progression, as seen in figure 1. Shown here is the mean gap size as a function of lesion grade.

Karyometry

It is not always possible to measure the required number of glands for a histometric progression index in a needle biopsy. Thus, the utility of karyometric features as indicators of lesion progression was investigated.

To derive a progression index for prostatic intraepithelial neoplasia (PIN) lesions based on karyometric variables, a subset of such variables was selected such that each showed a monotonic increase in value, from values seen in normal tissue to values seen in high-grade PIN lesions. Only secretory cell nuclei facing an intact basal cell layer were used in this procedure.

Next, a linear combination of these selected variables was formed such that the difference between the mean discriminant function score from normal nuclei and from high-grade PIN nuclei was maximized. Figure 2 shows the progression curve with the 95% confidence limits for the mean discriminant function scores. In this discriminant function, karyometric features descriptive of run length statistics, pixel optical density (OD) histogram and variance of pixel OD values carried the greatest weights.

Next the discriminant function was applied to nuclei no longer facing an intact basal cell layer. For both low-grade PIN and high-grade PIN lesions the observed discriminant function scores were lower. When applied to secretory cell nuclei from glands immediately adjacent to adenocarcinoma and from adenocarcinoma lesions themselves – i.e., also to nuclei no longer facing an intact basal

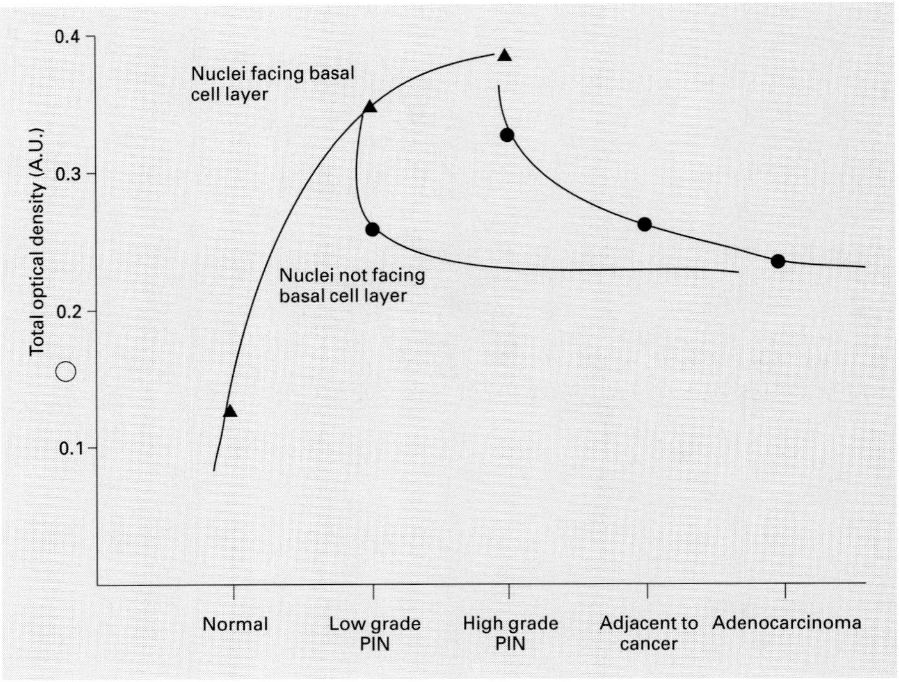

Fig. 3. Nuclear total optical density as a function of prostatic lesion progression.

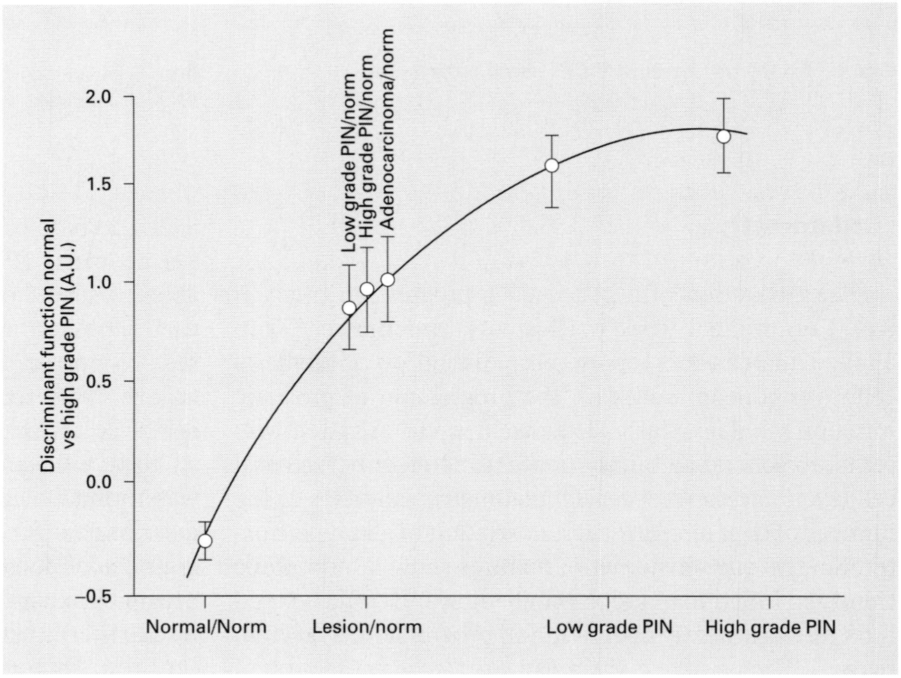

Fig. 4. Mean discriminant function scores in nuclei from histologically normal appearing tissue of prostates harboring low grade, high grade and adenocarcinoma lesions.

cell layer – it became apparent that a second trend is in effect in the progression from a PIN lesion to adenocarcinoma. The lowering of the discriminant function score for the nuclei no longer facing an intact basal cell layer is the first indication for this trend. This is shown in figure 3 for the total OD values.

Karyometric measurements thus were found to be able to detect some rather small differences for nuclei no longer facing an intact basal cell layer. The next question was whether even earlier changes could be detected in histologically normal appearing tissue from prostates harboring PIN or adenocarcinoma. These nuclei were to be compared to normal secretory cell nuclei from cystoprostatectomy specimens shown to have no prostatic lesions at all.

The above derived discriminant function was applied to these data sets and it could be shown that, indeed, a statistically significant change in karyometric variable values occurs long before a PIN lesion is visually detected. These changes can be seen in normal appearing tissue regions from prostates with low-grade PIN, high-grade PIN or adenocarcinoma. Figure 4 shows the mean discriminant function scores with their confidence limits.

In a subsequent study, the expression of these PIN and carcinoma-associated karyometric changes was examined as a function of distance from the margin of the PIN or adenocarcinoma lesion. It was found that the changes are evident up to the site at the largest examined distance of 10 mm, in a majority of nuclei measured at each location. Figure 5 shows the results.

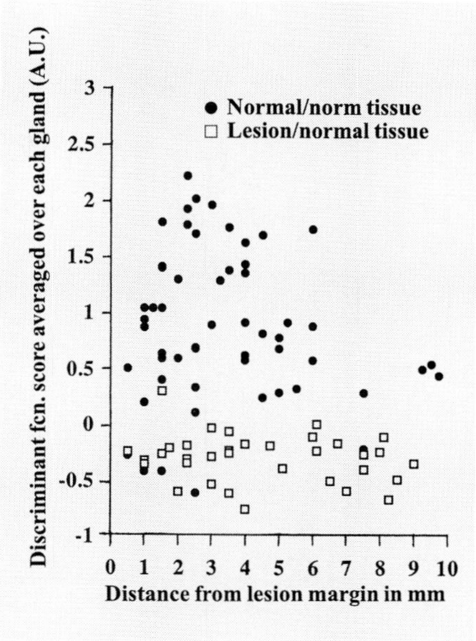

Fig. 5. Average discriminant function score per gland in normal prostatic tissue and in histologically normal appearing tissue from prostates with prostatic lesions, as a function of distance from the margin of the lesion.

Specific Characterization of Nuclei

Efforts to document progression of a prostatic lesion or regression in response to chemopreventive intervention invariably raise the issue of the nature of the variability observed among different cases. First is the effect of statistical randomness. Next, cases diagnostically grouped together as 'low-grade PIN' or 'high-grade PIN' each constitute fuzzy sets representing cases of different progression along the trend line shown in figure 1. Finally, one must consider that this reductionist mathematical/statistical analytic approach may not be fully appropriate when applied to patients. Individual patients are in their response to the disease greatly affected not only by a large number of influences, but by a multitude of feedback and control mechanisms, i.e. by characteristics inherent in complex systems. In short, a 'patient' cannot be adequately and fully described by a linear system. Rather, there is genuine diversity between patients, as a third reason for the observed case to case variability.

An effort was made, therefore, to develop methods that would allow a highly specific characterization of individual nuclei and of lesions, describing these in terms of representation by nuclei of different degrees of deviation from normal.

To characterize nuclei, a 'nuclear chromatin texture signature' was defined. The values of approximately 100 nuclear features descriptive of the statistical and spatial distribution of the nuclear chromatin were arranged in an arbitrarily chosen but consistent sequence. As sequencing criterion we chose the spatial order of dependence of pixel values that the features represented. First-order features are, e.g. the relative frequencies of occurrence of pixel OD values, which have no spatial dependence; second-order statistical features are the frequencies of occurrence of pairs of pixel OD values at adjacent pixel locations, from the co-occurrence matrix; the run-length features express higher order dependencies. In principle, one could have chosen any other sequencing of features to form a profile.

The feature values were standardized by dividing them by the standard deviation observed for each feature in a large set of normal nuclei serving as reference data set. The nuclear signature, or profile, thus is a set of z-values. Finally, some value limits were set to rein in the effects of extreme outliers. It can be shown that the nuclei from PIN lesions undergo a systematic change as a function of lesion progression, as seen in figure 6.

Also, the same changes in the nuclear chromatin texture signature can be observed in nuclei measured in the histologically normal appearing tissues from prostates harboring a PIN lesion or adenocarcinoma (fig. 7).

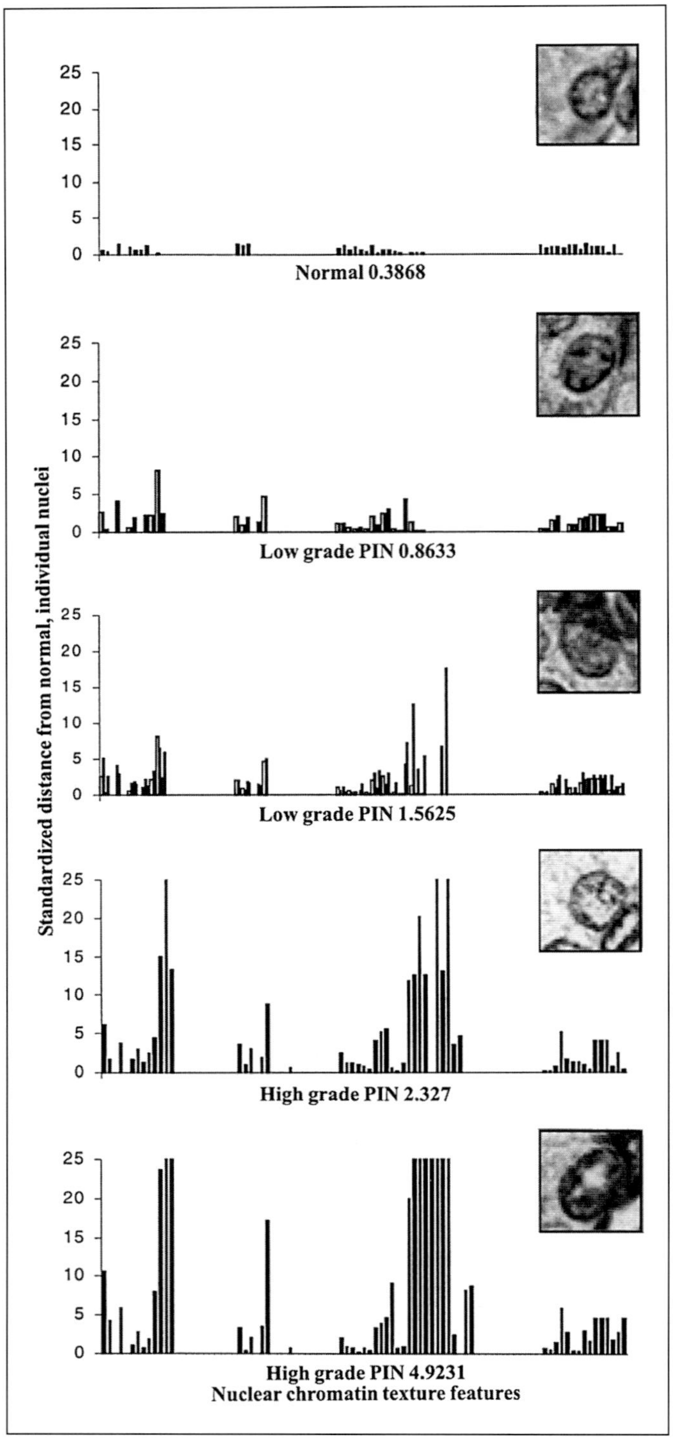

Fig. 6. Nuclear signatures of individual nuclei from PIN lesions.

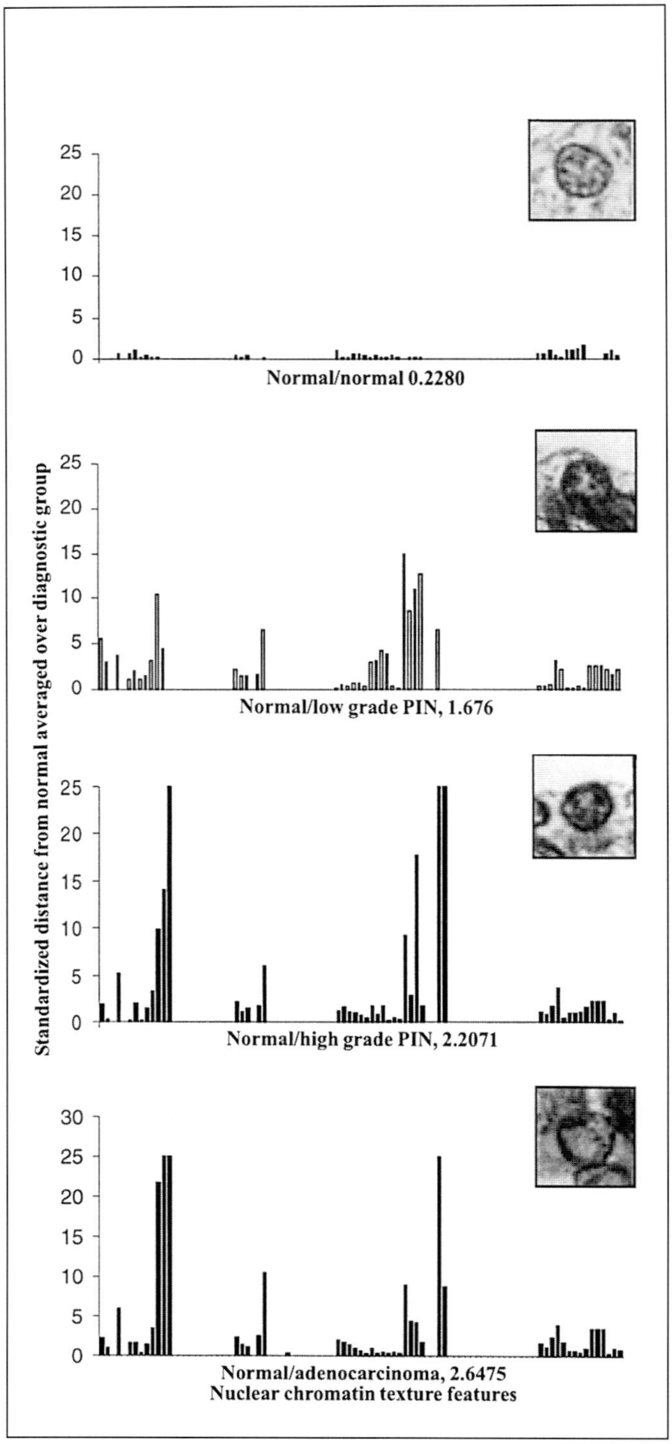

Fig. 7. Nuclear signature of individual nuclei from histologically normal appearing tissue of lesions of prostates with PIN and adenocarcinoma lesions.

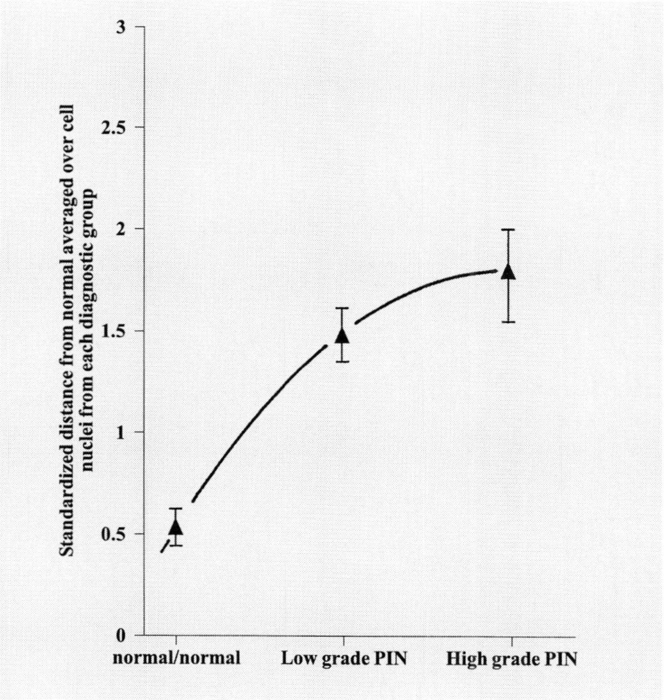

8

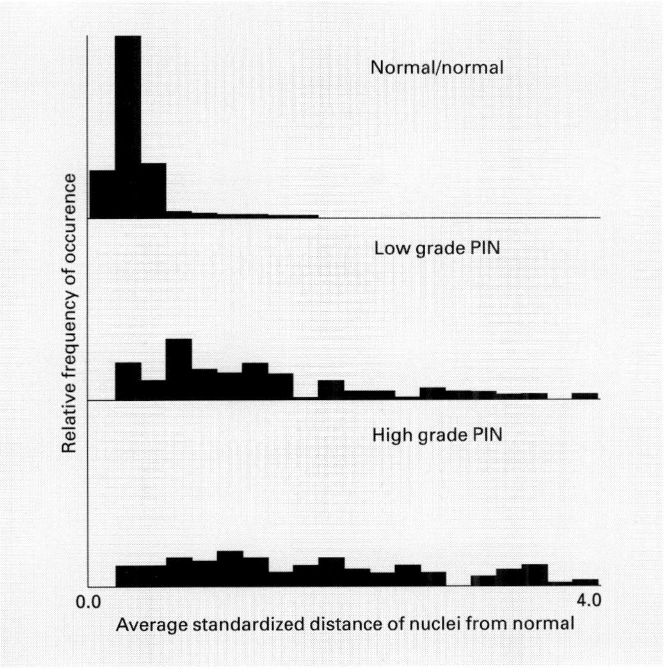

9

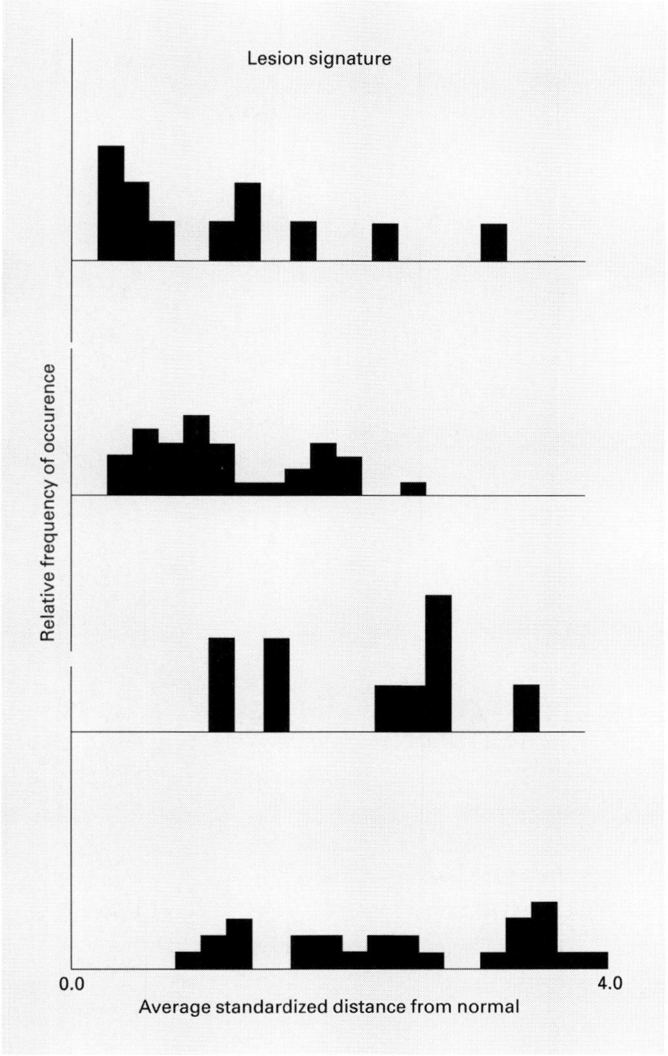

10

Fig. 8. Averaged standardized distance of nuclei as a function of PIN lesion grade.

Fig. 9. Lesion signatures: the distribution of frequency of occurrence of nuclei of different degree of abnormality.

Fig. 10. Lesion signatures for four cases of high grade PIN. Note the diversity in abnormality of the nuclei between cases.

Lesion Signatures

To characterize a specific lesion one may average the 100 values in the nuclear signature of a given nucleus and derive a single numeric value, as the average standardized deviation from normal. Figure 8 shows this plot. More informative than the mean values is the distribution of values within each of the diagnostic categories, as seen in figure 9. Of clinical interest due to its prognostic potential, though, is the substantial diversity of lesion signatures observed among cases within the same diagnostic grading. This is seen in figure 10.

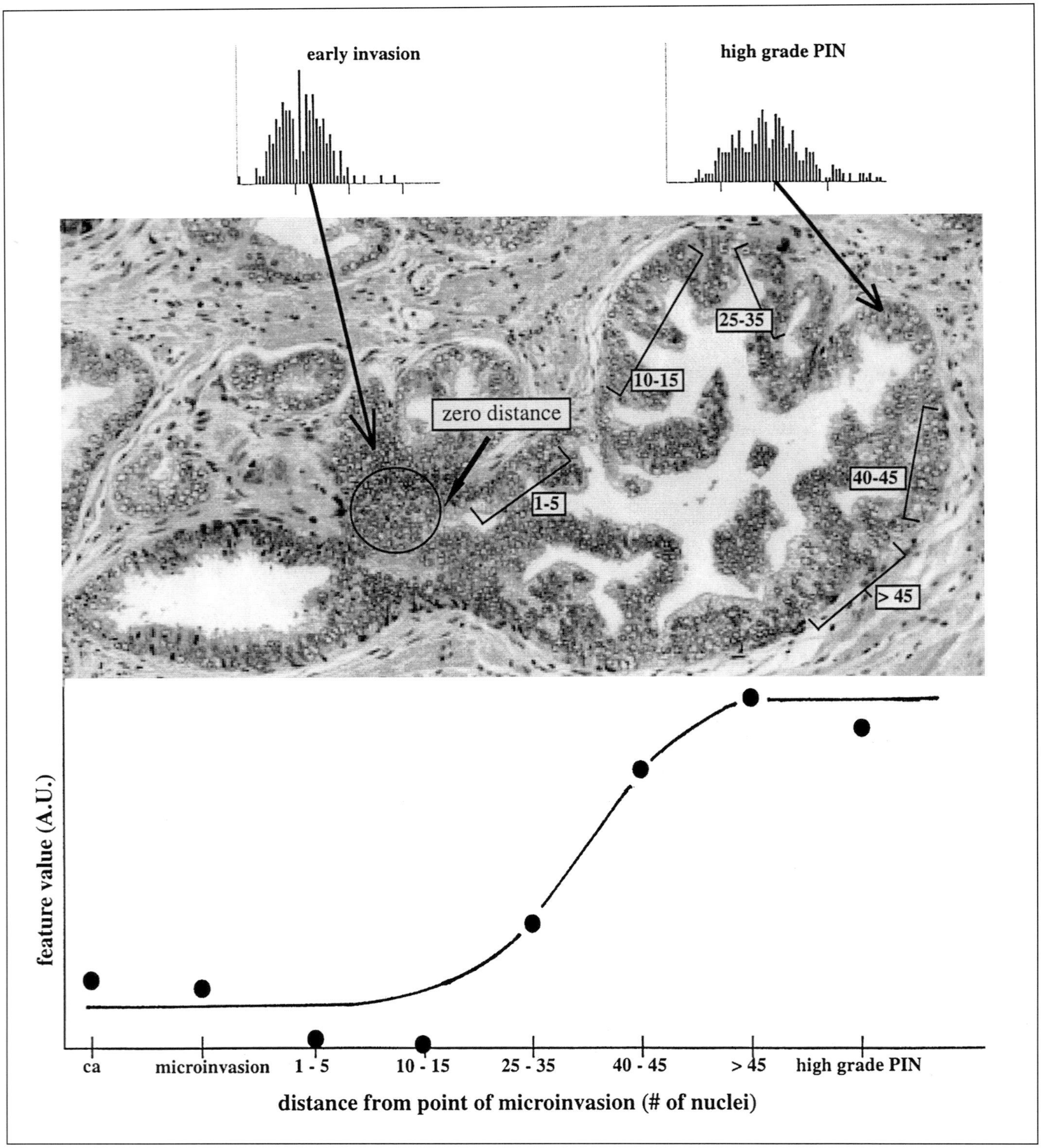

Fig. 11. Deviation of individual nuclei from normal plotted as a function of distance from the point of microinvasion. Note the high degree of aneuploidy in the high grade PIN region with a mode at approximately 4N at the upper right, and the near diploid stem lines seen in the area of microinvasion, centered around the 2N ploidy value.

Microinvasion

The specific characterization of individual nuclei by a nuclear signature has been applied to an analysis of microinvasion [8]. Histopathologic sections from high-grade PIN lesions were selected which showed a region of microinvasion emanating from a gland with high-grade PIN. The chromatin texture signatures of nuclei were recorded for the area of microinvasion, and along the secretory cell layer, as a function of distance into the high-grade PIN gland. It can be seen that the high-grade PIN nuclei undergo a gradual change in their chromatin texture, beginning at a distance of about 40–50 nuclear locations from the point of microinvasion. At a distance of 5–10 nuclear locations the secretory cell nuclei are indistinguishable in their signature from the nuclei of the microinvasion, as seen in figure 11.

Note that the distribution of total OD values in high-grade PIN is highly aneuploid, whereas nuclei in the area of microinvasion show near diploid stemlines. Microinvasion may be due to outgrowth of a clone of lower ploidy.

Summary Discussion

Micromorphometric features derived from image analysis provide markers for the progression or regression of prostatic lesions. These markers can be documented in numeric form and secured in value on a statistical basis. Thus, the detection of very small changes or differences is possible. Micromorphometric analysis allows the detection of change in histologically seemingly normal appearing tissue, i.e., at a very early stage of a pathologic process, and at a time when chemopreventive intervention might be effective.

Acknowledgements

This research has been supported by a grant from the National Institutes of Health. National Cancer Institute, Bethesda, Md., R35 CA53877 (P.H.B.). The content of this paper is solely the responsibility of the authors and does not necessarily represent the official views of the National Cancer Institute. Further support was provided by CAPES, Brasília, Brazil.

References

1 Bartels PH, Montironi R, Thompson D, Vaught L, Hamilton PW: Statistical histometry of the basal cell/secretory cell bilayer in prostatic intraepithelial neoplasia. Anal Quant Cytol Histol 1998;20:381–388.

2 Bartels PH, Montironi R, Hamilton PH, Thompson D, Vaught L, Bartels HG: Nuclear chromatin texture in prostatic lesions. I. PIN and adenocarcinoma. Anal Quant Cytol Histol 1998;20:389–396.

3 Bartels PH, Montironi R, Hamilton PH, Thompson D, Vaught L, Bartels HG: Nuclear chromatin texture in prostatic lesions. II. PIN and malignancy-associated changes. Anal Quant Cytol Histol 1998;20:397–406.

4 Bartels PH, da Silva VD, Montironi R, Hamilton PW, Thompson D, Vaught L, et al: Chromatin texture signatures in nuclei from prostate lesions. Anal Quant Cytol Histol 1998;20:407–416.

5 Bartels PH, Thompson D, Bartels HG, Montironi R, Scarpelli M, Hamilton PW: Machine vision-based histometry of premalignant and malignant prostatic lesions. Pathol Res Pract 1995;191:935–944.

6 Bartels PH, Gahm T, Thompson D: Automated microscopy in diagnostic histopathology: From image processing to automated reasoning. Int J Imaging Syst Technol 1997;8:214–223.

7 Bostwick DG, Brawer MK: Prostatic intra-epithelial neoplasia and early invasion in prostate cancer. Cancer 1987;59:788–794.

8 DaSilva VD, Montironi RM, Thompson D, Bartels HG, Vaught L, Hamilton PW, Bartels PH: Chromatin texture in high-grade prostatic intraepithelial neoplasia and early invasive carcinoma. Anal Quant Cytol Histol, in press.

European Urology

Eur Urol 1999;35:492–495

Reversibility of Prostatic Intraepithelial Neoplasia: Implications for Chemoprevention

David G. Bostwick Roxann Neumann Junqi Qian Liang Cheng

Department of Laboratory Medicine and Pathology, Mayo Clinic, Rochester, Minn., USA

Key Words

Chemoprevention · Prostatic intraepithelial neoplasia · Prostate neoplasms · Prostatic carcinoma · Androgen deprivation therapy · Hormonal therapy · Radiation therapy

Abstract

High-grade prostatic intraepithelial neoplasia is the most likely precursor of prostatic adenocarcinoma, according to virtually all available evidence. It has a high predictive value as a marker for adenocarcinoma, and its identification in biopsy specimens of the prostate warrants further search for concurrent invasive carcinoma. Androgen deprivation therapy and radiation therapy decrease its prevalence and extent, suggesting a role in chemoprevention.

The genetic events associated with initiation and progression of prostate cancer are poorly understood. Carcinogenesis apparently involves multiple genetic changes, including activation of dominantly acting oncogenes that promote cell proliferation and loss of tumor suppressor genes that negatively regulate cell proliferation.

High-grade prostatic intraepithelial neoplasia (PIN) is the earliest accepted stage in prostatic carcinogenesis, possessing most but not all of the phenotypic and biochemical changes of cancer [1]. Like prostatic carcinoma, PIN is usually multifocal and genotypically heterogeneous [2, 3]. Genetic events in PIN have been linked to the development of prostatic carcinoma, and the remarkable morphologic heterogeneity of prostatic carcinoma is reflected at the genetic level.

Androgen Deprivation Therapy Reverses High-Grade PIN

All modes of hormonal treatment alter the prostatic epithelium, causing acinar atrophy and apoptosis (programmed cell death). This therapy also induces significant histologic changes in PIN and prostatic adenocarcinoma [4–10].

The histopathologic effects are remarkably similar for most forms of androgen deprivation, with varying degrees of acinar and stromal atrophy (table 1, fig. 1) [11]. Squamous metaplasia and glycogenic acanthosis are common findings after orchiectomy and diethylstibestrol (DES), but are uncommon after contemporary forms of treatment. Combination therapy, sometimes referred to as total androgen blockade, is particularly effective in induc-

KARGER

Fax + 41 61 306 12 34
E-Mail karger@karger.ch
www.karger.com

0302–2838/99/0356–0492$17.50/0

Accessible online at:
http://BioMedNet.com/karger

David G. Bostwick, MD
Department of Pathology, Mayo Clinic
200 First St. S.W., Rochester, MN 55905 (USA)
Tel. +1 507 284 1870, Fax +1 507 284 1599
E-Mail bostwick.david@mayo.edu

Table 1. Effect of androgen deprivation therapy on the benign prostate and PIN

Architecture
Prominent acinar atrophy
Decreased ratio of acini to stroma
Basal cell hyperplasia in benign epithelium
Foci of epithelial hyperplasia
Stromal edema in early stages; fibrosis in late stages
Squamous metaplasia
Decrease in extent of PIN
Cytology
Prominent clear cell change
Nuclear shrinkage
Nuclear hyperchromasia
Nucleolar shrinkage

There is some variability in these changes depending on the method of therapy.

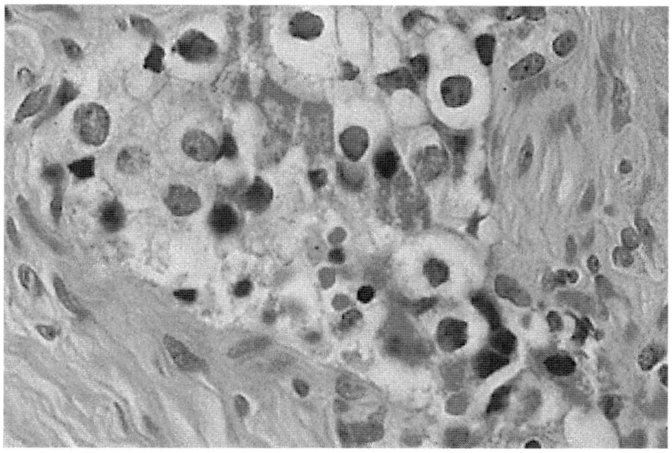

Fig. 1. Androgen deprivation therapy changes in prostatic adenocarcinoma, including nuclear shrinkage and hyperchromasia in association with cytoplasmic clearing.

ing changes. Androgen deprivation causes regression of high-grade PIN, with a decrease in prevalence and extent [12–14]. This decrease is accompanied by epithelial hyperplasia, cytoplasmic clearing, and prominent acinar atrophy, with decreased ratio of acini to stroma. These findings indicate that the dysplastic prostatic epithelium is hormone-dependent. Treated dysplastic epithelial cells separate from the basal cell layer and exfoliate into the acinar lumen.

A short-term prospective, double-masked, placebo-controlled, phase II chemoprevention trial utilizing low-dose flutamide with cancer incidence as an endpoint was begun at our institution in 1997 in patients with high-grade PIN without cancer [15, 16]. Chemoprevention trials designed to reverse high-grade PIN may be confounded by the presence of underlying but undetected prostate cancer. This problem is addressed by requiring a second biopsy without cancer before entry into the study (preferably sextant or more biopsies with special attention to areas of abnormality on ultrasonogram or digital rectal examination) and by including enough subjects in the study and control groups to equalize the risk of coexistent cancer between the two groups. PIN is routinely monitored by repeat biopsy in contemporary urologic practice, with recommended repeat evaluation every 6 months for 2 years and annually thereafter. These study methods are consistent with current urologic practice and would allow other promising chemopreventive agents to be evaluated in a comparable design. The information gained could provide the basis for additional clinical trials directed toward the prevention and elimination of the prostate cancer in other high-risk target populations and in the general population.

Blockade of 5α-reductase with finasteride appears to have less effect on PIN than other forms of androgen deprivation therapy, according to the limited available evidence. The incidence of PIN was unchanged in one study after 1 year of finasteride, and there was a significant increase in the number of patients with subsequent cancer on biopsy after this treatment [17].

Radiation Therapy Reverses High-Grade PIN

The prevalence and extent of PIN is decreased after radiation therapy [18]. However, one study paradoxically noted a higher incidence (70%) of PIN after radiation therapy than expected [19], but they failed to employ accepted diagnostic criteria for PIN, so their results are not comparable with others (tables 2, 3).

Following radiation therapy, PIN retains the features characteristic of untreated PIN, and is readily recognized in tissue specimens (fig. 2) [18]. The key pathologic features include nuclear crowding, nuclear overlapping and stratification, nuclear hyperchromasia, and prominent nucleoli. The basal cell layer is present, but often fragmented. The most common patterns of PIN are tufting and micropapillary, similar to those reported in untreated PIN [18].

The main differential consideration of high-grade PIN after radiation therapy is atypical basal cell hyperplasia (ABCH) [20, 21]. The proliferation of basal cells in ABCH is often eccentrically located with partial involvement of acini, retaining the overlying columnar or cuboidal secretory cells. These atypical basal cells have enlarged nuclei and nucleoli, fine powdery chromatin, occasional nuclear grooves, and an absence of apocrine blebs. Nuclear 'bubble' artifact or intranuclear vacuoles may be seen. In difficult cases, the use of immunostaining for high-molecular-weight cytokeratin is helpful for distinguishing ABCH from high-grade PIN, and this is our favored application of this antibody.

The long-term efficacy of radiation treatment may depend on eradication of cancer as well as precancerous lesions that may otherwise lead to evolution of secondary metachronous invasive cancers. Identification of residual or recurrent cancer portends a worse prognosis. The ques-

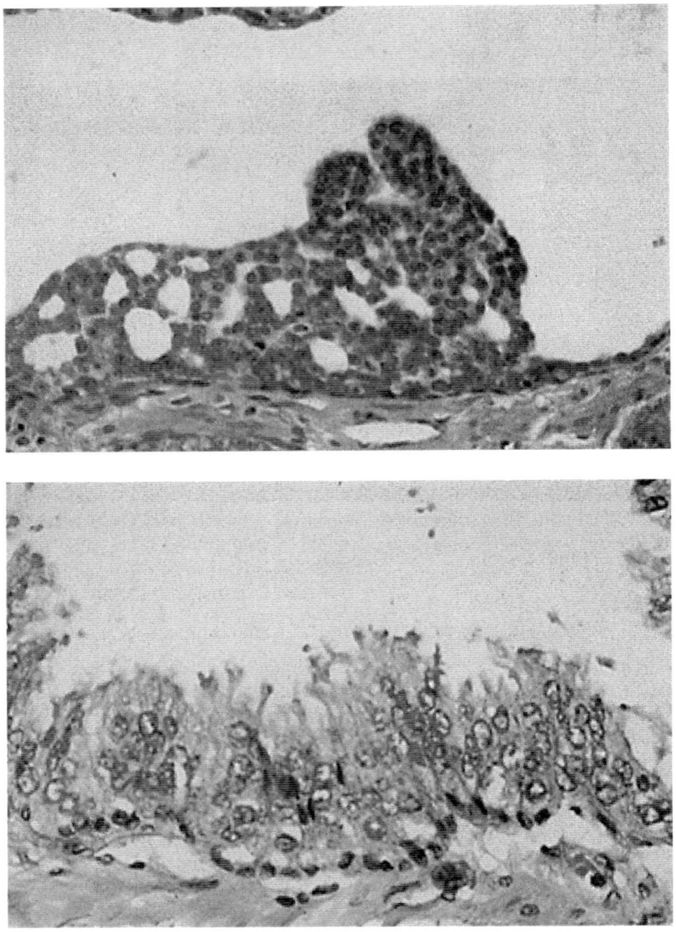

Fig. 2. PIN following radiation therapy. **a** There is partial acinar involvement by the cribriform pattern of high-grade PIN. **b** The nuclei show some artifactual clearing, but the proliferative changes are evident and scattered prominent nucleoli are present.

Table 2. Effect of radiation therapy on the benign prostate and PIN

Architecture
Prominent acinar atrophy and distortion
Decreased ratio of acini to stroma
Basal cell hyperplasia in benign epithelium
Foci of epithelial hyperplasia
Squamous and squamoid metaplasia
Stromal fibrosis with smooth muscle atrophy
Decrease in extent of PIN
Cytology
Nuclear hyperchromasia
Marked variation in nuclear size and shape
High nucleus:cytoplasmic ratio
Variable nucleolar enlargement
Decreased secretory activity of cells

Table 3. Comparative distribution of high-grade PIN in radical prostatectomies as primary treatment for cancer and salvage prostatectomies after radiation therapy failure

	No radiation therapy[a]		Radiation failure[b]	
	cases	%	cases	%
PIN (minimum distance from cancer)				
≤2 mm from cancer	156	93	50	94
>2 mm from cancer	11	7	3	6
Number of foci of PIN, % (in cases with PIN)				
One	58	35	16	30
More than one	109	65	84	70
Volume of PIN, cm^3				
<0.05 (including 0)	29	15	23	43
0.05–0.09	2	1	10	19
≥0.1	164	84	20	38

a Unpublished data from Qian et al. [22].
b Data from Cheng et al. [18].

tions remain whether recurrent cancer after irradiation is due to regrowth of incompletely eradicated tumor or progression from incompletely eradicated PIN. Further studies of salvage prostatectomy specimens and postradiation therapy needle biopsies are justified in an attempt to establish the significance of high-grade PIN as a source of long-term treatment failure among these patients. If PIN is associated with treatment failure, adjuvant chemoprevention strategies that ablate this lesion may reduce the risk of late cancer recurrence.

References

1 Bostwick DG: Prospective origins of prostate carcinoma: Prostatic intraepithelial neoplasia and atypical adenomatous hyperplasia. Cancer 1996;78:330–336.

2 Bostwick DG, Shan A, Qian J, Darson M, Maihle NJ, Jenkins RB, Cheng L: Independent origin of multiple foci of prostatic intraepithelial neoplasia: Comparison with matched foci of prostate cancer. Cancer 1998;83:1995–2002.

3 Bostwick DG, Pacelli A, Lopez-Beltran A: Molecular biology of prostatic intraepithelial neoplasia. Prostate 1996;29:117–134.

4 Tetu B, Srigley JR, Boivin JC, Dupont A, Monfette G, Pinault S, Labrie F: Effect of combination endocrine therapy (LHRH agonist and flutamide) on normal prostate and prostatic adenocarcinoma. Am J Surg Pathol 1991;15:111–120.

5 Murphy WM, Soloway MS, Barrows GH: Pathologic changes associated with androgen deprivation therapy for prostate cancer. Cancer 1991;68:821–828.

6 Civantos F, Marcial MA, Banks ER, Ho CK, Speights VD, Drew PA, Murphy WM, Soloway MS: Pathology of androgen deprivation therapy in prostate carcinoma. A comparative study of 173 patients. Cancer 1995;75:1634–1641.

7 Smith DM, Murphy WM: Histologic changes in prostate carcinomas treated with leuprolide (luteinizing hormone-releasing hormone effect). Distinction from poor tumor differentiation. Cancer 1994;73:1472–1477.

8 Armas OA, Aprikian AG, Melamed J, Cordon-Cardo C, Cohen DW, Erlandson R, Fair WR, Reuten VE: Clinical and pathological effects of neoadjuvant total androgen ablation therapy on clinically localized prostatic adenocarcinoma. Am J Surg Pathol 1994;18:979–991.

9 Ellison E, Chuang SS, Zincke H et al: Prostate adenocarcinoma after androgen deprivation therapy: A comparative study of morphology, morphometry, immunohistochemistry, and DNA ploidy. Pathol Case Rev 1996;2:36–46.

10 Montironi R, Bartels PH, Thompson D, Valli M, Prete E: Androgen-deprived prostate adenocarcinoma. Evaluation of treatment-related changes vs. no distinctive treatment effect with a Bayesian belief network. Eur Urol 1996;30:307–315.

11 Bostwick DG, Dundore PA: Biopsy Pathology of the Prostate. London, Chapman & Hall, 1997.

12 Vaillancourt L, Tetu B, Fradet Y, Dupont A, Gomez J, Cusan L, Suburu ER, Diamond P, Candas B, Labrie F: Effect of neoadjuvant endocrine therapy (combined androgen blockade) on normal prostate and prostate carcinoma. A randomized study. Am J Surg Pathol 1996;20:86–93.

13 Ferguson J, Bostwick DG, Ellison E, Zincke H: Decrease of prostatic intraepithelial neoplasia following androgen deprivation therapy in patients with stage T3 prostatic adenocarcinoma. Urology 1994;44:91–95.

14 Montironi R, Magi Galluzzi C, Fabris G: Apoptotic bodies in prostatic intraepithelial neoplasia and prostatic adenocarcinoma following total androgen ablation. Pathol Res Pract 1995;191:873–880.

15 Aquilina JW, Lipsky JJ, Bostwick DG: Androgen deprivation as a strategy for prostate cancer chemoprevention. J Natl Cancer Inst 1997;89:689–696.

16 Bostwick DG, Burke HB, Wheeler T, Chung LWK, Bookstein R, Pretlow TG et al: The most promising surrogate end-point biomarkers for screening candidate chemopreventive compounds for prostatic adenocarcinoma in short-term phase II clinical trials. J Cell Biochem 1994;19(suppl):283–289.

17 Slem CE, Cote RJ, Skinner EC et al: The effect of finasteride on prostate gland peripheral zone histology and proliferation rates in men at high risk for prostate cancer. J Urol 1997;157:228–232.

18 Cheng L, Cheville JC, Pisansky TM, Slezak J, Bergstralh EJ, Sebo TJ et al: Prevalence and distribution of prostatic intraepithelial neoplasia in salvage radical prostatectomy specimens after radiation therapy. Cancer 1999, in press.

19 Arakawa A, Song S, Scardino PT, Wheeler TM: High-grade prostatic intraepithelial neoplasia in prostates removed following irradiation failure in the treatment of prostatic adenocarcinoma. Pathol Res Pract 1995;191:868–872.

20 Devaraj LT, Bostwick DG: Atypical basal cell hyperplasia of the prostate. Immunophenotypic profile and proposed classification of basal cell proliferations. Am J Surg Pathol 1993;17:645–659.

21 Qian J, Wollan P, Bostwick DG: The extent and multicentricity of high-grade prostatic intraepithelial neoplasia in clinically localized prostatic adenocarcinoma. Hum Pathol 1997;28:143–148.

Surrogate Endpoint Biomarkers for Clinical Trials of Prostate Cancer Chemoprevention

European Urology

Eur Urol 1999;35:496–497

Evolution of Isolated High-Grade Prostate Intraepithelial Neoplasia in a Mediterranean Patient Population

Ferran Algaba

Fundació Puigvert, Universitat Autònoma de Barcelona, Spain

Key Words

Prostatic intraepithelial neoplasia · Prostatic cancer · Prostate biopsy

Abstract

The discovery of high-grade prostatic intraepithelial neoplasia (HGPIN) in prostatic needle biopsies is of clinical importance. Previous studies have shown prostate cancer to develop in 27–100% (average 55%) of the cases after HGPIN was diagnosed. Our preliminary findings in a Mediterranean population (Barcelona, Spain) revealed a prevalence of HGPIN of 4.4%, and an incidence of prostate cancer of 28.7% in cases in whom isolated HGPIN was identified at the first biopsy. The majority (64%) of these cases were diagnosed at the first biopsy after HGPIN diagnosis, and 52% within the first year. HGPIN persisted in 46.6% of the cases. The total mean serum prostate-specific antigen (PSA) was 9.9 ± 6.6 ng/ml in the prostate cancer cases, compared with 8.8 ± 7.5 in the cases without cancer. The low incidence of isolated HGPIN and subsequent cancer occurrence may be due to local factors or insufficient follow-up.

Introduction

Over the last decade, numerous studies have shown an interrelationship between high-grade prostatic intraepithelial neoplasia (HGPIN) and prostatic cancer (PC), particularly prostate cancer beginning at the peripheral zone [1–4]. Therefore, it is not surprising to find HGPIN in PC specimens. This suggests that the finding of isolated HGPIN may imply either the presence of a concomitant cancer not demonstrated on the material under study, or the later likely occurrence of some neoplastic process in the patient's prostate. In the literature available there is considerable disagreement over the evolution of isolated HGPIN. This may be due to the use of different methodology, to interpathologist reproducibility problems or to real geographical differences. The purpose of this study is to look at a Mediterranean population of patients with an isolated HGPIN.

Patients and Method

From November 1990 to June 1997, a total of 3,316 prostate biopsies were performed in 2,807 patients at our center (Fundació Puigvert). One hundred and twenty-six of them showed isolated HGPIN. Eighty-seven patients out of the 126 with isolated HGPIN underwent repeat biopsy. In 87 patients undergoing multiple prostate biopsies, the patient's history has been reviewed focusing on baseline serum PSA, number of biopsies performed, follow-up time and occurrence or nonoccurrence of carcinoma.

KARGER

Fax + 41 61 306 12 34
E-Mail karger@karger.ch
www.karger.com

0302–2838/99/0356–0496$17.50/0

Accessible online at:
http://BioMedNet.com/karger

Ferran Algaba, MD
Fundació Puigvert, Department of Pathology
calle Cartagena 340–350
E–8025 Barcelona (Spain)
Tel. +34 93 416 9700, Fax +34 93 416 9730

Results

HGPIN prevalence is 4.4%. Of the 87 patients undergoing multiple biopsies, 21 (24.1%) showed a subsequent PC and 4 (4.6%) had highly atypical glands suggestive of cancer. Therefore, it could be assumed that overall 25 patients (28.7%) had cancer subsequently.

In patients with subsequent PC, in 16 (64%) cancer was demonstrated at a second biopsy, in 6 (24%) at a third biopsy and 3 (12%) required more than three biopsies. Average time between first HGPIN biopsy and PC diagnosis biopsy was 364 days. It must be borne in mind that 52% of patients were diagnosed a PC within the first year, 32% within the first 2 years and 16% 2 years after HGPIN diagnosis. Baseline serum PSA in these patients was 9.9 ± 6.6 ng/ml.

The 62 patients who exhibited no subsequent PC had a variable follow-up (780 ± 408 days), with a modal value of 21.63 months. Forty (64.5%) patients have undergone one more biopsy, 17 two biopsies apart from the first one, and 5 (8.1%) have had more than two biopsies. In 29 patients (46.6%) new isolated HGPINs were identified in subsequent biopsies. Baseline serum PSA in these patients was 8.8 ± 7.5 ng/ml.

Comment

The first finding worthy of comment is the low prevalence of isolated HGPIN in our population, comparing to the figures up to 11% [5] reported in the USA literature. However, when PC incidence rates for different geographical areas are compared, it turns out that prevalence is 70.1 in 100,000 inhabitants among USA population with European ancestry [6], 35.2 in 100,000 inhabitants in the European Community [7] and 22.2 in 100,000 inhabitants in Spain [8]. We might, thus, conclude that since our PC incidence is only a third of the USA's, it is not surprising that our prevalence of isolated HGPIN is also a third. The incidence of carcinoma secondary to isolated HGPIN is 28.7%, which falls within the lower range of values reported in the literature (from 100 to 27%, with a mean of 55%) [9–11].

In most patients with subsequent carcinoma, this is identified within 2 years of diagnosing an isolated HGPIN (84%). This observation together with a higher baseline serum PSA (9.9 ± 6.6 ng/ml) suggests that in the majority of patients with an initial HGPIN who later exhibit a PC, prostate cancer was already present at the time of HGPIN diagnosis [12].

Conclusions

The occurrence of an isolated HGPIN implies that the patient is at risk of having a PC, particularly when serum PSA is increased. In our setting, the prevalence of isolated HGPIN accounts for only a third of the value reported in the USA literature, but it corresponds with the lower PC prevalence in our geographical area. Subsequent cancer occurrence rate is only 28.7%, which is also a low incidence rate. This (having ruled out reproducibility problems) may be due to insufficient follow-up time or to the fact that those factors contributing to a lower PC prevalence also result in a less aggressive biological evolution.

Obviously, the number of patients under study should be increased and follow-up time as well, in order to confirm such a perceived trend.

References

1 Bostwick DG, Pacelli A, López-Beltrán A: Molecular biology of prostatic intraepithelial neoplasia. Prostate 1996;29:117–134.

2 De la Torre M, Haggman M, Brandstedt S et al: Prostatic intraepithelial neoplasia and invasive carcinoma in total prostatectomy specimens: Distribution, volume and DNA ploidy. Br J Urol 1993;72:207–213.

3 Aboseif S, Shinohara K, Weidner N et al: The significance of prostatic intra-epithelial neoplasia. Br J Urol 1995;76:355–359.

4 Algaba F, Trias I, López L et al: Relación del carcinoma prostático de la zona periférica con la atrofia glandular y la neoplasia intraepitelial prostática. Actas Urol Esp 1997;21:40–43.

5 Palapattu GS, Kattan M, Scardino PT, Wheeler TM: The association of selected pathologic features with prostate cancer in a single needle biopsy accession. J Urol 1997;157:120–124.

6 Seidman H, Mushinski MH, Gelb SK et al: Probabilities of eventually developing or dying of cancer – United States 1985. CA Cancer J Clin 1985;35:36–56.

7 Moller JE et al: Cancer in the European Community and its member states. Eur J Cancer 1990;26:1167–1256.

8 Arrizabalaga M, Navarro M, Moral J et al: Incidencia de los principales carcinomas urológicos en el área sanitaria VII de Madrid. LIX Congreso Nacional de la asociación Española de Urologia, 1994.

9 Langer JE, Rovner ES, Coleman BG et al: Strategy for repeat biopsy of patients with prostatic intraepithelial neoplasia detected by prostate needle biopsy. J Urol 1996;155:228–231.

10 Brawer MK et al: Significance of prostatic intraepithelial neoplasia on prostate needle biopsy. Urology 1991;38:103–107.

11 Chéchile GE, Algaba F, Solsona E et al: Lesiones premalignas de la próstata en lesiones premalignas de los tumores urológicos. Valoración clínico, patológico y molecular p-98. LXIII Congreso Nacional de Urologia, 1998.

12 Epstein JI, Grignon DJ, Humprey PA et al: Interobserver reproducibility in the diagnosis of prostatic intraepithelial neoplasia. Am J Surg Pathol 1995;19:973–986.

Surrogate Endpoint Biomarkers for Clinical Trials of Prostate Cancer Chemoprevention

European Urology

Eur Urol 1999;35:498–503

Clinical Evolution of Prostatic Intraepithelial Neoplasia

A.R. Zlotta C.C. Schulman

Department of Urology, Erasme Hospital, University Clinics of Brussels, Belgium

Key Words

Prostatic neoplasms · Prostatic intraepithelial neoplasia

Abstract

High-grade prostatic intraepithelial neoplasia (PIN) is most likely a precursor of prostate cancer and is frequently associated with it whereas the direct link between low-grade PIN and cancer is not established. The clinical evolution of isolated high-grade PIN has been the object of much concern because of the possibility of undiagnosed prostate cancer or the evolution of this premalignant lesion in invasive carcinoma. Parameters predictive of the later finding of prostate cancer on repeat biopsy in patients with PIN are of evident interest and we have reviewed our experience and recent data from the literature on this topic as well as on the clinical management of these patients. Low-grade PIN is not by itself a risk of later cancer found on repeat biopsy unless other factors such as PSA increase the cancer suspicion. Patients with low-grade PIN and high serum PSA should therefore undergo repeat biopsies. Patients with low-grade PIN and without additional factors should be followed. Patients with high-grade PIN should systematically be rebiopsied. If a second set is still consistent with PIN, they should undergo additional biopsies again within 3–6 months because they are likely to have an undiagnosed cancer.

The clinical importance of high-grade prostatic intraepithelial neoplasia (PIN) has been underlined in recent years. Prostate cancer is now the most frequent form of cancer and the second killer in western men, and high-grade PIN represents its most likely precursor. PIN is now found in men as early as in their 30s and 40s [1, 2]. Since the natural course of prostate cancer is generally slow and the rate of progression from the intraepithelial stage of development to invasion is highly variable but is probably months to years, PIN might potentially be used as a biomarker of latent or occult prostate cancer and several authors have suggested that PIN may be an ideal candidate for chemoprevention strategies in order to reduce its progression to invasive cancer and ultimately reduce cancer death rates [3].

If PIN are now classified in two grades (low- and high-grade PIN) along a continuum of increasing severity, many pathologists currently use the term PIN to indicate high-grade PIN because low-grade PIN most probably is

KARGER

Fax + 41 61 306 12 34
E-Mail karger@karger.ch
www.karger.com

0302–2838/99/0356–0498$17.50/0

Accessible online at:
http://BioMedNet.com/karger

Dr. A.R. Zlotta, MD
Department of Urology, University Clinics of Brussels
Erasme Hospital, Route de Lennik 808
B–1070 Brussels (Belgium)
Tel. +32 2 555 36 14, Fax +32 2 555 36 99

not a precancerous lesion and several authors think that the distinction between low-grade PIN and normal epithelium is somewhat subjective [4–7].

In contrast, numerous works have pointed out that high-grade PIN is in frequent spatial association with prostate carcinoma [8, 9], has phenotypic similarities to invasive prostate cancer and that both pathological entities have similar genetic changes [10–12]. For instance, using down-regulation of the cyclin-dependent kinase inhibitor p27Kip1 to identify cells capable of entering the proliferative phase of the cell cycle, De Marzo et al. [13] examined the expression of p27Kip1 in relation to its role in the development of prostatic carcinoma. Consistent with the fact that cancer cells are capable of cell division, all cases of high-grade PIN and invasive carcinoma showed down-regulation of p27Kip1 as compared with the surrounding normal-appearing secretory cells.

High-grade PIN has been identified in approximately 4–14% of prostate needle biopsies [14–16]. Evaluating pathology trends of 62,537 first-time prostate needle-core biopsies submitted by office-based urologists, processed at a single pathology laboratory, isolated high-grade PIN was diagnosed in 4.1% of the biopsies, a number which probably reflects the real incidence of this entity in general practice as opposed to reference centers [16]. The diagnosis of PIN on prostate needle biopsy without associated prostatic carcinoma raises a difficult clinical problem and remains a clinical dilemma. Indeed high-grade PIN does not necessarily mean that prostatic carcinoma is concomitantly present but a major concern exists that prostate cancer might not have been detected in prostate biopsy specimens with PIN due to sampling limitations. Therefore, the definition of parameters that can be predictive of the later finding of prostate cancer on repeat biopsy in patients with PIN is of evident clinical interest.

PIN grade is undoubtedly an important predictive factor of later cancer since patients with isolated high-grade PIN had carcinoma of the prostate found on subsequent biopsy in 33–100% of cases [4–6, 17–20] (table 1). In low-grade PIN, the situation is quite different. Indeed, the cancer detection rate in low-grade PIN patients was shown to be identical to the one in patients who underwent rebiopsy for persistently elevated serum prostate-specific antigen (PSA) [5, 20].

In a community practice of 1,009 prostate needle biopsy specimens, diagnosis of an atypical focus suspicious for malignancy was made in 48 (4.8%), among which there were 17 cases with high-grade PIN (31%). Twenty-five patients (46%) underwent additional sampling of the prostate, and 15 of these (60%) were found to have adenocarcinoma; the remaining 30 patients did not undergo a subsequent biopsy [21].

Table 1. Cancer detection on subsequent biopsies in patients with initial isolated PIN

Reference (first author)	Low-grade PIN	High-grade PIN
Brawer [4]	2/11 (18%)	10/10 (100%)
Ellis [18]	–	5/5 (100%)
Aboseif [6]	2/12 (16.6%)	19/24 (79.1%)
Weinstein [19]	–	10/19 (53%)
Keetch [5]	4/19 (19%)	19/37 (51%)
Davidson [20]	–	35/100 (35%)
Markham [17]	3/23 (13%)	13/32 (40%)
Raviv [22, 23]	6/45 (13.3%)	23/48 (47.9%)

In our own study [22–24], analyzing 93 patients with a diagnosis of isolated PIN without concurrent carcinoma, cancer detection rate on repeat biopsy or operated specimen increased with PIN grades [25, 26]. In each PSA subgroup (0–4, 4.1–10, >10 ng/ml) the subsequent cancer detection rate was higher for high-grade PIN than for low-grade PIN. Nearly 50% of patients with isolated high-grade PIN were found to have prostate cancer on repeat biopsy, compared to 13% of patients with low-grade PIN.

Serum PSA, PSA Density, Percent Free PSA, PIN and Later Cancer

The correlation between serum PSA level and PIN remains controversial. However, PSA seems clearly to be an important factor to take into consideration when dealing with patients with PIN, especially high-grade PIN [6, 25, 27]. High-grade PIN alone does not appear to increase PSA levels [26]. Keetch et al. [5], using logistic regression analysis, did not find that PSA level was a significant predictor of later cancer found on repeat biopsy. Weinstein and Epstein [19] noted that serum PSA levels were elevated in 90% of patients with high-grade PIN and cancer compared to 50% of those with PIN without associated cancer at the time of initial diagnosis. Serum PSA may be useful in distinguishing which patients with PIN will have cancer detected on repeat biopsy [19]. Brawer et al. [4] found that PSA was higher in patients who were shown to have prostate cancer on repeat biopsy.

In the study by Raviv et al. [22, 23], the group of patients that later developed cancer had a significantly

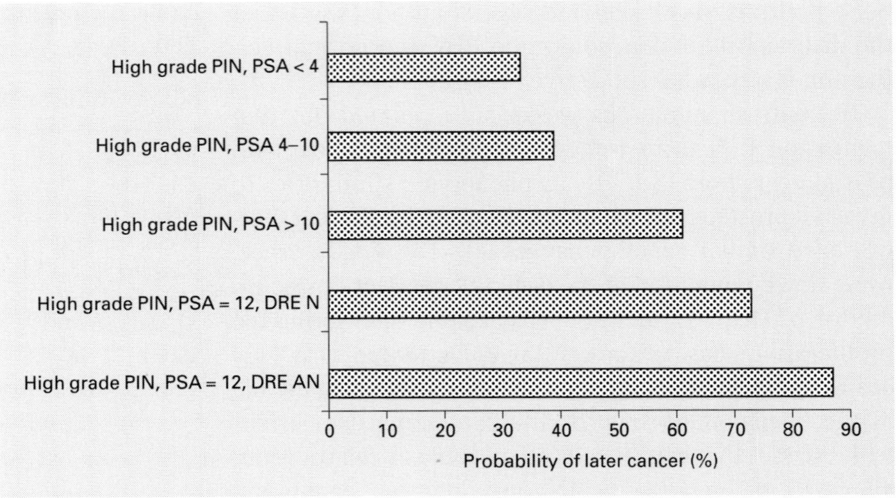

Fig. 1. Probability of later cancer found on repeat biopsy in isolated high-grade PIN, multivariate analysis.

higher PSA compared to patients without later cancer found on repeat biopsy. In high-grade PIN, the incidence of later cancer was respectively 33 and 69% when PSA was <4 or >10 ng/ml [23]. Therefore, all subgroups of patients with high-grade PIN, but especially those with elevated PSA, should undergo repeat biopsy. Low-grade PIN was associated with subsequent cancer in 42.8% of cases when PSA was >10 ng/ml, in 10.7% when PSA was between 4 and 10 ng/ml and in none of the cases when PSA was ≤4 ng/ml [23]. Low-grade PIN should cause no further action unless other factors such as an elevated PSA increase the suspicion of prostate cancer and should prompt repeat biopsies. The high detection rate of later cancer when PSA is >10 ng/ml in low-grade PIN is similar to Cooner's report [24] on the detection of prostate cancer without reference to PIN. When PSA is >10 ng/ml and whatever PIN grade, it seems clear that the high detection rate is more a reflection of the undetected presence of cancer than the presence of PIN (fig. 1).

If PSA density did not help in the strategy decision in either high/or low-grade PIN [23, 26], the decreased serum-free PSA/total PSA (fPSA/tPSA) ration obtained at the time of initial diagnosis of PIN without concurrent carcinoma was recently suggested as a predictive factor to distinguish patients in whom carcinoma will be found on subsequent biopsies from those with PIN not associated with cancer on repeat biopsy [28]. Determining the relationship between PIN and fPSA/tPSA ratios in 46 patients with PIN, in 15 patients with benign prostatic hyperplasia (BPH) and 16 patients with localized prostatic carcinoma assay, the fPSA/tPSA ratios decreased from BPH to prostate cancer but there was no significant difference between prostate cancer and high-grade PIN [28]. Additional studies are mandatory at this stage to further define the precise role of percent free PSA in PIN.

Digital Rectal Examination, Transrectal Ultrasound, PIN and Later Cancer

Transrectal ultrasound (TRUS) has currently very limited value in the diagnosis of PIN and even its role in invasive cancer is decreasing, at least with conventional TRUS. The appearance of PIN on TRUS has been reported as being hypoechoic as in cancer [6], but this has been refuted as well [29]. Lee et al. [25] and Bostwick et al. [14] have identified around 10% of PIN out of ultrasound-guided biopsies in hypoechoic lesions. Aboseif et al. [6] observed that 64% of PIN lesions were hypoechoic and this finding was more common in patients who subsequently had cancer.

Brawer et al. [4] found no differences between the sonographic appearance of PIN lesions associated with cancer and those without associated cancer on subsequent biopsy. Logistic regression analysis did not point out TRUS as an independent factor [22]. It remains to be proved whether PIN is actually giving rise to an hypoechoic zone, or may represent undetected associated carcinoma. Reports on digital rectal examination (DRE) influence on later prostate cancer findings in patients with isolated PIN are conflicting. DRE was found to be a predictor of later cancer in the study by Keetch et al. [5], and in the study by Raviv et al. [22] for high-grade PIN only, but not in other studies [6]. DRE should certainly be taken into account but most probably the grade of PIN is the important parameter.

Influence of a Second Set of Biopsies

The diagnostic yield of repeat biopsies depends on evidence of the number of biopsies performed. It has become clear that the usual sextant method is not necessarily the best technique in all cases and that the number of biopsies is dependent upon the size of the prostate. Recent works have usually increased the number of biopsies, sometimes up to 13 and sometimes more [30].

Investigating the role of performing two consecutive sets of TRUS-guided sextant biopsies of the prostate in a single office visit as the protocol for detecting prostate cancer in men presenting for the first time with an abnormal DRE and/or elevated serum PSA in a total of 137 consecutive men presenting for the first time with a clinically localized prostate nodule on DRE and/or elevated serum PSA based upon age-specific reference, adenocarcinoma of the prostate was diagnosed in 43 of the patients (31%) undergoing biopsy [31]. Adenocarcinoma of the prostate was diagnosed in only the second set of biopsies in 13 cases (10%). High-grade PIN without adenocarcinoma of the prostate was observed in 18 of the first set of biopsies (15%). High-grade PIN without adenocarcinoma of the prostate was the only pathological diagnosis in the second set of biopsies in 3 cases. The second set of biopsies provided important new clinical information related to prostate cancer in 20 cases (28%) and increased the number of cancers detected by 30%. In addition, 14 patients with high-grade PIN who would have required a second set of biopsies were found not to have adenocarcinoma of the prostate. Prostate cancer was detected in 43, 27 and 24% of men with prostate volumes <30, 30–50 and >50 cm^3, respectively. The percentage of prostate cancers detected only in the second set of biopsies was not significantly related to prostate size. The benefits of increasing the number of biopsies may include increasing the detection of adenocarcinoma of the prostate and providing the recommended second set of biopsies for high-grade PIN without increased morbidity or cost.

Clinical Recommendations

The clinical relevance of isolated PIN is based on the association of high-grade PIN and invasive prostate cancer. In order to predict the relative risks of later cancer found on repeat biopsy, probability values both for low- and high-grade PIN have been calculated by Zlotta et al. [24]. Logistic regression analysis for predicting carcinoma in patients with isolated PIN showed significant predictive value for PIN grade, DRE and serum PSA level only. There was a 33.3% probability to find cancer later in patients with high-grade PIN and PSA <4 ng/ml but this risk increased to 87% if DRE was abnormal and PSA at 12 ng/ml. This implies to combine PIN grade, DRE and TRUS when considering a management decision tree in patients with PIN. However, the age of the patient and its general health condition are important as well. Indeed, as recommended by several consensus meetings, further investigation of a PIN should logically be restricted to patients who would benefit from a radical treatment [12]. High-grade PIN in those patients, irrespective of DRE, TRUS or PSA, should prompt repeat biopsies. Since a substantial number of repeat biopsies yield PIN only and no cancer, radical surgery for isolated PIN cannot be advocated. If the second biopsy following isolated high-grade PIN does not indicate prostate cancer, a third biopsy should be performed at 3–6 months.

In low-grade PIN, the situation seems to be quite different. If the probability of later cancer appears very low when PSA is <4 ng/ml, it is nearly as high as in high-grade PIN when PSA is >10 ng/ml. These later patients should also be rebiopsied systematically since high PSA probably reflects the presence of undetected carcinoma.

Conclusions

Most experts agree that high-grade PIN is clearly a preneoplastic lesion because it fulfils all requirements for such a lesion. If the incidence of later cancer is 'only' 33% when PSA is <4 ng/ml in patients with isolated high-grade PIN, when PSA is >10 ng/ml and if DRE and/or TRUS are abnormal, it seems obvious that isolated PIN on prostate biopsy means that there is a very high probability that concurrent prostate cancer was missed [24]. Therefore, high-grade PIN, especially when associated with high PSA or abnormal DRE or TRUS, should be taken as a signal of high to extremely high probability of prostate cancer found on repeat biopsy and repeat biopsies should be performed [24, 32]. If these are still consistent with PIN, a third set of biopsies should be performed within 3–6 months [12]. If a second and a third set of biopsies do not show prostate cancer, then high-grade PIN might be considered for chemoprevention trial, based either on dietary modifications or pharmaceutical compounds. For low-

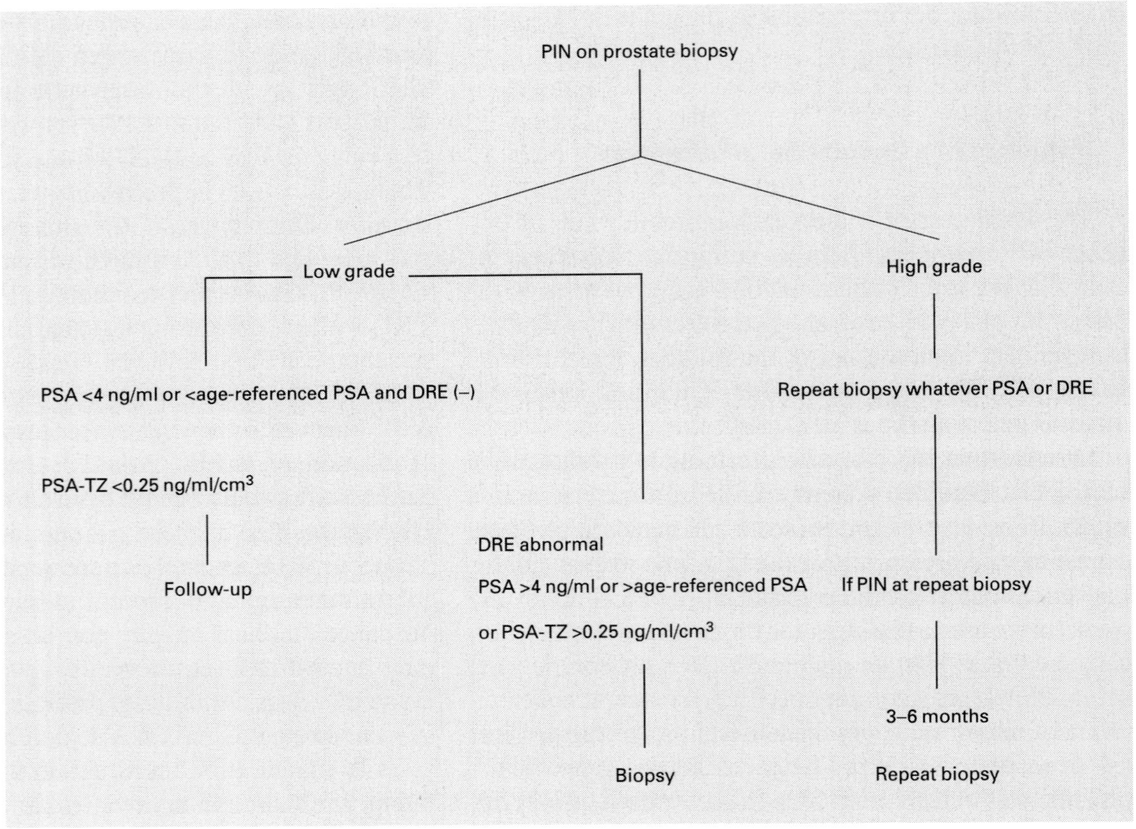

Fig. 2. Proposed management of PIN. PSA-TZ: PSA density of the transition zone [33].

grade PIN, other factors such as PSA, DRE, age reference PSA or PSA-TZ should be considered to perform biopsies [33] (fig. 2).

Future studies will tell us whether it might be possible to interfere at this precancerous stage with the transformation into an invasive carcinoma. Additional studies over longer periods of time are also required to determine the natural history of untreated isolated PIN found on prostate biopsies.

References

1 Sakr WA, Haas GP, Cassin BJ, Pontes JE, Crissman JD: Frequency of carcinoma and intraepithelial neoplasia of the prostate in young male patients. J Urol 1993;150:379–385.
2 Sakr WA, Grignon DJ, Haas GP, Heilbrun LK, Pontes JE, Crissman JD: Age and racial distribution of prostatic intraepithelial neoplasia. Eur Urol 1996;30:138–144.
3 Nelson PS, Gleason TP, Brawer MK: Chemoprevention for prostatic intraepithelial neoplasia. Eur Urol 1996;30:269–278.
4 Brawer MK, Bigler SA, Sohlberg OE, Nagle RB, Lange PH: Significance of prostatic intraepithelial neoplasia on prostate needle biopsy. Urology 1991;38:103–107.
5 Keetch DW, Humphrey P, Sthal D, Smith DS, Catalona WJ: Morphometric analysis and clinical follow-up of isolated prostatic intraepithelial neoplasia in needle biopsy of the prostate. J Urol 1995;154:347–351.
6 Aboseif S, Shinohara K, Weidner N, Narayan P, Carroll PR: The significance of prostatic intraepithelial neoplasia. Br J Urol 1995;76: 355–359.
7 McNeal JE, Villers A: Microcarcinoma in the prostate: Its association with duct acinar dysplasia. Hum Pathol 1991;22:644–652.
8 Brawer MK: Prostatic intraepithelial neoplasia: A premalignant lesion. Hum Pathol 1992; 23:242–248.
9 Bostwick DG, Brawer MK: Prostatic intraepithelial neoplasia and early invasion in prostate cancer. Cancer 1987;59:788–794.
10 Myers RB, Grizzle WE: Biomarker expression in prostatic intraepithelial neoplasia. Eur Urol 1996;30:153–166.
11 Qian J, Jenkins RB, Botswick DG: Potential markers of aggressiveness in prostatic intraepithelial neoplasia detected by fluorescence in situ hybridization. Eur Urol 1996;30:177–184.
12 Häggman MJ, Macoska JA, Wojno KJ, Oesterling JE: The relationship between prostatic intraepithelial neoplasia and prostate cancer: Critical issues. J Urol 1997;158:12–22.

13 De Marzo AM, Meeker AK, Epstein JI, Coffey DS: Prostate stem cell compartments: Expression of the cell cycle inhibitor p27Kip1 in normal, hyperplastic, and neoplastic cells. Am J Pathol 1998;153:911–919.
14 Bostwick DG, Qian J, Frankel K: The incidence of high-grade prostatic intraepithelial neoplasia in needle biopsies. J Urol 1995;154: 1791–1794.
15 Green J, Feneley MR, Young M, Peeling B, Kirby R, Parkinson C: The prevalence of prostatic intraepithelial neoplasia in biopsies from hospital practice and pilot screening: Clinical implications. J Urol 1996;155(suppl):A1260.
16 Orozco R, O'Dowd G, Kunnel B, Miller MC, Veltri RW: Observations on pathology trends in 62,537 prostate biopsies obtained from urology private practices in the United States. Urology 1998;51:186–195.
17 Markham CW: Prostatic intraepithelial neoplasia: Detection and correlation with invasive cancer in fine-needle biopsy. Urology 1989; 35(suppl):57–61.
18 Ellis WJ, Brawer MK: Repeat prostate needle biopsy: Who needs it? J Urol 1995;153:1496–1498.
19 Weinstein MH, Epstein JL: Significance of high-grade prostatic intraepithelial neoplasia on needle biopsy. Hum Pathol 1993;24:624.
20 Davidson D, Siroky M, Rudders R, Qian J, Oesterling J, Bostwick D, Stilmant M: Prostatic intraepithelial neoplasia is a risk factor for adenocarcinoma: Predictive accuracy in needle biopsy of the prostate. J Urol 1995;154:347–351.
21 Cheville JC, Reznicek MJ, Bostwick DG: The focus of 'atypical glands, suspicious for malignancy' in prostatic needle biopsy specimens: Incidence, histologic features, and clinical follow-up of cases diagnosed in a community practice. Am J Clin Pathol 1997;108:633–640.
22 Raviv G, Janssen TH, Zlotta AR, Descamps F, Verhest A, Schulman CC: Prostatic intraepithelial neoplasia: Influence of clinical and pathological data on the detection of invasive prostate cancer, in patients initially diagnosed on previous needle biopsy. J Urol 1996;156: 1050–1055.
23 Raviv G, Zlotta AR, Janssen TH, Descamps F, Verhest A, Schulman CC: Does prostate-specific antigen and prostate-specific antigen density enhance the detection of prostate cancer in patients initially diagnosed to have prostatic intraepithelial neoplasia? Cancer 1996;77: 2103–2108.
24 Zlotta AR, Raviv G, Schulman CC: Clinical prognostic criteria for later diagnosis of prostate carcinoma in patients with initial isolated prostatic intraepithelial neoplasia. Eur Urol 1996;30:249–255.
25 Lee F, Torp-Pedersen ST, Carroll JT, Siders DB, Christensen-Day C, Mitchell AE: Use of transrectal ultrasound and prostate-specific antigen in diagnosis of prostatic intraepithelial neoplasia. Urology 1989;34(suppl):4–8.
26 Ronnett BN, Carmichael MJ, Carter HB, Epstein JI: Does high-grade prostatic intraepithelial neoplasia result in elevated serum prostate specific antigen levels. J Urol 1993;150:386–389.
27 Brawer MK: Prostatic intraepithelial neoplasia and prostate specific antigen. Urology 1989; 34(suppl):62–65.
28 Kilic S, Kukul E, Danisman A, Guntekin E, Sevuk M: Ratio of free to total prostate-specific antigen in patients with prostatic intraepithelial neoplasia. Eur Urol 1998;34:176–180.
29 Shinohara K, Scardino PT, Carter SSC, Wheeler TM: Pathologic basis of the sonographic appearance of the normal and malignant prostate. Urol Clin North Am 1989;16:675.
30 Zlotta AR, Schulman CC: Prostate cancer; in Shah J (ed): Urology Highlights 1997. Oxford, Health Press, 1997, pp 12–22.
31 Levine MA, Ittman M, Melamed J, Lepor H: Two consecutive sets of transrectal ultrasound guided sextant biopsies of the prostate for the detection of prostate cancer. J Urol 1998;159: 471–475.
32 Langer JE, Rovner ES, Coleman BV, Yin D, Arger PH, Malkowicz SB, Nisenbaum HL, Rowling SE, Tomaszewski JE, Wein AJ: Strategy for repeat biopsy of patients with prostatic intraepithelial neoplasis detected by prostate needle biopsy. J Urol 1996;155:228–231.
33 Zlotta AR, Djavan B, Marberger M, Schulman CC: Prostate-specific antigen density of the transition zone: A new effective parameter for prostate cancer prediction. J Urol 1997;157: 1315–1321.

Surrogate Endpoint Biomarkers for Clinical Trials of Prostate Cancer Chemoprevention

European Urology

Eur Urol 1999;35:504–507

PIN I–III: When Should We Interfere?

Don Newling

Department of Urology, Academic Hospital, Vrije University, Amsterdam, The Netherlands

Key Words
PIN I/III · Timing treatment · Prostate cancer

Abstract
The identification of 2 or 3 different grades of prostate intraepithelial neoplasia has led to a number of difficult concepts and treatment possibilities. Postmortem examination of the prostates of men over the age of 20, who have died of other causes, mainly road traffic accidents, have been examined and the earliest signs of intraepithelial neoplasia can be seen in some of them. The most common age for prostate cancer to present clinically is between 60 and 65 years and because the majority of men do not develop clinical prostate cancer, there must be a very large number who never progress further than PIN I or II. It is very rare for the early stages of intraepithelial neoplasia to be associated with frank carcinoma. However, it is known that PIN III is frequently found in the presence of carcinoma elsewhere in the gland and this stage is seen as a premalignant development. PIN III in the presence of prostate carcinoma is treated by whatever modality is used to treat the carcinoma. In the absence of carcinoma, there are urologists who consider that it should be regarded as a T1 tumor and radical prostatectomy or radiotherapy with delayed hormonal therapy are definite alternatives. From a certain amount of anecdotal evidence, it seems that the transition from PIN III to a focal carcinoma may take in the order of 2–3 years. Whether this transition can be definitely postponed by the early use of hormonal therapy is not known. Prostate intraepithelial neoplasia may also be treated by other modalities such as anti-angiogenesis agents, gene therapy, anti-metastatic agents, or metalloproteinase inhibitors. The effects of these treatments can be examined histologically by repeated biopsies to ensure that the process remains arrested. If the process of intraepithelial neoplasia can be identified at early stages, dietary modifications may well reduce mitogenic influences and slow down the process or even halt it altogether.

Introduction

Prostate intraepithelial neoplasia (PIN) is widely regarded as a premalignant condition. Formally divided into three different grades, it is now reduced to two, these being low-grade PIN and high-grade PIN. The simultaneous association of high-grade PIN with areas of neoplasia has been clearly established and the subsequent development of neoplasia in the peripheral zone of the prostate gland, where PIN has been diagnosed by prostate biopsy, is of the order of 60%. Examination of the microscopic appearance of PIN confirms that many of the cellular and tissue changes seen in PIN are reflected in similar aberrations in prostate cancer cells. What is as yet unknown is whether it is possible with dietary, hormonal or other

KARGER

Fax + 41 61 306 12 34
E-Mail karger@karger.ch
www.karger.com

0302–2838/99/0356–0504$17.50/0

Accessible online at:
http://BioMedNet.com/karger

Prof. Don Newling
Academic Hospital, Vrije University
Polikliniek Urologie, Postbus 7057
NL–0117 MB Amsterdam (The Netherlands)
Tel. +31 204 440272, Fax +31 206 425085

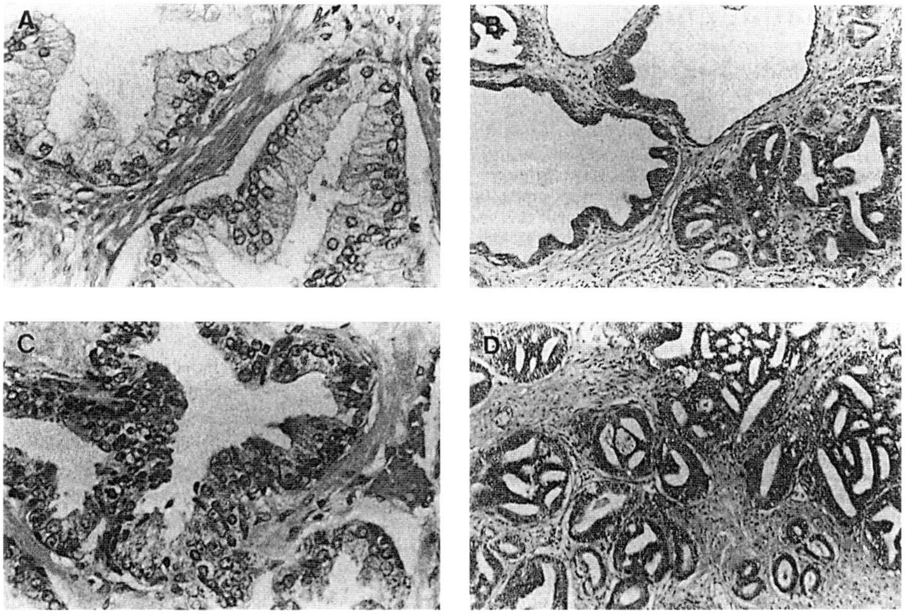

Fig. 1. A Normal prostatic epithelium. Note two epithelial layers lining normal prostatic acini and ductules and the cuboidal lumenal layer with basally-oriented small nuclei. **B** Low-power magnification shows an acini lined with high-grade PIN (lower left) and a gland (upper middle section) with PIN on the left aspect, atrophic epithelium on the right, and invasive prostatic carcinoma (lower right). **C** High-grade PIN. Note proliferation and dysplasia of the luminal cell layer and scattered basal cells present, particularly in the lower left. Note prominent nucleoli in the majority of the nuclei. **D** The cribiform variant of Gleason grade 3 adenocarcinoma. Note the similarity to acini and ductules lined with high-grade PIN, which makes the differential diagnosis of these two conditions sometimes problematic. Cribiform carcinoma is devoid of a basal cell layer, which can be an important discriminatory consideration.

pharmacological interventions to reverse high-grade PIN and so prevent cancer. The alternative is to regard high-grade PIN as the earliest form of cancer and to offer patients radical therapy.

Pathology of PIN

PIN is characterized by cellular crowding and stratification. There is an inequality in cell and nuclear size. Hyperchromatism is frequently seen with an enlarged nucleus, often containing prominent nucleoli lines. These changes are also seen in Gleason grade 1–4 prostate carcinoma [1]. The fact that the changes of PIN are most commonly seen in the periphery of the gland is also an indication that this is almost certainly a premalignant condition. Only 5% of PIN changes are seen in the transitional zone of the gland. Although in low-grade PIN, formerly PIN I, only 0.7% show evidence of basal cell layer disruption, in high-grade PIN more than 50% of abnormal cells are seen to have disrupted the basal cell layer of the acini. Biochemically, the cells of PIN show changes in the cytoskeletal proteins, secretory proteins and nuclei, which are shared with established prostate malignancies. There is also evidence of aneuploidy and an increase in microvascular density both frequently regarded as evidence of aggressiveness in established prostate cancer [2] (fig. 1).

What Is the Recommended Treatment of PIN?

Shepherd et al. [3] have suggested that the diagnosis of any grade PIN should lead to a repeated biopsy after 6 months. If in the first instance the biopsy showed high-grade PIN, almost 60% of the patients, after 6 months, were shown to have prostate cancer present in their specimens. Brawer et al. have shown that high-grade PIN is often associated with a PSA above normal levels, in other words PIN grade III should probably be regarded as T1c prostate cancer. Traditional therapeutic strategies, including radical prostatectomy and radiotherapy, are at the present time regarded by many urologists as inappropriate for the management of patients with PIN. The presence of a PSA above normal range is almost certainly indicative of at least basal layer penetration and therefore disruption of the normal architecture of the prostate gland or even capsular penetration not detectable by transrectal ultrasound and guided biopsies. Although low-grade PIN, on subsequent biopsies 6 months later, only showed carcinoma to be present in 24% [3], if this finding occurred in a patient in his early 50s then it would seem logical to assume that before the age of 60 he would have at least high-grade PIN or possibly invasive prostate cancer. There are a number of alternatives to radical therapy.

Table 1. Therapeutic methods for treatment of prostatic cancer

Matrix metalloproteinase inhibitors
Differention therapies
Antiangiogenesis therapies
Gene therapy
Immunotherapy
Early hormonal therapy
Vitamin D analogues

What Is Recommended in Place of Radical Therapy?

In the past 10 years, a number of interesting new therapeutic modalities have appeared for the treatment of prostatic cancer. These include those listed in table 1. Patients with PIN, either low grade or high grade, would seem to be ideal candidates for the use for these, at present experimental therapies. The effect of such therapeutic interventions could be assessed by repeated biopsy or on subsequent radical prostatectomy specimens [4].

Matrix Metalloproteinase Inhibitors, Antimetastatic Agents

It is known that matrix metalloproteinases play an important role in the invasion of the basement membrane of the prostate gland and therefore early invasion into lymphatic and perineural spaces. Marmorinstat is an important MMP inhibitor which has been effective in preventing metastases of LinCap cells in nude mice. It is at present being evaluated in phase I and phase II studies in advanced prostate cancer, where it is most unlikely to have a significant role. This is one of many agents which will probably only be effective in early stage prostate cancer and therefore is unlikely to show a significant effect on advanced, measurable, hormone escaped disease [5].

Antiangiogenesis Agents

Following penetration of the basal cell layer and invasion into the stroma of the prostate gland, the next step is the development of new blood vessels. The changes that occur in PIN III leading to focal carcinoma include neoangiogenesis and the use of agents that prevent this, such as thalidomide and platelet growth factor 4, could be a very important therapeutic intervention at this stage. Sequential examination of prostate biopsy and subsequent radical prostatectomy specimens would be a method of assessing the effectiveness of these agents [6].

Differentiation Therapies

Retinoids and vitamin D antagonists are known to improve differentiation of epithelial cells, including prostate epithelium. The development of invasiveness, as seen in the latest stages of PIN III, are characteristic of loss of adhesion facilities and dedifferentiation with aneuploid nuclear characteristics, which may be sensitive to differentiation therapies using retinoids or vitamin D antagonists [7].

Hormonal Therapy

The recent development of relatively nontoxic antiandrogen therapies has led to the increasing use of hormonal therapy at earlier stages of prostate cancer than formerly. Although hormonal therapy is always regarded as being palliative, it is possible that in the early stages of prostate cancer, and even in PIN, that it can prevent the development of invasive cancer for prolonged periods of time [8].

Gene Therapy and Immunotherapy

In prostatic cancer, genetic and immunotherapies are still experimental. The introduction of antisense nucleotides, herpes virus complexes and PSA linked to liposomes, are still in very early stages. Nevertheless, it is in the treatment of PIN at all stages that these may prove to be therapeutically advantageous. Again, serial examination of prostate biopsies and subsequent prostatectomy specimens may give an indication of the effectiveness of these agents.

Finally, there are an increasing number of urologists who think that the diagnosis of high-grade PIN is an indication for more radical therapy, i.e. radical prostatectomy or radiotherapy. The sound evidence that within 6 months of the first biopsy showing high-grade PIN, invasive prostate cancer is present has persuaded many people to offer radical prostatectomy or radiotherapy to this group of patients. Although this stand can be defended, it would seem logical that there be seen a progression in cytological and histological changes before such radical therapy is offered [9].

Conclusion

There is an increasing body of evidence that PIN is a premalignant condition. Patients diagnosed with such a condition, in their 6th and 7th decade, should probably be offered experimental or radical therapy. In those developing this condition in the 8th decade, knowing that the development of symptomatic prostate cancer will probably only occur after 8–10 years, a policy of watchful waiting could be recommended.

References

1 Bostwick DG, Amin MB, Dundore P, Marsh W, Schultz DS: Architectual patterns of high-grade prostatic intraepithelial neoplasia. Hum Pathol 1993;24:298.

2 Bostwick DG: High-grade prostatic intraepithelial neoplasia. Urology 1989;34(suppl):16.

3 Shepherd D, Keetch D, Humphrey PA, Smith DS, Stahl D: Repeat biopsy strategy in men with isolated prostatic intraepithelial neoplasia on prostate needle biopsy. J Urol 1996;156: 460–463.

4 Newling DWW, Fosså SD, Andersson L, Abrahamsson PA, Aso Y, Eisenberger M, Khoury S, Kozlowski JS, Kelly K, Scher H, Hartley-Asp B: Assessment of hormone refractory prostate cancer. Urology 1997;49(suppl 4A):46–53.

5 Thompson IM, Coltman Cam, Brawley OW: Chemoprevention of prostate cancer. Semin Urol 1995;13:122–129.

6 Ferrer FA, Miller LJ, Andoawir RI, et al: Cytokine regulation of angiogenesis factors in human prostate cancer (abstract). J Urol 1995; 155(suppl 5):189.

7 Mahler C, Denis L: Treatment of hormone refractory disease. Semin Surg Oncol 1995;11: 770–783.

8 Tyrrell CJ, Denis L, Newling DWW, et al: Casodex 10–200 mg daily, used as monotherapy for the treatment of patients with advanced prostate cancer – An overview of the efficacy, tolerability and pharmacokinetics from three phase II dose-ranging studies. Eur Urol 1998; 33:39–54.

9 Sanda MG: Biological principles and clinical development of prostate cancer gene therapy. Semin Urol Oncol 1997;15:43–55.

Surrogate Endpoint Biomarkers for Clinical Trials of Prostate Cancer Chemoprevention

European Urology

Eur Urol 1999;35:508–510

Prostatic Intraepithelial Neoplasia and Endocrine Manipulation

Th.H. van der Kwast F. Labrie B. Têtu

Department of Pathology, Erasmus University, Rotterdam, The Netherlands, and Centre Hospitalier Université de Québec, Canada

Key Words

Prostatic intraepithelial neoplasia · Endocrine therapy · Histopathology · Chemoprevention · Proliferative activity

Abstract

Prostatic intraepithelial neoplasia (PIN) is the most common precursor lesion of prostatic adenocarcinoma. In 50- to 70-year-old participants of a randomized screening program for prostate cancer (Rotterdam section of the ERSPC) the frequency of high-grade PIN as an isolated finding in sextant prostatic needle biopsies was estimated to be about 1%. As yet, data in literature on the impact of androgen deprivation on PIN lesions are limited, showing discrepant outcomes. In part this may be the consequence of the application of different criteria for the identification of PIN under conditions of androgen deprivation. Foci of PIN could be distinguished in the majority of radical prostatectomy specimens of men treated for 3 or 6 months with combined endocrine therapy. Endocrine manipulation led to architectural changes (remodelling) in residual PIN which were more pronounced at 6 months of endocrine therapy. This is consistent with a prolonged effect of androgen deprivation on this precursor lesion. The presence of MIB-1 immunopositive nuclei in PIN lesions suggests that they still have the potential to expand after cessation of therapy.

Introduction

Prostatic intraepithelial neoplasia (PIN) is regarded as the most likely precursor lesion for prostatic adenocarcinomas arising in the peripheral zone of the prostate [1, 2]. The histological and cytological characteristics of high-grade PIN are now well established. An important feature of high-grade PIN is the presence of prominent nucleoli in the majority of the dysplastic cells [3]. High-grade PIN is found in association with prostatic adenocarcinoma in 80–90% of radical prostatectomy specimens [2, 4]. It has been reported that in 5–16% of diagnostic needle biopsies, high-grade PIN is diagnosed in the absence of accompanying adenocarcinoma [5, 6]. The incidence of high-grade PIN as an isolated finding may be influenced by the nature of the population under study and the needle biopsy strategy. Data on the frequency of high-grade PIN in a nonselected population are limited [6]. The detection of an isolated high-grade PIN in men with elevated PSA levels could mean that a focus of adenocarcinoma has been missed owing to a sampling error, particularly if a limited number of biopsies was taken. Nevertheless, its presence in men with low PSA levels is also frequently associated with the finding of an adenocarcinoma in subsequent biopsies [7, 8]. This has been interpreted as evidence for the commonly held view that prostatic adenocarcinoma may evolve from high-grade PIN.

After androgen deprivation both the benign peripheral and transitional zone prostatic glands and adenocarcino-

KARGER

Fax +41 61 306 12 34
E-Mail karger@karger.ch
www.karger.com

0302–2838/99/0356–0508$17.50/0

Accessible online at:
http://BioMedNet.com/karger

Prof. Dr. Th. H. van der Kwast
Department of Pathology, Erasmus University
Postbox 1738, NL–3000 DR Rotterdam (The Netherlands)
Tel. +31 10 4087924, Fax +31 10 4366660
E-Mail vanderkwast@path.fgg.eur.nl

mas show regressive changes associated with a considerable reduction in prostatic size and tumor volume [9–11]. Characteristically, the benign luminal cells undergo vacuolization and shrinkage, while the basal cells become relatively more prominent [9, 10]. Recently, we demonstrated that these luminal cells retain the potential to proliferate, although this proliferative activity does not match cell loss as a consequence of programmed cell death [12]. Since the dysplastic cells in PIN share morphological and biochemical features with prostatic secretory epithelial cells, it may be anticipated that androgen deprivation leads to comparable morphological and functional changes. Several studies have reported a decrease in the incidence and extent of PIN following 3 months of androgen deprivation therapy [9, 11, 13–15]. This observation has been attributed both to the real loss of PIN lesions and to a loss of features helping to distinguish high-grade PIN from normal luminal cells [11].

In untreated prostatectomy specimens, at least four histological patterns of PIN can be distinguished: tufting and micropapillary in the majority of cases and cribriform and flat in a minority [16]. Analogous to the remodelling of benign prostatic glands observed after androgen deprivation, it is conceivable that the architecture of PIN lesions undergo similar changes. The availability of prostatectomy specimens of patients randomized to a 3- or 6-month regimen of neoadjuvant endocrine combination therapy allowed us to study the effects of androgen deprivation on (1) the frequency of residual PIN lesions, (2) the morphological changes of PIN-involved glands and (3) the potential of dysplastic cells of residual PIN to proliferate.

Materials and Methods

Tissue Specimens and Patient Material

The presence of isolated high-grade PIN in sextant needle biopsies of 3,607 men was recorded. The men were aged between 55 and 75 years with a PSA level >3 ng/ml and participated in a randomized screening program on prostate cancer (Rotterdam section of the ERSPC study).

Prostatectomy specimens of men with clinically localized prostate cancer were randomized at the Centre Hospitalier Université Laval, Québec, Canada, to 3 months (group A) and 6 months (group B) of neoadjuvant combined androgen blockade. Patients received either daily injections of a luteinizing hormone-releasing hormone agonist [*D*-Trp^6,des-Gly-NH_2^{10}]LHRH ethylamide (Tryptal) or monthly depot injections (Lupron). In addition, oral flutamide (Eulexin, 250 mg, 3 times/day) was given.

Processing and Histopathology of Prostatectomy Specimens

The prostatectomy specimens were fixed overnight in buffered formalin (pH 7.2), completely embedded in paraffin and processed to allow histopathological examination of tissue sections stained with hematoxylin and eosin. All slides, retrieved from the archives of the Hôtel Dieu de Québec, Canada, were reviewed by one pathologist (ThvdK) who was unaware of the treatment group. The presence and architectural pattern of PIN was recorded.

Immunohistochemistry

Proliferative activity was assessed by immunostaining with monoclonal antibody MIB-1 (Immunotech, France). Five-micrometer-thick sections were deparaffinized in toluene and rehydrated in ethanol. Endogenous peroxidase activity was quenched by 20 min treatment with methanol-0.3% H_2O_2 while rehydration was completed by rinsing in running tap water. Antigen retrieval was done by microwave treatment in 0.01 *M* citric acid (adjusted to pH 6.0). For visualization of primary antibody binding an avidin-biotin peroxidase complex method (Dako, Denmark) was used.

Results

In the ERSPC study, a total of 36 men were found to have isolated high-grade PIN corresponding with an incidence of 1% in men with a PSA level >3 ng/ml.

In radical prostatectomy specimens of patients treated for 3 or 6 months with endocrine therapy, PIN could be identified at high-power magnification on the basis of nuclear crowding, increased nuclear size, and disordered or irregular arrangement of nuclei.

The proportion of prostatectomies with PIN dropped from 72% at 3 months to 59% at 6 months. Strikingly, tufted PIN was much more frequent in 3-month- (48%) than in 6-month-treated cases (10%). Flat PIN was present in nearly all radical prostatectomy specimens which contained PIN lesions.

Immunohistochemical staining of 6-month-treated PIN-containing prostatectomy specimens revealed that some MIB-1-labeled nuclei were present in most PIN lesions, but no mitotic figures were detected.

Discussion

Here we show that in a nonselected population the incidence of high-grade PIN detected by sextant needle biopsies is rather low, i.e. 1%. The treatment of isolated high-grade PIN is not established as yet. It has been suggested that in the absence of detectable cancer after repeat biopsies, androgen deprivation therapy might be a suitable approach [15]. In the literature, the percentage of residual PIN during androgen deprivation varies from 6 to 83% [9, 11, 13–15]. Variation may be the consequence of different treatment regimens, but some of the discrepancies can be attributed to inter-observer variation among pathologists. Indeed, if the presence of large prominent nucleoli was considered as a prerequisite for a diagnosis of PIN, very few prostatic glandular lesions in treated prostatectomies would fit within this category.

It is well established that most residual prostatic adenocarcinomas lose the typical inclusion-like nucleoli as a consequence of androgen deprivation [11]. Therefore, we consider it very likely that loss of nucleoli as observed in regressive adenocarcinoma also occurs in PIN during androgen deprivation. In our opinion, (high-grade) PIN under endocrine therapy can still be identified by other criteria, namely increased nuclear size, nuclear crowding, and anisonucleosis. It is well established that androgen deprivation leads to a remodeling of benign prostatic glands, both in the peripheral and transitional zone [9, 10]. The alterations in the frequency of the various architectural patterns of PIN observed after 3 and 6 months of combined androgen blockade indicate that PIN-involved glands undergo the same set of changes as benign glands.

The finding of MIB-1-positive dysplastic cells in the majority of PIN lesions, even after 6 months of combined endocrine therapy, implies that these cells still have the potential to replicate. This corresponds with our recent finding that under the condition of low androgen levels, luminal but not basal cells of benign prostatic glands show increased proliferative activity as defined by MIB-1 antibody immunostaining [12]. This further underlines the resemblance of dysplastic cells of PIN with benign prostatic secretory cells.

Chemoprevention of prostate cancer by reduction of androgen levels should act by elimination of PIN or by prevention of the transition of PIN to overt carcinoma. Given the observed slow decline in frequency of PIN after androgen deprivation, it can be concluded that eradication of PIN will require a very long androgen deprivation treatment.

References

1 Bostwick DG, Brawer MK: Prostatic intra-epithelial neoplasia and early invasion in prostate cancer. Cancer 1987;59:788–794.
2 McNeal JE, Bostwick DG: Intraductal dysplasia: A premalignant lesion of the prostate. Hum Pathol 1986;17:64–71.
3 Bostwick DG: High-grade prostatic intra-epithelial neoplasia: The most likely precursor of prostate cancer. Cancer 1995;75:1823–1836.
4 Qian J, Wollan P, Bostwick DG: The extent and multicentricity of high-grade prostatic intraepithelial neoplasia in clinically localized prostatic adenocarcinoma. Hum Pathol 1997;28:143–148.
5 Bostwick DG, Qian J, Frankel K: The incidence of high grade prostatic intraepithelial neoplasia in needle biopsies. J Urol 1995;154:1791–1794.
6 Mettlin C, Lee F, Drago J, Murphy GP: Investigators of the American Cancer Society National Prostate Cancer Detection Project. The American Cancer Society National Prostate Cancer Detection Project: Findings on the detection of early prostate cancer in 2,425 men. Cancer 1991;67:2949–2958.
7 Keetch DW, Humphrey P, Stahl D, Smith DS, Catalona WJ: Morphometric analysis and clinical follow-up of isolated prostatic intraepithelial neoplasia in needle biopsy of the prostate. J Urol 1995;154:347–351.
8 Raviv G, Janssen T, Zlotta AR, Descamps E, Verhest A, Schulman CC: Prostatic intraepithelial neoplasia: Influence of clinical and pathological data on the detection of prostate cancer. J Urol 1996;156:1050–1054.
9 Montironi R, Magi-Galluzi C, Muzzonigro G, Prete E, Polito M, Fabris G: Effects of combination endocrine therapy on normal prostate, prostatic intra-epithelial neoplasia, and prostatic adenocarcinoma. J Clin Pathol 1994;47:906–913.
10 Tetu B, Srigley JR, Boivin JC, Dupont A, Monfette G, Pinault S, Labrie F: Effect of combination endocrine therapy (LHRH agonist and flutamide) on normal prostate and prostatic adenocarcinoma. A histopathologic and immunohistochemical study. Am J Surg Pathol 1991;15:111–120.
11 Vaillancourt L, Têtu B, Fradet Y, Dupont A, Gomez J, Cusan L, Suburu ER, Diamond P, Candas B, Labrie F: Effect of neoadjuvant endocrine therapy (combined androgen blockade) on normal prostate and prostatic carcinoma: A randomized study. Am J Surg Pathol 1996;20:86–93.
12 Van der Kwast ThH, Têtu B, Suburu ER, Gomez J, Lemay M, Labrie F: Cycling activity of benign prostatic epithelial cells during long-term androgen blockade: Evidence for self-renewal of luminal cells. J Pathol 1998;186:406–409.
13 Armas OA, Aprikian AG, Melamed J, Cordon-Cardo C, Cohen DW, Erlandson R, Fair WR, Reuter VE: Clinical and pathobiological effects of neoadjuvant total androgen ablation therapy on clinically localized prostatic adenocarcinoma. Am J Surg Pathol 1994;18:979–991.
14 Civantos F, Marcial MA, Banks ER, Ho CK, Speights VO, Drew PA, Murphy WM, Soloway MS: Pathology of androgen deprivation therapy in prostate carcinoma. A comparative study of 173 patients. Cancer 1995;75:1634–1641.
15 Ferguson J, Zincke H, Ellison E, Bergstrahl E, Bostwick DG: Decrease of prostatic intra-epithelial neoplasia following androgen deprivation therapy in patients with stage T3 carcinoma treated by radical prostatectomy. Urology 1994;44:91–95.
16 Bostwick DG, Amin MB, Dundore P, Marsh W, Schultz DS: Architectural patterns of high-grade prostatic intraepithelial neoplasia. Hum Pathol 1993;24:298–310.

Surrogate Endpoint Biomarkers for Clinical Trials of Prostate Cancer Chemoprevention

European Urology

Eur Urol 1999;35:511–514

The Utility of Prostate-Specific Antigen as a Surrogate Marker for Identification of High-Risk Cohorts and Assessing Response in Chemoprevention Trials

E.D. Crawford

University of Colorado Health Sciences Center, Denver, Colo., USA

Key Words

Chemoprevention · PSA as surrogate marker

Abstract

Serum prostate-specific antigen (PSA) is the most important tumor marker in oncology practice. It may assume a similar role in chemoprevention strategies. It is a simple and reproducible blood test that can both identify a high-risk cohort and provide meaningful information regarding the response to intervention. A wealth of information is available regarding the relationship of PSA to age, race and velocity. Free and total values may serve to further define high-risk cohorts and provide a barometer for response and disease presence in chemoprevention trials.

Introduction

During the past two decades there have been a number of significant advances in the diagnosis and treatment of cancer. Several important discoveries have improved our diagnosis and treatment of tumors such as lymphoma and seminoma leading to excellent cure rates over a wide range of disease stage. The concept of cancer prevention has been around for a long time, however it is not until relatively recently that a better understanding of tumor biology has led to an increased interest in this field.

Along with the interest in cancer chemoprevention, have come a number of new challenges including the identification of high-risk groups as well as assessing response to intervention. The ability to identify these high-risk cohorts substantially reduces the number of subjects necessary to design prospective randomized trials. Most cancer clinical trials utilize death as the definitive endpoint. Improvement in survival is easy to judge and widely accepted. In many cancer clinical trials, death is a reasonable endpoint since most patients live 3–5 years. However, in chemoprevention studies, survival may not be an acceptable endpoint because of the extended interval between the intervention and death. Therefore other 'intermediate endpoints' which are a surrogate for progression and death are sought. This article will review the utilization of serum prostate-specific antigen (PSA) as a surrogate marker both to identify high-risk cohorts and to assess the effects of chemoprevention strategies.

Surrogate endpoints are based on the concept that an observable and measurable phenomenon that occurs in a

KARGER

Fax + 41 61 306 12 34
E-Mail karger@karger.ch
www.karger.com

0302–2838/99/0356–0511$17.50/0

Accessible online at:
http://BioMedNet.com/karger

E. David Crawford, MD
University of Colorado Health Sciences Center
4200 East Ninth Avenue, Box C-319
Denver, CO 80262 (USA)
Tel. +1 303 771 36 89, Fax +1 303 721 65 89

high-risk population is reflective of what occurs in the general population. This permits the design of very specific short-term trials [1].

Prostate Cancer

Prostate cancer is a prime target for chemopreventive studies. The cancer has a long latency period and autopsy series demonstrate that prostatic intraepithelial neoplasia (PIN), the probable precursor to prostate cancer, is identifiable decades before presence of the disease. Sakr et al. [2] reported that this premalignant condition can occur in men as young as 30 years of age. Because there is such a long time between the precursor lesion to development of clinically significant disease, therapies that do not reverse the premalignant condition but merely delay its presentation may be sufficient to improve survival.

The importance of the hormonal milieu in both the development and progression of prostate cancer has been known for 60 years. Men with congenital 5α-reductase deficiency and eunuchs provide us with insight as to the role of androgens in the genesis of cancer. These patients do not develop any significant prostate disease including cancer [3]. Interfering with androgen balance may have an effect on the development of prostate disease. Numerous drugs interfere with androgens including: estrogens, antiandrogens, LHRH agonists and 5α-reductase inhibitors. Of these there is significant morbidity and side effects for most except 5α-reductase inhibitors. Most of the agents above will have an effect on serum PSA by suppressing its production. The value of PSA as a marker will be altered unless there are methods to account for the changes. Other agents, such as differentiation agents, will have an opposite affect in that the serum PSA will be elevated.

Prostate Specific Antigen

PSA is the most useful tumor marker in clinical practice [4]. The natural history of changes in PSA might make it a useful surrogate endpoint for prostate cancer in the setting of chemoprevention trials. PSA levels may be able to identify high-risk cohorts for chemoprevention trials. Since PSA is not exclusive of cancer and since most diseases of the prostate can elevate it, techniques to increase its sensitivity and specificity are desirable.

PSA is a serine protease of the kallikrein family with a molecular weight approaching 65 kDa. Seminogelin, a major protein is seminal fluid, it is cleaved by PSA aiding in the liquefaction of semen [5]. Most PSA remains in the lumen of the prostate glands but a small portion can be detected in serum. Normal levels are <4 ng/ml, which is about 10^{-6} less than in seminal fluid. It is important to consider that even though PSA is associated with prostate tissue growth, it is not exclusive. Therefore, elevations in PSA represent a spectrum of changes that include tumor size, grade, inflammation as well as growth factors. These complexities may make the interpretation of results more difficult. Review of PSA nuisances is important.

Age-Specific PSA Reference Ranges

Serum PSA increases with age. This has been generally attributed to an increase in prostate size. However, other factors need to be considered. These are: prostate infections, prostate infarction, microscopic prostate cancer and 'leaking' of the prostate epithelium. Age-specific reference ranges (ASRR) help establish baseline data for patients undergoing chemoprevention trials. The data gathered from Prostate Cancer Awareness Week for 1993–1994 suggests that PSA variance increases with age. Hence younger subjects have less variation in their PSA values and make this a more useful biomarker for the chemoprevention of cancer in the 30- to 50-year age range [6]. We also compared PSA by race. It was found that the greatest variability occurred among African-Americans (table 1). This may complicate the usefulness of PSA in this subset of high-risk subjects.

PSA Velocity

PSA velocity (PSAV) represents the changes in time of several measurements of PSA. Data from the Baltimore Longitudinal Study on Aging suggest that increments of 0.04 ± 0.02 ng/ml/year are normal. BPH accelerates the rate to 0.07 for men up to 60 years, 0.15 for men up to 70 years and 0.23 for men up to 80 years old [7]. Prostate cancer is associated with increments of 0.1 ng/ml/year, which rise exponentially before diagnosis. In addition, PSAV rises in a steeper fashion for advanced cases than for localized or regionally advanced cases of prostate cancer. Important limitations to PSAV are intraindividual PSA variations and sampling variability. These variations can be as high as 30% when the same assay is used on a different day [8]. To consider the usefulness of PSAV in chemoprevention trials, the frequency of determinations and careful assay variability analysis is required.

Table 1. ASRR in various ethnic groups

Age	PSA, ng/ml			
	White	Black	Latino	Asian
40–49	2	2.3	2.1	1.9
50–59	3.3	3.8	3.7	3.8
60–69	4.8	5.4	5.2	5.1
70–79	5.7	6.2	5.4	6.4

Table 2. High-risk cohorts

Age
Race, African-American
Genetics, family history
High-grade PIN
? PSA level

Free, Complex and Total PSA

Analysis of the forms of PSA in serum has revealed that up to 85% of PSA is bound to α_1-antichymotrypsin, one of the major serine protease inhibitors formed by the liver [9]. It has also been observed that the proportion of free (unbound) PSA to complexed PSA is different in some patients with cancer and BPH. The proportion of free to total PSA is lower in patients with cancer than those with BPH. There is considerable controversy as to how much lower. It is generally accepted that a ratio of <0.20 is associated with cancer. The value of this assay in the setting of chemoprevention trials is not known.

PSA Reverse Transcription-Polymerase Chain Reaction Assay

Polymerase chain reaction (PCR) techniques multiply vast quantities of a specific segment of DNA from a template. When reverse transcription (RT) is used, the template (cDNA) is made from mRNA. The PSA RT-PCR assay demonstrates the signal for PSA (i.e. mRNA) in the circulation [10]. In theory the finding of mRNA for PSA in peripheral blood implies that there are cells producing PSA circulating in peripheral blood. The sensitivity of these assays is exquisite and various techniques have added to the power of this test. However, at this time, its use in the management of prostate cancer is investigational [11]. Certainly if the role of RT-PCR in prostate cancer is not completely understood it is difficult to apply this concept to chemoprevention studies. Further studies are indicated to evaluate the role, if any, of this technique.

PSA appears to be a useful surrogate for following patients on chemoprevention trials. A rising level increases the risk of progression and/or the development of prostate cancer. However, age-related changes, velocity, racial differences should be accounted for in these trials. In addition, certain interventions may have an effect of the serum level, raising it in the case of differentiation agents, while lowering the level when hormonally active agents are utilized. Methods to adjust for these variations are imperative if the marker is used for a surrogate of disease.

Value of PSA to Identify High-Risk Cohorts for Chemoprevention Trials

Table 2 lists a number of accepted risk factors of identifying men with a high risk of development of prostate cancer. Inclusion of such patients serves to reduce the number of subjects required in trials to evaluate chemopreventive strategies. As an example, if men with familial prostate cancer are included, where the risk approaches nearly 50%, only several hundred men would be required in a trial to demonstrate a 20–30% reduction in the incidence of prostate cancer. Whereas if the general population were studied, the required number would exceed 10,000 subjects in a randomized trial. Another example is HGPIN where the risk is also substantial. The challenges facing such a trial with high-risk patients is not only recruitment but also that the group may not represent the general population. Nevertheless, strategies are being developed to study these cohorts.

It is recognized that the risk of prostate cancer parallels PSA level. Men with an initial PSA of >10 ng/ml have nearly a 50% risk of the disease [6]. We have recently investigated the utilization of serum PSA levels to define a high-risk cohort by studying men who participated in yearly screening for 3 years [12]. From our Prostate Cancer Awareness Week database of 55,000 men, we extracted the records of 6,804 men who had an initial PSA level of <4 ng/ml (IMx assay) and had a normal digital rectal examination. An additional criterion was that they

Table 3. Advantages and disadvantages of PSA as surrogate for high-risk cohorts

Advantages	Disadvantages
Blood test	Racial variability
Frequent monitoring	Age variability
Inexpensive	Affected by hormones
Reproducible	Affected by differentiation agents

returned for screening examination for a total of 3 years. We were able to identify groups at high- and low-risk of developing an abnormality of their PSA during the follow-up period. Those that had a level of <2 ng/ml had a very low risk of an abnormal PSA within 3 years (<3%), while those with a level of 2.1–4.0 ng/ml experienced nearly a 34% chance of developing an abnormal PSA during the follow-up. This group seems to represent an ideal cohort to include in chemoprevention trials. The average age of the entire group was 64.6 years. Those in the high-risk category had a mean age of 69.

There are several advantages of utilizing the initial serum PSA level in defining high-risk cohorts for chemoprevention clinical trials (table 3), the primary one being the ability to utilize an inexpensive noninvasive method of selection. The disadvantage is that this group does not represent the normal population and that as many as 20% already have prostate cancer [13]. However, the same criticism can be directed to employing patients with HGPIN into such trials. A substantial number have existent cancer even if their repeat biopsies are negative [14].

References

1 Conti CJ, Gimenez-Conti IB: Molecular genetic alterations as intermediate end points in chemoprevention studies. IARC Sci Publ 1996; 139:249–460.

2 Sakr WA, Haas GP, Cassin BF, Pontes JE, Crissman JD: The frequency of carcinoma and intraepithelial neoplasia of the prostate in young male patients. J Urol 1993;150:379–385.

3 Imperato-McGinley J, Guerrero L, Gautier T, Peterson RE: Steroid 5α-reductase deficiency in man: An inherited form of male pseudohermaphroditism. Science 1974;186:1213–1215.

4 Oesterling JE: Prostate-specific antigen: A critical assessment of the most useful tumor marker for adenocarcinoma of the prostate. J Urol 1991;145:907–923.

5 Lilja JA: Kallikrein-like serine protease in prostatic fluid cleaves the predominant seminal fluid protein. J Clin Invest 1985;76:1899–1903.

6 DeAntoni EP, Crawford ED, Stone NN, Blum DS, Berger ER, Eisenberger MA, Gambert SR, Staggers F: Prostate cancer awareness week, summary of key findings. Clin Invest Med 1994;16:448–457.

7 Carter HB, Epstein JI, Chan DW, Fozard JL, Pearson JD: Recommended prostate-specific antigen testing intervals for the detection of curable prostate cancer. JAMA 1997;277: 1456–1460.

8 Stamey TA: Second Stanford Conference on international standardization of prostatic-specific antigen immunoassays. Urology 1995;45: 173–184.

9 Tchetgen MB, Oesterling JE: The role of prostate-specific antigen in the evaluation of benign prostatic hyperplasia. Urol Clin North Am 1995;22:333.

10 Gomella LG, Raj GV, Moreno JG: Reverse transcriptase-polymerase chain reaction for prostate-specific antigen in the management of prostate cancer. J Urol 1997;158:326–337.

11 Goodman GE: The clinical evaluation of cancer prevention agents. Proc Soc Exp Biol Med 1997;216:253–259.

12 Leewansantong S, Crawford ED, Gordon ST, Baier M, Holthaus K, Stone N: Three-year follow-up of men with normal prostate-specific antigen and normal digital rectal exam: Is yearly screening necessary? N Engl J Med 1999, submitted.

13 Harris CH, Dalkin BL, Martin E, Marx PC, Ahmann FR: Prospective longitudinal evaluation of men with initial prostate-specific antigen level of 4 ng/ml or less. J Urol 1997;157: 1740–1743.

14 Crawford ED, Hirano D, Werahera PN, Lucia MS, DeAntoni EP, Daneshgari F, Brawn PN, Speights VO, Stewart JS, Miller GJ: Computer modeling of prostate biopsy: Tumor size and location – not clinical significant – determine cancer detection. J Urol 1998;159:1260–1264.

Clinical Trial Designs for Chemoprevention of Prostate Cancer

European Urology

Eur Urol 1999;35:515–518

Practical Aspects of Clinical Trials on Chemoprevention of Prostate Cancer

Adrian P.M. van der Meijden

Department of Urology, Bosch Medical Center, 's-Hertogenbosch, The Netherlands

Key Words

Chemoprevention · Prostate cancer · Practical aspects

Abstract

In addition to the normal aspects of organizing clinical trials, the launch of a chemoprevention trial on prostate cancer needs extra effort. The sample size and duration of follow-up is so extensive that such a trial should be organized as an intergroup study, preferably worldwide. For that a central data center and data management is mandatory. Because healthy individuals are involved, refusal, loss to follow-up and inadequate adherence may be substantial. The choice of the study endpoint presence of prostate cancer or death due to prostate cancer will lead to completely different sample sizes and length of follow-up. Of criteria leading to the diagnosis of prostate cancer (PSA, DRE and transrectal ultrasound), at least two are rather subjective. The drug involved might affect the criteria for diagnosis. Because of the high incidence of clinically nonsignificant prostate cancer of men over 55, a large number of nonrelevant prostate cancers will be detected in both arms. Due to the long follow-up and alterations in the state of the art of detection and therapy of prostate cancer, the completion of such a study might be hampered. If the average price per patient involved in a clinical trial is currently between USD 1,000 and 2,000, one may calculate that for 30,000 men, USD 20–40 million are needed, not including the hospital visits, examinations and biopsies. Economic considerations thus play a major role in organizing trials on the chemoprevention of prostate cancer.

Introduction

Early detection and treatment of cancer have improved for some malignancies but the outcome in several solid tumors is disappointing including prostate cancer. The high incidence of many cancers is not yet under control nor have the survival rates been improved. Therefore, new approaches to prevent cancer have been developed and one of these is chemoprevention. Chemoprevention can be defined as the use of specific natural or synthetic chemical agents to reverse, suppress or prevent carcinogenic progression to invasive lethal cancer [1]. The attitude of many people in Western countries towards the fight against cancer has been changed during the last two decades. Many believe that healthy food, water and clean air play an important role in preventing many diseases, including cancer. However, it is very hard to find the scientific evidence that a certain food compound or a synthetic drug is able to prevent cancer or to reverse the multistep process of carcinogenesis. Epidemiologic studies and laboratory evidence in animal models do not necessarily translate to the human situation. Therefore, the method to investigate the efficacy of chemoprevention drugs parallels the way to investigate chemotherapeutic drugs in humans. This is done through phase I, II and III trials [1].

KARGER

Fax + 41 61 306 12 34
E-Mail karger@karger.ch
www.karger.com

0302–2838/99/0356–0515$17.50/0

Accessible online at:
http://BioMedNet.com/karger

Adrian P.M. van der Meijden
EORTC-GU Group Chairman
Department of Urology, Bosch Medical Center, PO Box 90153
NL–5200 ME 's-Hertogenbosch (The Netherlands)
Tel. +31 73 616 2407, Fax +31 73 616 2373

Carcinogenesis is extremely complex. There may be a long latency between exposure and disease. Many exogenous and endogenous factors may enhance or inhibit the process to the evaluation of a malignant tumor. Complex cellular, genetic and biochemical processes are involved and the cascade of events necessary for the establishment of a life-threatening malignant tumor are not only sequentially but simultaneously and interacting in an unknown way. Many tumors derive from epithelium. Large areas of epithelium surface are exposed to carcinogens delivered from the environment. Solar ultraviolet irradiation, bile acids and fatty acids for colon epithelium, tobacco smoke carcinogens for mouth, esophagus and respiratory tract are hitting epithelium layers continuously. By this, multiple primary cancers may develop concurrently. This phenomenon is named field cancerization [2].

For bladder cancer this concept might be applied too as carcinogenic agents are excreted by the urine. For prostate cancer however, no hard evidence exists that urine plays an important role although many investigators believe that chemical compounds of urine might penetrate through acini and ducts and cause a bacterial prostatitis. The link to prostate cancer development has not been identified. Until now the progress on the treatment of prostate cancer was predominantly achieved by conducting phase I, II and III clinical trials.

The multistep carcinogenis process might take such a long time that the endpoint development of invasive cancer is not feasible. To gain time, intermediate endpoints might be chosen. Intermediate endpoints include changes in histologic premalignant lesions and in biochemical and molecular markers [5]. Such intermediate biomarkers should have the following characteristics [6]: (1) detectable in small specimens of tissue (e.g. in prostate needle biopsies); (2) high specificity and sensitivity, and (3) low range of spontaneous change.

Unfortunately it seems that no reliable biomarker has been validated in such a way that they can be used for replacement of definitive endpoints: the expression of cancer [1].

These problems make it difficult to determine a reliable sample size of subjects to be investigated in a phase II setting. For already existing tumors this is totally different and this is why in phase II chemotherapeutic trials often less than 50 patients are needed to obtain reliable results.

The real answer whether chemoprevention works has to come from phase III randomized clinical trials. These are conducted to establish long-term efficacy in reducing cancer. Many disadvantages compared to chemotherapeutic phase III randomized trials exist. All of them lead to practical aspects which should be considered before conducting chemoprevention trials.

Design of Chemoprevention Trials

Because progress in cancer treatment has to come from evidence-based medicine, the design for chemoprevention trials largely parallels the design used in therapeutic trials [3]. This means that promising new agents detected in laboratory and epidemiologic studies should be tested in phase I trials with the objective to determine toxicity. Phase I testing includes investigation of drug metabolism, drug interaction, tissue distribution, pharmacokinetics, etc. In the phase I testing, escalation schedules are used to establish the appropriate dose with minor toxicity. The drug to be tested should preferentially be given to subjects who are at high risk to develop the tumor. For prostate cancer such a high-risk population has been identified [4]. Because of familiar or genetic predisposition, certain men have a 4- to 8-fold higher risk to develop prostate cancer than average men.

The next step is to conduct phase II trials. Here the activity of the drug is evaluated. For chemoprevention drugs this is difficult.

Chemoprevention in Practice

Ideally, the incidence of cancer should be the endpoint. However, 5, 10 or even more years might be necessary to reach this endpoint testing a chemoprevention drug. If a reliable intermediate endpoint would exist in phase II, such an endpoint could also be used in phase III trials. Considering the long study period of subjects, intermediate endpoint biomarkers could reduce the study period considerably. The ongoing chemoprevention trial in prostate cancer using finasteride has a definitive endpoint: the incidence of prostate cancer [7]. A study period of 7 years is foreseen. Such a long time leads to a potential long-term toxicity of the drug to be investigated [1]. Furthermore, subjects are prone to long-term intervention and recurrent investigations.

To assess the long-term toxicity and safety of the investigational drug, a so-called vanguard cohort of subjects from the phase II study can be used [8]. Normally it takes 2–4 years to complete a phase II study, before embarking on phase III. However, the phase I/II study population can be kept on study in the phase III setting to monitor toxicity. Identified difficulties in the vanguard cohort may provide the basis for modifying the intervention in the phase III trial. Furthermore, substantial time benefit can be achieved. Because the activity of the drug to be tested may be rather low and because many compounds used for chemoprevention are widespread, the amount of bias is potentially substantial. Many chemoprevention agents are on the market as multiple vitamins, minerals and nutrient supplements. Although the incidence of prostate cancer has increased during the past two decades, not every man will develop prostate cancer.

To find a difference between the subjects taking the chemoprevention drug or placebo of 25% reduction in period prevalence, 18,000 men are needed [7]. If the estimated difference is smaller, study populations of 30,000 or 50,000 men would be necessary. These enormous sample sizes can only be achieved when chemoprevention studies are done on a global basis.

Study Population

Chemoprevention can be applied to a study population which is at high risk for developing the investigational tumor. Such increased risk might be genetically determined or acquired. [5]. Another high-risk population is formed by patients who have been cured from a cancer previously but are still at risk because the organ involved is still present. An example of this are patients who had a hemicolectomy for colon cancer [9].

The ultimate goal however for chemoprevention trials is to show efficacy of the drug in the general healthy population. Here the impact is much larger than in a small cohort of patients who are genetically more at risk. This is the reason to conduct chemoprevention trials in the general population.

It is often difficult to explain to a patient with an existing prostate cancer that he should be randomized to a phase III study. It is however much harder to convince healthy subjects to be randomized in a chemoprevention trial. Study entry and compliance are motivated by a subject's perception of risk to develop the disease [8]. For such perception a certain level of education, social and economic circumstances are necessary.

The perception of risk may differ considerably from the actual risk. Ultimately only 10–15% of the highest risk individuals will be enrolled in a chemoprevention study [9]. Moreover, there will be a difference in compliance between the intervention and the control arm. This affects the validity of study results. To improve compliance a run-in phase of 2–4 months is advised. Noncompliers will be identified particularly in the first 4 months of study entry and randomization of noncompliers will be avoided.

The number of subjects that will drop out before randomization in phase III trials is approximately 10–15% [10]. Until now about 40 randomized phase III chemoprevention trials have been reported. They have produced significant activity in reversing colon, oral and skin cancer. For prostate cancer the finasteride trial is ongoing. Chemoprevention trials to investigate the prevention of cancer incidence in general have also been designed and executed.

In 1982 the Physicians Health Study started in the USA. In this trial, using a factorial design, two assumptions were tested. Can β-carotene prevent cancer and can low-dose aspirin prevent cardiovascular disease? Eleven years later the aspirin results have been published [11] but not the results of β-carotene effects. The sample size consists of 22,071 male physicians. An even larger challenge is the Women's Health Study Investigation on β-carotene, vitamin E and aspirin in preventing cancer and cardiovascular disease. For this, more than 40,000 female nurses have to be recruited [12].

As in chemotherapeutic trials, an Independent Data Monitoring Committee should be involved in chemoprevention trials. This committee is responsible to assess adverse events which is particularly important with regard to potential long-term toxicity. The relation between toxicity and efficacy as well as changes in the state-of-the-art treatment have to be considered as well. The problem that not every prostate cancer is clinically important remains actual because a chemoprevention trial in prostate cancer will inevitably generate a number of prostate cancers in both arms which undetected and untreated would never harm the patient [13].

Economical Aspects

To run a phase III trial in the EORTC the average price per patient involved is between USD 1,000 and 2,000. One may calculate that for a sample size of 30,000 men, USD 20–40 million are needed, not including the hospital visits, examinations and biopsies. Economic considerations play a major role and sponsoring of such trials will be the largest obstacle in the future.

Nevertheless, chemoprevention is a new challenge for basic and clinical researchers and a logical extension in the struggle against malignant disease. This novel approach should be incorporated in medical educations and it should be explored on a global basis.

References

1 Lippman SM, Benner SE, Waun KH: Cancer chemoprevention. J Clin Oncol 1994;12:851–873.

2 Slaughter DP, Southwick HW, Smejkal W: Field cancerization in oral stratified squamous epithelium. Clinical implications of multicentric origin. Cancer 1953;6:963–968.

3 Bertram JS, Kolonel LN, Meyskens FL: Rationale and strategies for chemoprevention of cancer in humans Cancer Res 1987;47:3012–3031.

4 Spitz MR, Currier RD, Fueger JJ, Babaian RJ, Newell GR: Familial patterns of prostate cancer: A case-control analysis. J Urol 1991;146:1305.

5 Lippman SM, Lee JS, Lotan R et al: Biomarkers as intermediate end points in chemoprevention trials. J Natl Cancer Inst 1990;82:555–560.

6 Boone CW, Kelloff GJ, Steele VE: Natural history of intraepithelial neoplasia in humans with implications for cancer chemoprevention strategy. Cancer Res 1991;52:1651–1659.

7 Feigl P, Blumenstein B, Thompson I et al: Design of the Prostate Cancer Prevention Trial (PCPT). Control Clin Trials 1995;16:150–163.

8 Goodman GE: The clinical evaluation of cancer chemoprevention agents: Defining and contrasting phase I, II and III objectives. Cancer Res 1992;52(suppl):2752–2757.

9 Vogelstein B, Fearon ER, Hamilton SR: Genetic alterations during colorectal tumor development. N Engl J Med 1988;319;525–532.

10 Slovic P: Perception of risk. Science 1987;236:280–285.

11 Freedman LS: The effect of partial noncompliance on the power of the clinical trial. Control Clin Trials 1990;11:157–168.

12 Gann PH, Manson JE, Glynn RJ: Low-dose aspirin and incidence of colorectal tumors in a randomized trial. J Natl Cancer Inst 1993;85;1220–1224.

13 Buring JE, Hennekens CH: The Women's Health Study: Summary of the study design. J Myocard Ischemia 1992;4:27–29.

14 Holund B: Latent prostatic cancer in a consecutive autopsy series. Scand J Urol Nephrol 1980;14:29–35.

European Urology

Eur Urol 1999;35:519–522

Statistical Considerations of Chemoprevention Clinical Trials in Prostate Cancer

Richard Sylvester   Laurence Collette

EORTC Data Center, Brussels, Belgium

Key Words

Prostate cancer · Chemoprevention · Statistical considerations · Endpoints

Abstract

The design and analysis of chemoprevention trials in prostate cancer is more complicated than that of an ordinary treatment efficacy trial. The following issues must be taken into account when designing prospective randomized chemoprevention trials: (1) The choice of the primary endpoint: biopsy-proven prostate cancer or mortality from prostate cancer? The choice of the endpoint has a major impact on the design of the trial, its overall duration, and the number of patients required. (2) The sample size calculation which depends on the event rate in the control group, the size of the difference to be detected, the size of the type I and type II errors, the non-adherence and crossover rates, and the duration of patient entry and follow-up. (3) The possible confounding between the intervention and ascertainment of the endpoint. What is the effect of the intervention on the sensitivity and specificity of prostate screening tests? What are its implications on trial design? (4) The effect of 'noncompliance' on intent-to-treat analyses: nonadherence or treatment refusal, crossovers, loss to follow-up, biopsy refusal, and intercurrent deaths. (5) The assessment of side effects, both acute and long term.

Introduction

Since prostate cancer incidence and mortality rates continue to increase [1], effective prostate cancer prevention strategies are needed. Prevention might entail reducing the exposure to risk factors, modifying risk-taking behaviors, or as considered here, the administration of agents designed to prevent the disease.

Over the past 20 years there has been an ever-growing literature dealing with the design and analysis of phase III clinical trials in the treatment of prostate cancer [2]. While many of the same concepts also apply to chemoprevention trials, such studies are considerably more complicated and there is less experience in their conduct. The Prostate Cancer Prevention Trial (PCPT) has highlighted many of the difficulties which exist in the design and analysis of chemoprevention trials [3].

Design of Chemoprevention Studies

A number of issues must be considered in designing a chemoprevention study.

Choice of the Design

Similar to a clinical trial in patients with prostate cancer, the objective of a chemoprevention study is to compare two or more agents for efficacy and patient accept-

KARGER

Fax + 41 61 306 12 34
E-Mail karger@karger.ch
www.karger.com

0302–2838/99/0356–0519$17.50/0

Accessible online at:
http://BioMedNet.com/karger

Richard Sylvester, ScD
EORTC Data Center, 83, ave E.-Mounier, Bte 11
B–1200 Brussels (Belgium)
Tel. +32 2 774 1613, Fax +32 2 772 3545, E-Mail rsy@eortc.be

ability. While the design should be kept as simple as possible in order to encourage enrollment, necessary precautions must be taken to minimize bias. The trial should be prospective, randomized, and when feasible double blind. A run-in or enrollment period prior to randomization may be used to identify early dropouts and patients with poor compliance.

Choice of Treatments to Be Compared

The ideal agent should be effective in preventing the development of prostate cancer, have low toxicity (high benefit to risk ratio), be easy to administer and inexpensive [4, 5]. In addition, the agents studied should not affect the sensitivity or specificity of prostate cancer screening tests, otherwise biased comparisons may result.

Choice of the Patient Population

Patients with a normal PSA and no significant urinary obstructive symptoms, but at high risk of developing clinically important prostate cancer, should be included. Different factors that one might take into account include age, family history, genetic factors, racial and ethnic background, dietary fat consumption, and the presence of prostatic intraepithelial neoplasia (PIN). Patients may be stratified at entry for study site and one or two of the above factors.

Choice of the Primary Endpoint

One of the most critical aspects in designing a chemoprevention study is the choice of the primary endpoint. While a reduction in the disease incidence rate would appear to be the ultimate goal, the detection of early stage disease is not necessarily a clinically meaningful event in a patient population where many may die due to other causes. A more meaningful endpoint might be disease-specific survival or the development of distant metastases. Treatment acceptability in terms of both side effects and quality of life should also be assessed.

These endpoints all require a large number of patients and a potentially long follow-up period. It is important that patients in all the treatment groups are followed and assessed at the same frequency. In order to shorten this period or decrease the number of patients, the use of intermediate (surrogate) endpoints such as the development of premalignant lesions or the increase of PSA has sometimes been proposed. While their use may permit an earlier evaluation of the agents being tested, they must be used with extreme caution since they are not necessarily predictive for the primary endpoint and their assessment may be influenced by the agents under study. For example, if the treatment alters the PSA level, then use of PSA as an intermediate endpoint may be biased.

An Example of a Prostate Cancer Chemoprevention Trial: The PCPT

The PCPT [3] is a randomized double-blind chemoprevention trial comparing finasteride to placebo. The primary endpoint was to determine whether participants treated with finasteride for 7 years have a lower period prevalence of biopsy-proven prostate cancer than those treated with placebo. Annual digital rectal examinations (DREs) and serum PSA determinations were carried out, with eventual prostate biopsies. Since finasteride reduces serum PSA levels, it may influence detection of the disease. If uncorrected serum PSA levels are used as a criteria for biopsy, fewer finasteride patients would undergo prostate biopsy than those on placebo. Thus the disease detection rate would be artificially low on finasteride as compared to placebo and the effect of the drug would be overestimated.

Endpoints

Initially three possible primary endpoints were considered in this trial:

(1) Diagnosis of prostate cancer of any stage: Since uncontrolled PSAs could bias the endpoint, a central PSA laboratory was set up. Several different strategies were considered:

Withhold PSA levels from investigators: In this case DRE would be the chief clinical indicator for biopsy. However, DRE is not sensitive in detecting early stage disease and its use might bias detection since finasteride decreases prostate volume. It was also thought that study accrual might suffer if PSA information was withheld.

Use PSA indexing: Different cut-off levels of PSA would be used in the two treatment groups in order to adjust for the lowering of PSA values on finasteride. In this way the biopsy rates in the two groups would be the same, however it has the potential problem of using an indexed PSA as the basis for diagnosis when diagnosis is the primary endpoint.

Conduct multiple biopsies in a small (10%) sample (vanguard approach): Data from a small sample would be used to determine cut-off PSA levels to trigger biopsies in future patients. This approach is not attractive because of the possibility of a high dropout rate after one or two biopsies. In addition, only a few prostate cancers would be

Table 1. Assumptions in designing the PCPT trial

p_0 = 7-year event rate in the control arm if perfect compliance	6%
p_1 = 7-year event rate in the experimental arm if perfect compliance	4.2%
d_0 = % contamination of the control arm by the experimental arm	5%
d_1 = % nonadherence in the experimental arm	14%
p_{0r} = adjusted 7-year event rate in the control arm	5.91%
p_{1r} = adjusted 7-year event rate in the experimental arm	4.45%
b = % patients having known prostate cancer status	60%
α = size of the type I error	0.05
β = size of the type II error (power = 1 – β)	0.08 (0.92)
One- or two-sided test of significance	two-sided

detected each year in the vanguard group so that estimates of PSA sensitivity would not be very precise.

(2) Death from prostate cancer or diagnosis of metastatic disease: A large simple trial would be conducted where there would be no attempt to standardize either the diagnostic procedures or treatment. Since finasteride decreases the PSA level, the use of PSA as a monitoring tool may lead early on to more patients on placebo either taking finasteride or having biopsies with a resultant increased tumor detection rate. One might be tempted to stop the trial early simply because of an increase in the tumor detection rate even if it is not the primary endpoint. There is also the question of the potential impact of subsequent treatment on the study groups. Adoption of this approach in the PCPT would have required the randomization of 51,000 men in a 15-year study in order to detect a 26% reduction in prostate cancer deaths based on a two-sided test at error rates $\alpha = 0.05$ and $\beta = 0.10$.

(3) Seven-year period prevalence: The endpoint actually used was the prevalence of prostate cancer at 7 years: biopsy-proven prostate cancer prior to or immediately after 7 years of treatment. Absence of prostate cancer could only be determined by a negative biopsy at 7 years.

Determination of the sample size: Taking the 7-year period prevalence as the primary endpoint, the sample size in the PCPT trial depended on a number of factors as indicated in table 1. The contamination and nonadherence rates d_0 and d_1 dilute the size of the treatment difference, making the treatments appear to be more similar than they actually are. Under the above assumptions the resulting adjusted event rates are:

$$P_{0r} = (1 - d_0)p_0 + d_0p_1 = 5.91\%$$
$$P_{1r} = d_1p_0 + (1 - d_1)p_1 = 4.45\%$$

Thus the absolute and relative differences of 1.8 and 30% with no contamination become smaller adjusted differences of 1.46 and 24.7% under the above assumptions. It was estimated that 40% would not have known prostate cancer status at 7 years: 17% mortality (other than prostate cancer), 18% loss to follow-up, and 5% biopsy refusal. Based on these assumptions, a total of 18,000 men were required.

Possible confounding between the endpoint and the intervention (bias ascertainment): Since finasteride reduces PSA levels and decreases the size of the prostate gland, the use of PSA and DRE to select patients for biopsy may yield misleading and biased results. The following assumptions were to be verified during the trial: (1) Finasteride results in a simple downward shift of PSA values so that based on an arm-specific threshold, comparable groups of patients in the two arms are biopsied prior to 7 years. (2) Finasteride nonadherence which could affect PSA interpretation can be adequately monitored. (3) The distribution of and reasons for nonbiopsy are the same in the two arms. (4) Finasteride does not affect the sensitivity or specificity of the DRE or transrectal ultrasonography (TRUS) or the sensitivity of the prostate biopsy (untestable). (5) Biases resulting from TURPs for BHP, which may be more frequent on the placebo arm, are negligible.

Analysis and Monitoring of Chemoprevention Studies

Besides the classical analyses of treatment efficacy and side effects/quality of life, additional analyses must be carried out to verify the design assumptions.

Effect of Noncompliance

Intent-to-treat analyses must be carried out since the exclusion of randomized patients, whatever the reason, may bias the results. Nevertheless, additional analyses assessing the degree and impact of noncompliance are required.

Assessment of Side Effects/Quality of Life

An important factor in these trials is the acceptability of long-term use of the agent by healthy participants. In the PCPT, every 6 months it was planned to closely monitor side effects in the first 20% (3,600) of the patients randomized, with special attention being paid to sexual function. This provides a power of 99% to detect a difference in the rates of side effects of 5% on finasteride versus 2% on placebo based on a one-sided test at $\alpha = 0.01$.

Data and Safety Monitoring Committee (DSMC)

A data and safety monitoring committee was set up to monitor the PCPT, meeting every 6 months after 1 year, to suggest whether or not changes in the trial's design might be required. The DSMC plays a very important role by assessing participant safety, side effects (sexual functioning), and violations of the assumptions given above. During patient entry, data will not yet be available to monitor the primary endpoint so that an early stopping rule for treatment efficacy is not possible.

Conclusions

The design of prostate cancer chemoprevention trials poses special problems not found in treatment efficacy studies, especially if there may be a confounding between the treatment and ascertainment of the endpoint. The effect of noncompliance further complicates the trial's design and interpretation. It is thus mandatory that the statistical issues related to the trial's design and analysis be thoroughly discussed and resolved early on in the planning of the study.

References

1 Cancer Facts and Figures – 1996. Atlanta, American Cancer Society, 1996.

2 Andersson L (ed): Design of clinical trials on prostate cancer. Urology 1997;49:1–76.

3 Feigl P, Blumenstein B, Thompson I, Crowley J, Wolf M, Kramer BS, Coltman CA, Brawley OW, Ford LG: Design of the prostate cancer prevention trial (PCPT). Control Clin Trials 1995;16:150–163.

4 Nelson PS, Brawer MK: Chemoprevention of prostate carcinoma. Urol Int 1997;4:7–9.

5 Ellis WJ, Brawer MK: Prostate cancer: Chemoprevention strategies; in Raghavan D, Scher HI, Leibel SA, Lange PH (eds): Principles and Practice of Genitourinary Oncology. Philadelphia, Lippencott-Raven, 1997, pp 437–441.

Clinical Trial Designs for Chemoprevention of Prostate Cancer

European Urology

Eur Urol 1999;35:523–538

Prostate Cancer Screening in Tyrol, Austria: Experience and Results

W. Horninger A. Reissigl H. Rogatsch H. Volgger M. Studen H. Klocker G. Bartsch

Department of Urology, University of Innsbruck, Austria

Key Words

Prostate-specific antigen · Free prostate-specific antigen · Prostate-specific antigen transition zone density · Transitional zone cancer · Stage migration · Organ-confined tumors · PSA screening · Probability of prostate cancer

Abstract

Background: This article summarizes the experience and results of different prostate carcinoma screening projects using total prostate-specific antigen (PSA) and percent free PSA as the initial test. ***Methods:*** The twelve projects studied included: (1) a mass screening study using PSA as the initial test in 21,079 volunteers; (2) an investigation of the usefulness of normal and age-referenced PSA cut-offs in 1,618 men; (3) a PSA-based screening study of 2,272 asymptomatic blood donors; (4) an investigation of the evidence and significance of transition zone carcinoma in 340 men with negative digital rectal examination findings; (5) determination of percent free PSA in one retrospective and two prospective studies to determine the appropriate cutpoints for percent free PSA; (6) evaluation of the diagnostic benefit of PSA transition zone density in 308 screening volunteers; (7) a study of the impact of PSA-based screening on the percentage of incidental prostate carcinoma in 1,543 men undergoing transurethral resection of the prostate; (8) an evaluation of the changes in total PSA and pathologic stages in radical prostatectomy over 5 years in a PSA-based mass screening program; (9) a study evaluating the probability of having prostate cancer given the patient's age, total PSA and digital rectal examination findings; (10) an evaluation of the correlation between preoperative predictors and pathologic features in radical prostatectomy specimens; (11) an investigation of the correlation of total PSA with pathologic stage and tumor volume in patients undergoing radical prostatectomy with low PSA cut-off level, and (12) a study whether age has an impact on the extension of prostate cancer. ***Results:*** (1) of the 21,079 volunteers, 1,618 (8%) had elevated PSA levels. Of these men, 778 (48%) underwent biopsies; 197 biopsies were positive for prostate carcinoma and 135 underwent radical prostatectomy. Ninety-five were found to be organ-confined. (2) A PSA cut-off of 2.5 ng/ml in men aged 45–49 years and of 3.5 ng/ml in men aged 50–59 years resulted in an 8% increase in the detection rate of organ-confined disease. (3) Of the 2,272 men, 284 had elevated PSA levels and prostate carcinoma was detected in 62 men. All patients underwent radical prostatectomy and histologic examination revealed organ-confined tumor in all but 8 men. (4) Ninety-eight of

KARGER

Fax + 41 61 306 12 34
E-Mail karger@karger.ch
www.karger.com

0302–2838/99/0356–0523$17.50/0

Accessible online at:
http://BioMedNet.com/karger

Wolfgang Horninger, MD
Department of Urology, University of Innsbruck
Anichstrasse 35
A–6020 Innsbruck (Austria)
Tel. +43 512 504 4810, Fax +43 512 504 4873, E-Mail wolfgang horninger@uibk.ac.at

340 men had biopsies positive for carcinoma; 28 of these patients (28.5%) had carcinoma that originated in the transition zone only. (5) In the retrospective study, receiver-operating characteristic curve analysis showed that by using a percent free PSA of 18% as a biopsy criterion, 37% of the negative biopsies could be eliminated although 94% of all carcinomas would still be detected. In the first prospective study, 106 of 158 men with elevated PSA levels < 10.0 ng/ml were further evaluated and 37 prostate carcinomas were detected. By using a % free PSA of < 22% as a biopsy criterion, 30% of the negative biopsies could be eliminated although 98% of the carcinomas would still be detected. In the second prospective study, 120 of 465 men with total PSA levels between 1.25 and 6.49 ng/ml and a % free PSA < 18% were further evaluated and 27 (22.5%) were found to have prostate carcinomas. (6) Receiver-operating characteristic curve analysis for PSA transition zone density showed that by using a PSA transition zone density of > 22 ng/ml/cm^3 as a biopsy criterion, 24.4% of negative biopsies could be avoided without missing a single carcinoma. (7) In the prescreening era the incidence of T1a grade 1 and 2 carcinomas was 3.1% and the incidence of T1a grade 3 and T1b carcinoma was 2.3% whereas in the years after the establishment of PSA-based screening the incidence was 4.6 and 1.03% respectively. (8) The rate of organ-confined tumors increased from 28.7% in 1993 to 65.7% in 1997. (9) In this evaluation a new approach to proceed with a prostate biopsy based upon the individual risk of having prostate cancer rather than a single PSA cutpoint was developed. (10) High total PSA levels, PSA density and PSA transition zone density correlated significantly with high Gleason scores, capsular penetration, a high percentage of cancer in the prostatectomy specimen and a high cancer volume. (11) In this evaluation all of the 95 patients with PSA levels < 3.99 ng/ml who underwent radical prostatectomy showed clinically significant, organ-confined prostate cancer with negative surgical margins. (12) The results of this evaluation suggest that older men have larger tumor volumes compared to younger men with the same PSA levels. ***Conclusions:*** These data suggest that PSA-based screening with low PSA cut-off values increase the detection rate of clinically significant, organ-confined and potentially curable prostate cancer. Percent free PSA and PSA transition zone density provide an additional diagnostic benefit over total PSA.

Several studies have demonstrated that prostate-specific antigen (PSA)-based screening is the most effective screening method, however most of these studies were done in men referred to urological care settings because of signs and symptoms [1–3]. It is only recently that large-scale screening studies have been conducted in asymptomatic men within a limited time frame [4]. A mass screening project was carried out in the Tyrol, one of nine federal states of the Republic of Austria. The Tyrol is an alpine region in the western part of Austria with 631,410 inhabitants (324,161 females and 307,249 males) in an area of 12,647 km^2. The region is dominated by the mountains of the Central Alps, and the distances to Innsbruck, the capital, where the central health care unit is located, are not too long. This geographical situation, as well as the willingness of the general population to participate in preventive medical programs caused us to launch a state-wide mass screening program with PSA as the initial test for early detection of prostate cancer. Of the 307,249 male inhabitants, 65,000 were between 45 and 74 years of age. We recommended that men within this age range should undergo screening, and information to this effect was distributed to all Tyrolean males by press, radio and television.

The screening project was carried out in collaboration with general practitioners, medical officers, urologists, and the Tyrolean Blood Bank of the Red Cross. All coworkers were fully informed about the guidelines for withdrawal, storage, and shipping of the blood samples. PSA was assessed immediately upon arrival of the blood or serum samples. All volunteers and/or referring physicians were informed in writing about the results. In case of elevated PSA levels, the volunteers were invited to undergo further urological evaluation, while men with normal PSA levels were invited to have a repeat PSA test 1 year later.

Projects

The following twelve projects are summarized:

1 Results of a mass screening with PSA as the initial test – The Tyrol Project.
2 Comparison of different PSA cutpoints.
3 PSA study in blood donors.
4 Incidence and significance of transitional zone cancer.
5 Determination of the ratio of free/total PSA in screening volunteers to define the optimal range of total PSA and determine the appropriate cutpoints for percent free PSA within this range.
6 Evaluation of PSA transition zone density.

7 Reduction in the incidence of incidental prostate cancer by PSA screening.
8 Stage migration in a 5-year PSA-based screening program.
9 The probability of having prostate cancer given the patient's age, serum PSA value and digital rectal examination findings.
10 Correlation between preoperative predictors and pathologic features in radical prostatectomy specimens.
11 Correlation of total PSA with pathologic stage and tumor volume in patients undergoing radical prostatectomy with low PSA cut-off levels.
12 PSA-based screening with very low PSA cut-off values: Correlation between age and clinical and pathologic features in the 40- to 59-year age group.

The Tyrol Project

This mass screening project was conducted between October 1993 and September 1994 with PSA as the initial test for early detection of prostate cancer. About 65,000 Tyrolean males between 45 and 75 years of age were invited to participate in this screening program free of charge. 21,078 male volunteers (30%) responded to press releases, and radio and TV programs asking healthy men to participate in a PSA screening test for prostate cancer. None of them had a history of prostate cancer and males with a history of prostatitis were excluded from the study. All volunteers underwent determination of serum PSA concentration (Abbott IMX assay) in the same laboratory using age-referenced PSA levels [5].

Age-referenced PSA levels were defined according to the recommendations made by Oesterling et al. [5] (2.5 ng/ml for men aged 40–49, 3.5 ng/ml for men aged 50–59, 4.5 ng/ml for men aged 60–69, and 6.5 ng/ml for men aged 70–79). Age was defined as the subject's age on the day of PSA assessment. All males who – according to age-referenced levels – had elevated PSA concentrations were invited to undergo further urological evaluation including digital rectal examination (DRE) and ultrasound-guided biopsies. DRE and transrectal ultrasound (TRUS) examinations were performed by the same four urologists. With the help of three-dimensional (3D) ultrasound equipment, ultrasonography was performed in three planes (sagittal, horizontal, coronal), and biopsies were made under ultrasound guidance with an automatic biopsy gun and an 18-gauge needle (sextant biopsy).

Table 1. Age distribution and number of volunteers, biopsies and tumors

Age group years	Volunteers	Biopsies	Positive for carcinoma
45–49	2,054	28	3
50–59	9,541	142	28
60–69	7,601	401	109
70–75	1,882	207	57
Total	21,078	778	197

Of the 21,078 volunteers, 1,618 (18%) were found to have elevated PSA levels. The age distribution is shown in table 1. Overall, biopsies were obtained in 778 of 1,618 men (48%) with elevated PSA levels. In 197 (25%) of them the biopsies were positive for prostatic carcinoma. The overall cancer detection rate was 1.2%. 70% of these lesions were missed on DRE and were detected only by PSA determination. TRUS was normal in 65% of the cancer patients. Of the 197 males presenting with cancer, 135 (69%) underwent radical prostatectomy. Of these 135 pathologically staged tumors, 130 (96%) were judged to be clinically important with regard to stage, grade and volume.

Comparison of Different PSA Cutpoints

This study was designed to investigate the usefulness of normal and age-referenced PSA cut-offs in our mass screening study for early detection of prostate cancer. Previously most screening studies used a PSA concentration of 4.0 ng/ml as the upper limit of normal, while some reports suggested the use of age-specific PSA reference ranges [6].

In this mass screening project we used the age-referenced PSA levels described above. Furthermore, all men aged between 50 and 75 with PSA levels between 4 and 6.5 ng/ml, which were considered normal according to age-specific PSA reference ranges, were invited to undergo further urological evaluation as described above.

Of the 1,618 men with elevated PSA levels, 66 presented with levels >2.5 ng/ml but <4.0 ng/ml. Age distribution, PSA levels, number of biopsies and number of cancers detected are shown in table 2. The average age was 53.7 years and the average PSA level was 3.66 ng/ml. DRE findings were negative in all 66 subjects; all of them

Table 2. Age distribution, average value, number of biopsies and number of carcinomas in men with PSA levels between 2.5 and 4.0 ng/ml

Age group years	Volunteers	Average PSA ng/ml	Biopsies	Positive for carcinoma
45–49	18	3.2	18	2
50–59	48	3.8	48	14
Total	66	3.66	66	16

Table 3. Pathologic stage and grade of carcinoma in 6 patients (group 1)

Staging				Grade (Gleason score)			
organ-confined		advanced		4	6	7	8
pT2a	pT2b	pT2c	pT3				
1	3	1	1	1	1	3	1

underwent biopsy (100%). As a result, the biopsy rate increased by 8%. In 16 (24%) of these men the biopsies were positive for cancer. All 16 pathologically staged tumors (100%) were organ-confined, and none of the lesions were microscopically focal and well differentiated and hence possibly insignificant.

When the normal PSA cut-off of 4.0 ng/ml was used, 1,872 of the 21,078 volunteers had elevated PSA levels. 320 men with PSA concentrations >4.0 ng/ml but <6.5 ng/ml were further evaluated as described above. The average age was 72.5 years and the average PSA level was 6.12 ng/ml. Overall, 205 of the 320 men (64%) underwent biopsy. In 23 (11%) of these men the biopsies were positive for cancer. Seven of the 23 (30%) had positive findings on rectal examination. All 23 males underwent radical prostatectomy. Overall, 8 of the 23 pathologically staged tumors (35%) were organ-confined. Only 5 tumors were considered clinically significant with regard to stage, grade and volume.

These 205 biopsies represent 21% of the 983 biopsies performed in the study population. The 23 patients whose cancers would not have been detected, if age-specific reference ranges had been used, represent 0.1% of all participants in the study and 10% of all cancers detected. In the younger age groups (40–49 and 50–59) the number of biopsies did not increase significantly. In this cohort, 66 biopsies (8%) were performed and 16 (24%) cancers were detected. All cancers detected were organ-confined and clinically significant (100%). In the group older than 59, by comparison, only 5 (22%) cancers were considered to be of clinical importance. Thus, only a small number of life-threatening cancers was missed in this age group as a result of using age-specific reference ranges. The detection rates of organ-confined cancers showed a significant age-related difference ($p = 0.00004$); in the younger group (PSA 2.5–4.0 ng/ml) 16 out of 16 cancers and in the older group (PSA 4.0–6.5 ng/ml) 8 out of 23 tumors were detected. The results obtained from 21,078 screening participants support the clinical usefulness of age-specific reference ranges for serum PSA.

PSA-Based Screening Study in Blood Donors

Every year about 50,000 blood donors aged between 18 and 65 years are recruited by the regional Blood Bank at Innsbruck University Hospital. Donation of blood routinely involves a medical checkup which comprises various blood tests such as liver function tests, cholesterol, neopterin, human immunodeficiency virus (HIV) and other investigations. In 1991, PSA determination was also included and is now routinely performed in all male blood donors aged between 40 and 65 years. The study was launched on January 2, 1991 and carried out over a period of 3 years. PSA was measured with a commercially available immunoradiometric assay (Tandem-R-PSA; Hybritech Corp., San Diego, Calif., USA).

The volunteers were divided into two age groups: group 1 included men between 40 and 49 years, while group 2 comprised males aged between 50 and 65 years. PSA serum levels were determined at our laboratory in a total of 2,272 asymptomatic blood donors.

Age Group 1: 40–49 Years

In this screening group, volunteers presenting with serum PSA levels >4 ng/ml were invited to undergo further urological evaluation. In patients with abnormal findings on DRE, ultrasound-guided biopsies were performed to sample regions with palpable abnormalities and/or hypoechoic areas.

In view of their young age, patients in this group who had normal findings on DRE were not further evaluated. However, they were encouraged to return for annual PSA determination. 568 males showed a 20% increase in PSA; they underwent systematic sector biopsy under ultrasound guidance. 44 men (8%) presenting with serum PSA

Table 4. Pathologic stage and grade of carcinoma in 58 patients (group 2)

Staging								Grade (Gleason score)					
organ-confined					advanced			4	5	6	7	8	9
pT1a	pT1b	pT2a	pT2b	pT2c	pT3a	pT3b	pT3c						
1	1	22	18	8	3	4	1	2	5	24	21	5	1

levels >4 ng/ml were further evaluated by DRE (compliance rate 100%). Only 2 males (5%) who had suspicious findings on DRE underwent biopsy, the results of which, however, were negative for carcinoma.

Forty-two patients with PSA levels of >4 ng/ml and normal findings on DRE were encouraged to return annually for PSA assessment. Twelve of them showed a 20% increase in the concentration of PSA 1 year later. Among those biopsied, prostate cancers were detected in 4 males (33%). Two patients who despite suspicious DRE findings – had negative biopsies in the first year presented with an increase in PSA in the second year (4.1–6.2 and 4.8–5.8 respectively) and exhibited carcinoma when biopsied again.

Clinical staging in the 4 patients presenting with carcinoma revealed nonpalpable clinical stage B cancer in 2; their Gleason scores ranged from 4 to 8 (mean 5.2). Radical prostatectomy was performed in all 6 men. Table 3 provides information on the pathological stages. Five of the cancers detected were organ-confined. Only 1 patient had advanced disease with microscopically positive margins. None of the lesions was a possibly latent tumor.

Age Group 2: 50–65 Years

In this age group, PSA determination was performed in a total of 1,704 males. Men with serum PSA levels >4 ng/ml were referred for TRUS and, depending on the findings, random or ultrasound-guided biopsies of suspicious areas.

240 (14%) of the 1,704 males were found to have serum PSA levels >4 ng/ml; only 9% of them had suspicious findings on DRE. Biopsy specimens were obtained from all males presenting with elevated PSA levels (compliance rate 100%). In 58 (24%) of them the biopsies were positive for prostatic carcinoma. The overall cancer detection rate was 3.4%. 42 (73%) of these lesions were missed on DRE and detected solely by PSA. When used to confirm suspicious findings on DRE or PSA assessment, TRUS yielded false negative results in 48% of patients.

Table 5. Detection of organ-confined carcinoma (n = 50; group 2)

Results category		Pathologic stage				
DRE	PSA, ng/ml	pT1a	pT1b	pT2a	pT2b	pT2c
Negative	4.1–9.9	1	1	13	12	8
Negative	≥10.0	0	0	2	2	5
Positive	4.1–9.9	0	0	1	1	2
Positive	≥10.0 or more	0	0	2	0	2

In all 58 patients whose biopsy specimens had yielded prostatic lesions, clinical staging revealed nonpalpable or clinical stage B cancers (100%), with Gleason scores ranging from 4 to 9 (mean 5.5).

All of them underwent radical prostatectomy. Table 4 shows the pathological stages. Overall, 50 of the 58 pathologically staged lesions (86.2%) were found to be organ-confined. Of the 8 patients presenting with advanced cancer, 7 had microscopically positive margins, while only 1 showed invasion of the seminal vesicle; none of them had pelvic lymph node metastases. Only two tumors were microscopically focal and well differentiated and hence possibly clinically insignificant (5%).

By BSA-based screening a significantly higher percentage of organ-confined cancers could be detected (50 of 50; 100%) than by DRE (6 of 50; 12%). Of the organ-confined cancers, 44 (88%) were missed by DRE and detected solely by PSA (table 5). The higher the PSA level, the less likely was the chance of the lesion to be organ-confined.

Incidence and Clinical Significance of Transitional Zone Cancer

Approximately 20% of prostate cancers originate from the transitional zone (TZ) [7]. Although TRUS-guided biopsies in men with elevated PSA levels and negative rectal examination findings have improved the diagnosis

Table 6. Pathologic findings and PSA levels of TZ carcinomas

Patients (n = 28)	Pathologic stage	Gleason score	PSA = 2.5–9.9 ng/ml	PSA ≥ 10 ng/ml
1	pT1b	5	1	0
9	pT2a	4.7	7	2
10	pT2b	5	8	2
4	pT3a	5.5	2	2
4	pT3b	7	0	4

Table 7. Pathologic findings and PSA levels of carcinomas originating in the transition and peripheral zones

Patients (n = 5)	Pathologic stage	Median Gleason score	PSA, ng/ml
4	pT3c N0	7	8.5 (median)
1	pT3c N1	9	50

Table 8. Pathologic stages of 48 radical prostatectomy specimens

Stage	Patients
pT1b	1
pT2a	5
pT2b	10
pT2c	17
pT3a	9
pT3b	4
pT3c	2
N+	1

of peripheral zone cancer, the yield of carcinoma can be further improved by additional biopsies obtained from the TZ.

To evaluate the incidence and clinical significance of TZ cancers, two TZ biopsies were added to the routinely performed sextant biopsies in males with elevated PSA levels and negative findings on rectal examination. The study included 340 volunteers with negative rectal examination findings and clearly visible prostatic zones on 3D TRUS, who were recruited from our PSA screening program. Ultrasonography was performed in three planes (sagittal, horizontal, coronal).

The three sections of the prostate in the horizontal, sagittal and coronal planes are displayed simultaneously on the monitor of the system. Depending on the level of the horizontal section, the relative proportions of the transition and peripheral zones vary considerably. Cranially, the enlarged TZ dominates the horizontal plane, while the slightly hypoechoic peripheral zone forms a narrow band of tissue dorsal and lateral to the TZ. Caudal to the verumontanum, only the peripheral zone is seen. In the coronal plane the enlarged TZ and the hypoechoic central zone, which is displaced dorsally and cranially, can be demonstrated most clearly, and the regions of the apex of the prostate and the bladder neck can be visualized even better. This plane allows for better assessment of the topographical relationships not only between the prostatic zones but also between the prostate and its surrounding structures, thus facilitating precise delineation of the prostatic zones. The additional information provided by the coronal plane permits identification of the different prostatic zones in any section.

The ultrasound images were evaluated for abnormalities in the TZ before biopsies were made as described above. Following systematic sextant biopsy, all patients underwent two additional biopsies of the TZ. These biopsies were obtained from both the right and the left portion of the TZ.

The study group included 340 males. In 98 (29%) of them the biopsies were positive for prostate cancer. Of these 98 patients, 66 (67%) presented with peripheral cancers, which were detected by traditional sextant biopsies. 28 cancers (28%) originating from the TZ could only be detected by two additional TZ biopsies; 5 males (5%) presented with lesions which were located in the TZ and the peripheral zone. None of the patients showed palpable abnormalities on DRE. 18 men showed TZ abnormalities on ultrasound imaging; in 4 of them the biopsies were positive for TZ cancer. TZ abnormalities included hypoechoic areas and localized asymmetry at the junction of the prostatic capsule with the anterior fibromuscular stroma. 18 patients with proven TZ cancer had preoperative serum PSA levels ranging between 2.6 and 9.9 ng/ml (mean 5.6), while 10 patients presented with levels >10 ng/ml (mean 12.2). Of 33 patients undergoing radical prostatectomy, 28 presented with cancers arising solely from the TZ, while 5 had cancers originating from the peripheral zone as well as the TZ. The pathological stages and grades as well as the PSA levels are shown in tables 6 and 7. Of the prostatic carcinomas detected, 96% (27 of 28 cases) had a malignant potential, while only one tumor (4%) was microscopically focal and well differentiated and therefore possibly insignificant with regard to stage and grade. In the radical prostatectomy specimens the mean Gleason grade (score) was 7.2 (range 4–8) for TZ cancers and 7.4 (range 6–9) for cancers originating from the TZ as well as the peripheral zone. Overall, 71% of the pathologically staged cancers (20 of 28) were found to be organ-confined. All 5 combined TZ and peripheral zone cancers were advanced lesions showing invasion of the seminal vesicles in all men and, in addition, invasion of the pelvic lymph nodes in 1 patient. Altogether, 30% of the cancers detected were so-called TZ cancers, which corresponds to a 95% confidence interval (20–40%).

These data support the assumption that a significant subset of prostatic carcinomas originate from the TZ. These results further support the concept that cancers of TZ origin have a malignant potential.

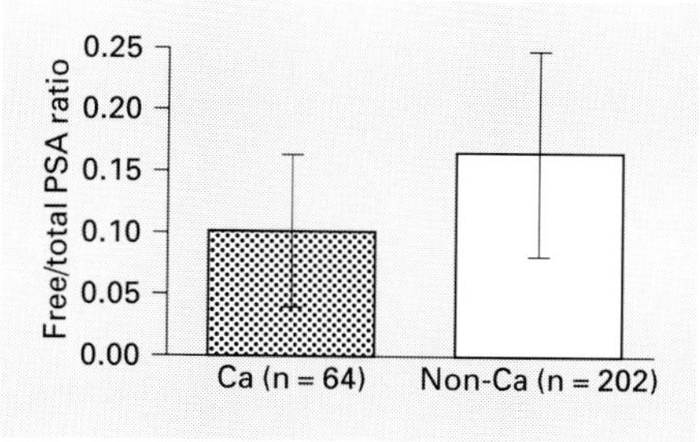

Fig. 1. Free/total PSA ratio in 64 patients with prostate carcinoma (Ca) and 202 patients with nonmalignant disease (Non-Ca). Difference is significant (p = 0.0001).

Evaluation of the Clinical Utility of the Free/Total PSA Ratio in Distinguishing Benign Prostatic Disease from Prostate Cancer in a Screening Population

Retrospective Study

This study was conducted with 266 screening volunteers who were identified to have elevated serum PSA levels by means of a conventional PSA determination kit (Abbott MEIA performed on an IMX equipment). Subsequently, their diagnosis was confirmed by biopsies. The serum samples of these 266 patients were stored at –80 °C for further measurement. Free and total PSA levels were determined with the DELFIA PSA dual-label free/total PSA kit (Wallac Oy, Turku, Finland). This kit uses two differently labeled antibodies, one specific for free PSA, the other one for complexed PSA, and allows for simultaneous equimolar measurement of free PSA and α_1-antichymotrypsin-complexed PSA. The assay was performed according to the recommendations of the manufacturer. A modular DELFIA system equipped with the Multicalc software (Wallac) was used to determine the two labels europium (Eu) and samarium (Sm), and to calculate the amounts of free and complexed PSA.

The mean age of the 266 men enrolled in this study was 63 years ranging from 45 to 75 years. In 64 (24%) men the biopsies were positive for prostate cancer, while 202 men were histologically free of cancer. Only 8 of the 64 patients with biopsy-proven cancer had suspicious findings on DRE. In 56 patients, clinical staging revealed nonpalpable or clinical stage T1c cancer. Radical prostatectomy was performed in 48 patients. Table 8 demonstrates the pathological stages. Overall, 33 of the 48 pathologically staged lesions were found to be organ-confined (69%). Of the 15 patients presenting with advanced cancer, 2 showed invasion of the seminal vesicles and 1 had pelvic lymph node metastases. The 64 cancer patients had a mean total PSA of 16.4 ng/ml (4.1–168.0), while the 202 patients who were histologically free of cancer had a mean total PSA of 7.5 ng/ml (2.6–28.2). The mean free/total PSA in the 64 patients with prostate cancer was 0.10. This differed significantly (p = 0.001) from the mean free/total PSA of the 202 men with negative biopsy results, which was 0.17 (fig. 1).

In order to clearly distinguish benign prostatic hyperplasia (BPH) patients from prostatic carcinoma patients, we chose a cut-off for the percentage of free/total PSA that would include virtually all prostate cancer patients with elevated total PSA, regardless of their DRE findings. Receiver-operating characteristic (ROC) curve analysis showed that by using a free/total PSA of <18% as a biopsy criterion in men with elevated PSA levels, 37% of negative biopsies could be eliminated while still detecting 94% of carcinomas. Figure 2 shows ROC curves for total PSA and the free/total PSA ratio. The main difference between the two ROC curves is in the region indicated by arrows. Only four prostate cancers (6%) showed free/total PSA ratios of >18%. All 4 patients had suspicious findings on rectal examination. Percent free/total PSA did not correlate with tumor stage (organ-confined disease versus extracapsular extension or lymph node involvement). In the group of men with elevated serum PSA levels of <10 ng/ml, a free/total PSA ratio of up to 0.18 as a criterion for biopsy would eliminate 42% of negative biopsies while still detecting 94% of carcinomas. By using this free/total PSA ratio (≤0.18) as a criterion for biopsy in the group with total PSA levels <20 ng/ml, 38% of negative biopsies

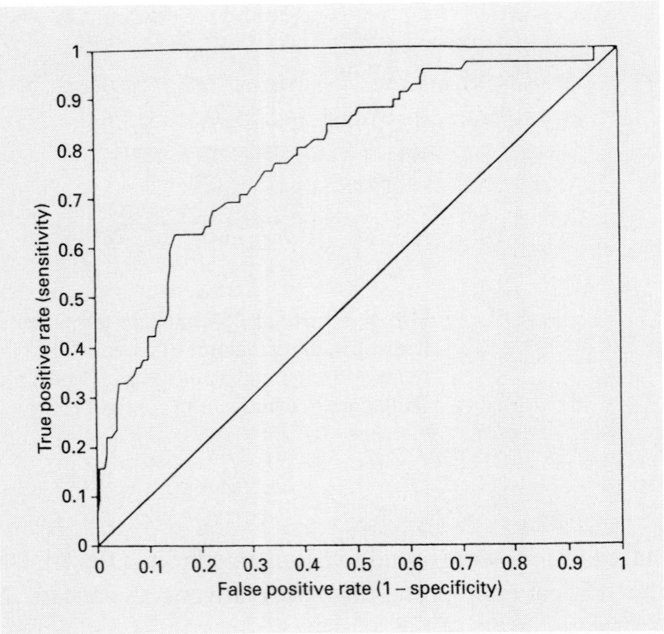

Fig. 2. ROC curve for free/total PSA of men with elevated PSA levels.

Table 9. Different free/total PSA cut-off values

Cut-off value	Total PSA ng/ml	Biopsy saving %	PCA loss %
18%	≤10	44	25
	>10	46	25
20%	≤10	36	10
	>10	31	9
22%	≤10	30	2
	>10	29	1

could be avoided while still detecting 98% of prostate cancers. The diagnostic specificity of our free/total PSA ratio measurements was evaluated by comparing them with those obtained by conventional measurement of serum PSA concentration. Age-referenced cut-offs for total serum PSA yielded a specificity of 25% and a sensitivity of 93%. When calculating specificity at a sensitivity level of 93% from a plot of free/total PSA ratios against total PSA concentrations, a significant increase in specificity (from 25 to 37%) was observed at a cut-off level of 0.18 for the free/total PSA ratio.

Prospective Study I

The results of our retrospective study encouraged us to incorporate assessment of free PSA into our current screening study. Between March 1995 and May 1996, total serum PSA levels were determined in 1,426 prostate cancer screening volunteers aged between 45 and 75 years. The study protocol was described previously [8]. All males who – according to age-specific reference ranges – had elevated total PSA levels (2.5–10.0 ng/ml) were entered into the study. Age was defined as the subject's age on the day of PSA assessment. A total of 158 men met the aforementioned selection criteria and were included in the current analysis. Measurement of free PSA was done immediately after obtaining the results of total PSA assessment.

The cut-off points for the free/total PSA ratio were determined on the basis of the data obtained in the retrospective study and other studies on the assessment of free PSA concentrations in males with elevated total PSA levels undergoing evaluation for prostate cancer. The free/total PSA ratio cut-off point chosen for this study group was 22%. All screening volunteers were further evaluated by DRE, TRUS and biospy as described above.

106 of the men studied showed PSA levels between 2.5 and 10.0 ng/ml. Biopsy specimens were obtained from all of them; 37 (35%) biopsies were positive for prostate cancer, while 69 were histologically free of cancer. Six of the 37 cancer patients had suspicious findings on DRE [9, 10]. The majority of the 37 patients (62%) had Gleason scores 5 or 6, 31% had Gleason scores 7 or 8, and 7% had Gleason score 4. The 37 cancer patients had a mean total PSA of 7.2 ng/ml (2.5–10.0), while the 69 patients with no evidence of disease had a mean total PSA of 5.4 ng/ml (2.5–10.0). The mean free/total PSA in the 37 cancer patients was 0.10, which differed significantly from the mean free/total PSA of the males without cancer (0.22). In order to determine whether assessment of the free/total PSA ratio in men with serum PSA levels of 2.5–10.0 ng/ml would help distinguish prostate cancer patients from patients with benign disease, a cut-off for the percentage of free/total PSA that would include virtually all prostate cancer patients was chosen.

Table 9 shows the percentages of cancers missed with different cut-offs for percent free PSA. The free/total PSA ratio ≤0.18 used in our retrospective study corresponded to a 25% loss of prostate cancers. By using a free/total PSA ratio of up to 0.22 as an indication for biopsy, 30% of negative biopsies could be eliminated while still detecting 98% of cancers independent of the findings on DRE.

Prospective Study II
(Using Halved Age-Referenced Ranges)

The two studies presented above address the usefulness of the free/total PSA ratio in the range of 2.5–10.0 ng/ml. Both studies have shown that percent free PSA significantly improves specificity with a minimal decrease in sensitivity [11, 12]. In the two studies the standard age-referenced ranges were used in combination with percent free PSA, therefore, we were unable to detect cancers in subjects whose total PSA levels were within the normal range. In the literature, 38–48% of patients with clinically significant organ-confined cancers are reported to have normal PSA levels [13, 14]. In addition, at least 30% of all prostate cancers detected are locally advanced with PSA levels between 4 and 10 ng/ml. Hence, reducing the upper limit of normal for PSA may improve detection of organ-confined prostate cancer. Our objective was to evaluate the clinical utility of the free/total PSA ratio in distinguishing benign prostatic disease from prostate cancer in screening volunteers with low total PSA levels.

This free/total PSA ratio was measured in 465 screening volunteers who had total serum PSA levels between 1.25 and 6.4 ng/ml according to our modified age-referenced ranges which had been reduced by 50%. Table 10 summarizes the halved age-referenced PSA levels. Our aim was to enhance detection of cancer (sensitivity) within the range of 1.25–6.4 ng/ml, although this is associated with an increase in the number of biopsies. Various free/total PSA ratio cut-off points were analyzed and finally a cutpoint of 18% was chosen.

120 of the 465 volunteers (25.8%) presented with percent free PSA levels of <18% and normal DRE findings; for this reason, they were further evaluated by ultrasound-guided prostatic biopsies.

Of the 120 men, 27 (22.5%) were found to have prostate cancer, while 2 showed isolated high-grade prostatic intraepithelial neoplasia. The mean total PSA level was 2.66 ng/ml for prostate cancer patients, and 2.45 ng/ml for males with no evidence of disease. The mean percent free PSA was 10.8% for prostate cancer patients, and 13.3% for men with benign disease. Table 11 summarizes the values for total and percent free PSA in the study group.

All 15 patients who underwent radical prostatectomy had organ-confined disease. Table 12 provides information on the pathological stages and grades.

In conjunction with halved total PSA ranges, percent free PSA proved a useful tool for detecting clinically significant and pathologically organ-confined prostate cancers in screening volunteers with negative rectal examination findings.

Table 10. Bisected age-specific reference ranges

Age, years	Range, ng/ml
40–49	0–1.25
50–59	0–1.75
60–69	0–2.25
70–79	0–3.25

Table 11. Mean total and percent free PSA

	All patients (PSA range, 1.25–6.4 ng/ml)		
	benign disease (n = 91)	prostate carcinoma (n = 27)	PIN (n = 2)
Total PSA, ng/ml			
Mean	2.45	2.66	2.55
Percent free PSA			
Mean	15.3	10.8	12.2

PIN = Prostatic intraepithelial neoplasia.

Table 12. Pathologic stage and grade in 15 radical prostatectomy specimens

Tumors	Pathologic stage	Gleason score
2	pT2a	3–5
3	pT2b	4–7
10	pT2c	5–8

Improvement of Early Detection of Prostate Cancer by Using PSA TZ Density and Percent Free PSA in Addition to Total PSA levels

As BPH almost exclusively results from hyperplasia of the TZ, the PSA production in the peripheral zone can be assumed to remain relatively constant as the gland enlarges [14]. Therefore, it can be reasoned that in BPH changes in PSA levels are atrributable to the TZ of the prostate.

In the following study the diagnostic benefit from PSA TZ density (PSA TZ density = total PSA/TZ volume)

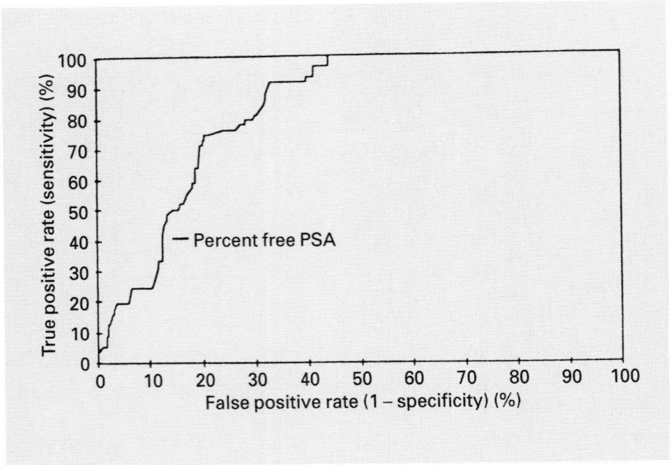

Fig. 3. ROC curves analysis for percent free PSA.

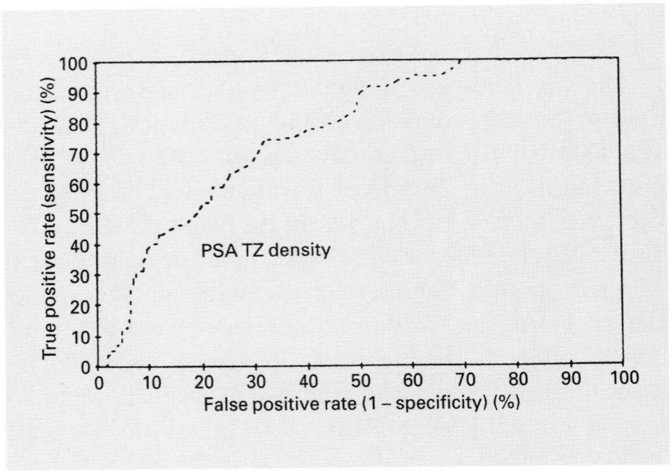

Fig. 4. ROC curves analysis for PSA TZ density.

Table 13. Mean values for total PSA, percent free PSA, and PSA TZ density

	BPH	PCA	Prostatitis
Total PSA, ng/ml	6.6 (2.5–10.0)	6.0 (3.1–10.0)	8.0 (2.5–9.7)
Free PSA, %	22 (4.7–43.2)	11.3 (4.1–19.1)	9.1 (4.6–20.2)
PSA TZ density, ng/ml/cm^3	0.35 (0.06–1.93)	0.56 (0.23–1.20)	0.50 (0.33–2.90)

alone and in combination with percent free PSA for the detection of early prostate cancer was evaluated.

Between August 1995 and May 1996, 308 consecutive screening volunteers with elevated total PSA levels ranging from 2.5 to 10.0 ng/ml were evaluated. All patients underwent DRE, TRUS and TRUS-guided biopsy of the prostate. Prior to these investigations, serum was obtained and total as well as free PSA levels were assessed with the DELFIA PSA dual-label free/total PSA kit (Wallac Oy) in one laboratory. TRUS using 3D ultrasound equipment with a 10-MHz endorectal transducer was performed in three planes. The volume of the entire prostate as well as the volume of the TZ were calculated for a prolate ellipsoid.

PSA TZ density was defined as follows:

PSA TZ density = total PSA (ng/ml)/TZ volume (cm^3).

The results for total PSA, percent free PSA and PSA TZ density were subjected to statistical analysis. The Mann-Whitney U-test was used to investigate whether there are significant differences between the groups. We evaluated the reciprocal relationship between sensitivity and specificity by plotting true positive (sensitivity) against false positive (1 – specificity) results in ROC curves. To check the validity of our findings the individual diagnostic tests were compared by means of the Youden Index.

Of the 308 screening volunteers undergoing transrectal biopsy, 228 had biopsy-proven BPH (74%), 22 had prostatitis with no evidence of hyperplastic tissue (7%) and 58 had biopsy-proven prostate cancer (19%).

The mean total PSA levels were 6.6 ng/ml (range 2.5–10.0) in the BPH group, 8.0 ng/ml (range 2.5–9.7) in the group with chronic inflammatory disease, and 6.0 ng/ml (range 3.01–10.0) in the cancer group. Mean percent free PSA levels in the BPH, prostatitis, and prostate cancer groups were 22.0% (range 4.7–43.2), 9.1% (range 4.6–20.2) and 11.3% (range 4.1–19.1), respectively. The differences between the BPH and prostate cancer groups and between the BPH and prostatitis groups were statistically significant, whereas the difference between the prostate cancer and prostatitis groups did not reach statistical significance.

Table 14. Youden Index for percent free PSA, PSA TZ density, and the combination of percent free PSA and PSA TZ density

	Youden Index	Free PSA	p value
Percent free PSA <20 ng/ml	0.560		
PSA TZ density >0.22	0.300	6.085	0.000
Percent free PSA <20 ng/ml and PSA TZ density >0.22	0.668	–2.496	0.013

The mean values for PSA TZ density were 0.35 ng/ml/cm^3 (range 0.06–1.93) in the BPH group, 0.50 ng/ml/cm^3 (range 0.33–2.90) in the prostatitis group, and 0.56 ng/ml/cm^3 (range 0.23–1.20) in the cancer group. The differences between the BPH and prostate cancer groups, between the BPH and prostatitis groups, and between the prostate cancer and prostatitis groups were statistically significant. The values for total PSA, free PSA and PSA TZ density are shown in table 13.

ROC curve analyses (fig. 3) show that by using percent free PSA <20% as a biopsy criterion in men with elevated PSA, 45.5% of negative biopsies could be eliminated while still detecting 100% of prostate cancers.

ROC curve analyses (fig. 4) for PSA TZ density show that by using a PSA TZ density of >0.22 ng/ml/cm^3 as a biopsy criterion, 24.4% of negative biopsies could be avoided without missing a single cancer. When combining these two diagnostic tests with the biopsy criteria mentioned above, 54.2% of negative biopsies could be eliminated.

In this study, percent free PSA proved to be a better predictor of prostate cancer than PSA TZ density, since it had the largest area under its ROC curve. In order to check the validity of our findings, the individual diagnostic tests were compared by means of the Youden Index (table 14). This statistical test confirmed that percent free PSA is a better predictor of prostate cancer than PSA-TZ density alone. However, the combination of percent free PSA and PSA TZ density is superior to free PSA alone.

In conclusion, our study demonstrated that, in addition to total and free PSA, PSA TZ density is an important diagnostic tool for calculating the probability of a patient developing prostate cancer. However, further prospective studies will be required to confirm the reproducibility and usefulness of PSA TZ density in PSA-based screening.

PSA-Based Screening and Incidental Prostate Cancer

PSA-based screening dramatically improves early detection of nonpalpable prostate cancer. In the discussion about the usefulness of screening programs, concerns have been raised about whether these programs would also lead to the detection of very small and well-differentiated prostate cancers requiring no therapy. The majority of well-differentiated A1 tumors are known to be clinically insignificant and therefore do not require further therapy, whereas patients presenting with dedifferentiated A1 grade III and A2 prostate cancers definitively need treatment.

In order to find out whether PSA-based screening has an impact on the incidence of incidental prostate cancer, 1,543 patients undergoing transurethral resection of the prostate (TURP) for suspected BPH at our department over the past 6 years were evaluated in a retrospective study. All patients older than 75 years were excluded as they did not participate in the screening program, and two different groups were distinguished. Group 1 comprising 868 patients aged 58–75 years who were operated on between 1990 and 1992 represented the pre-PSA era. Group 2 consisting of 675 consecutive patients aged 56–75 years who underwent TURP in the years 1993–95 represented the PSA screening era. The men in group 2 either had PSA levels in the normal range (according to age-specific reference ranges) or underwent TURP after TRUS-guided biopsy of the prostate.

The mean age of the patients in group 1 was 71.5 years as compared to 69.7 years in group 2. In the latter the mean PSA level for patients with stage A prostate cancer was 4.7 ng/ml. There was a significant difference in PSA levels between A1 and A2 cancer patients. Patients with A1 cancer had a mean PSA of 4.7 ng/ml, whereas patients with A1 grade III or A2 cancer had a mean PSA of 7.7 ng/ml.

The incidence of stage A tumors in the years before the introduction of PSA-based screening (group 1) was 5.2, 3.9 and 8.3%, respectively (mean 5.6; fig. 5). The incidence of A1 cancers in this group was 1.9, 2.3 and 5.5%, respectively (mean 3.1; fig. 6). The incidence of A1 grade III and A2 cancer was 3.2, 1.6 and 1.98% with an average of 2.3% (fig. 7).

In the years after establishing PSA-based screening (group 2) the incidence of stage A tumors was 7.2, 6.1 and 3.5%, respectively (fig. 5). Again the mean was 5.6%, however, the incidence of A1 and A2 tumors was completely different. We found an incidence of A1 prostate cancer of 7.2, 6.1 and 4.6%, respectively (fig. 6). The inci-

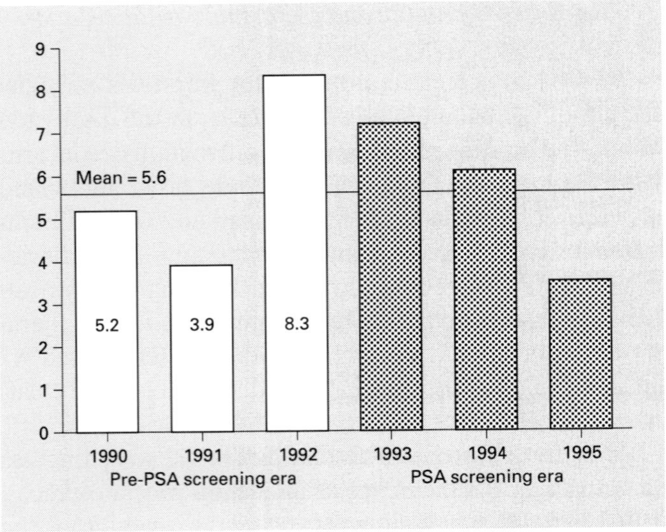

Fig. 5. Incidence of T1a,b prostate carcinoma.

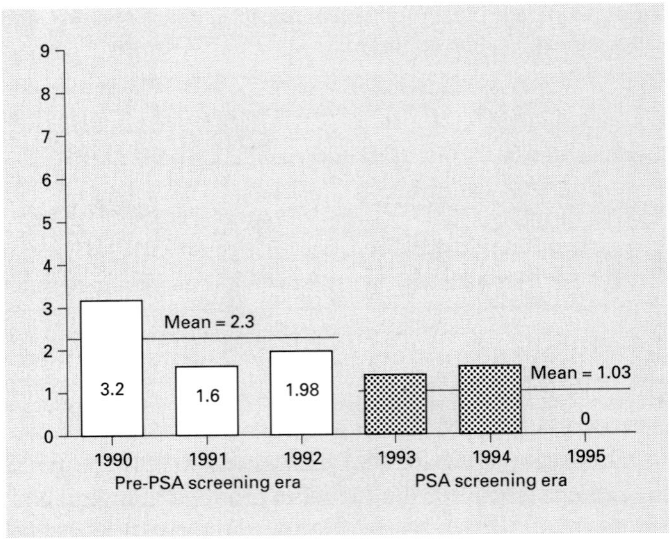

Fig. 7. Incidence of T1a grade III and T1b prostate carcinoma.

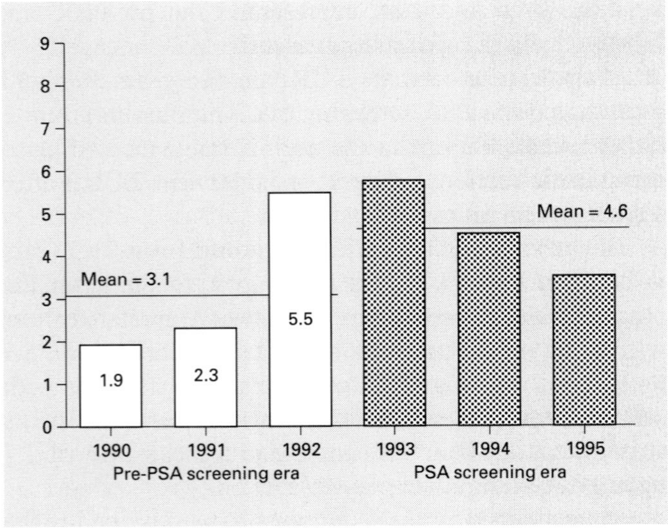

Fig. 6. Incidence of T1a grade I–II prostate carcinoma.

dence of A1 grade III and A2 cancer was 1.4, 1.6 and 0%, respectively (mean 1.03; fig. 7).

These data demonstrate that PSA-based screening for prostate cancer leads to a decrease in the incidence of dedifferentiated A1 grade III and A2 tumors, while there is no impact on the incidence of clinically insignificant A1 grades I and II prostate cancers.

Stage Migration in 5-Year PSA-Based Screening Program

Radical prostatectomy as a treatment for prostate cancer is potentially curative provided the tumor is still confined to the prostate at diagnosis [15, 16]. The following study was designed to evaluate changes in PSA levels and pathohistologic stages in radical prostatectomy specimens over a period of 5 years in a PSA-based mass screening program.

Between September 1993 and October 1997, the mean ages, mean total PSA levels, and rates of organ and nonorgan-confined tumors were evaluated in 595 patients undergoing biopsy and radical retropubic prostatectomy. Furthermore, the mean Gleason scores at biopsy were compared to those of the specimens obtained at radical prostatectomy. For statistical analysis the Mann-Whitney U-test was used to investigate whether there are significant differences for total PSA and pathologic stage between the different years.

The results of this evaluation show a statistically significant decrease in total PSA levels from a mean value of 14.9 ng/ml in 1993 to 8.6 ng/ml in 1997. In addition, the rate of organ-confined prostate cancers increased from 28.7% in 1993 to 65.7% in 1997, whereas a reciprocal decrease from 71.2% (1993) to 34.2% (1997) was observed for the rate of nonorgan-confined tumors (table 15).

Table 15. Change in total PSA, Gleason score and rate of organ-confined tumors in a 5-year PSA screening program

Year	Age	Mean PSA ng/ml	Histologic examination of biopsy specimen mean Gleason score	Radical prostatectomy specimen		
				organ-confined (%)	mean Gleason score	n
1993	63.7 (51.6–76.1)	14.9 (2.5–100)	4.9 (3–10)	23 (28.7)	5.0 (2–10)	80
1994	62.9 (49.4–74.3)	14.2 (0.4–55.0)	4.8 (3–10)	42 (27.6)	5.1 (2–9)	152
1995	62.5 (45.2–74.1)	12.7 (4.0–60.0)	4.6 (2–8)	37 (25.1)	5.2 (2–9)	147
1996	64.2 (46.5–74.7)	9.7 (1.3–30.0)	5.3 (2–8)	57 (55.8)	5.8 (2–9)	102
1997	64.9 (47.0–77.0)	8.6 (1.2–35.9)	5.5 (2–8)	75 (65.7)	5.8 (2–9)	114
						Σ = 594

Table 16. The probability (%) of having prostate cancer according to age, PSA and DRE findings

PSA range ng/ml	Age range							
	40–50 years		51–60 years		61–70 years		71–80 years	
	DRE–	DRE+	DRE–	DRE+	DRE–	DRE+	DRE–	DRE+
0.0–2.5	9	37	12	39	15	42	20	44
2.6–4.0	9	41	12	42	16	44	20	47
4.1–6.0	10	41	14	44	17	47	22	48
6.1–10.0	11	33	15	48	19	50	25	52
10.1–20.0	13	55	19	54	25	58	31	60
>20.0	22	82	45	74	43	81	59	84

These data indicate that between 1993, when PSA-based screening was introducted at our department, and 1997, a significant decrease in preoperative total PSA levels, a significant migration to lower stages and an increase in the number of organ-confined, potentially curable prostate cancers were observed. Long-term follow-up will show whether these trends will also have a positive impact on prostate cancer mortality rates.

The Probability of Having Prostate Cancer Given the Patient's Age, Serum PSA Value, and DRE Findings: Results from the Tyrol Screening Project

Traditionally, the decision to perform a prostate biopsy has been based upon whether the total serum PSA level is normal and abnormal (specific cutpoint) and the DRE findings [5, 6]. In the setting of a benign DRE, a 60-year-old man with a PSA level of 4.1 ng/ml would be encouraged to undergo a biopsy, whereas the same man with a PSA concentration of 3.9 ng/ml might be discouraged from having the procedure. Yet, in reality, there is little to no difference between the two PSA values. What might be more appropriate is informing the patient of the actual probability or risk of having prostate cancer and letting him, together with his physician, decide about proceeding ahead with a TRUS-guided prostate biopsy.

Using multivariate logistic regression analysis and data from the 2,054 men (mean age 64), most of whom were part of the Tyrol Screening Project in Innsbruck, Austria (screening volunteers 45–75 years of age) between September 1993 and October 1997, patient age, serum PSA level and DRE findings were identified as the three critical variables for determining the probability of having prostate cancer.

For men 40–80 years of age, the percentage of probability of having prostate cancer (with 95% confidence intervals) as a function of serum PSA and DRE findings are shown in table 16. By using this approach, the decision to proceed with a prostate biopsy is based upon the

Table 17. Correlation of total PSA with percent free PSA, age, tumor volume, Gleason score, pathological stage and surgical margin status

PSA	Free PSA, %	Age	Tumor volume, g	Gleason score	Pathologic stage	Surgical margin status
Group 1 (n = 5) (0.0–1.25)	14.7 (7.9–20.7)	61 (49–73)	0.80 (0.37–0.98)	5.6 (4–7)	Organ-confined	Negative
Group 2 (n = 27) (1.26–1.99)	14.1 (4.9–19.1)	57 (50–75)	0.43 (0.22–1.13)	5.9 (3–8)	Organ-confined	Negative
Group 3 (n = 30) (2.0–2.99)	15.1 (6.2–24.9)	61 (47–75)	0.92 (0.44–3.11)	5.6 (4–8)	Organ-confined	Negative
Group 4 (n = 33) (3.0–3.99)	12.9 (5.6–21.3)	61 (48–75)	0.79 (0.36–1.85)	5.4 (4–7)	Organ-confined	Negative

risk of having prostate cancer rather than a single cut-point. For one patient, a 22% risk warrants a biopsy; for another man it simply means a 78% chance of not having cancer, and watchful waiting is acceptable. Now, for the first time, the patient and the physician can make an informed decision as to whether a prostate biopsy is appropriate for that specific individual.

Correlation between Preoperative Predictors Obtained at PSA-Based Screening and Pathologic Features in Radical Prostatectomy Specimens

Measurement of percent free PSA, PSA density and PSA TZ density in addition to total PSA is known to improve the specificity of PSA-based prostate cancer screening. However, the value of total PSA in the preoperative staging of prostate cancer is controversial. Although studies by Stamey et al. [17] suggest it to be useful as a preoperative staging marker, other studies have not found it sufficiently reliable for predicting final pathologic stage on an individual basis [18]. In the following retrospective study the ability of total PSA, percent free PSA, PSA density and PSA TZ density to predict pathologic features in radical prostatectomy specimens was evaluated.

The levels of total PSA, percent free PSA, PSA density and PSA TZ density determined prior to the diagnosis of prostate cancer were correlated with the pathologic features of 102 prostate cancer specimens obtained at radical prostatectomy. The entire organs were examined histologically. The results obtained were subjected to statistical analysis. We evaluated the correlation between preoperative predictors and pathologic features in computing Pearson correlation coefficients. Independent predictors have been identified by means of stepwise logistic regression. The logistic model included only those predictors significantly identified within the univariant analysis. All p values of <0.05 were considered as significant, all stated p values are two-sided.

High total PSA, PSA density and PSA TZ density levels correlated significantly with high Gleason scores, capsular penetration, a high percentage of cancer in the prostatectomy specimen and a high cancer volume. Free PSA was found to correlate well with a higher Gleason score, a greater percentage of cancer and cancer volume but not with capsular penetration.

The four predictors were evaluated by means of logistic regression, which showed that only percent free PSA and total PSA were significant predictors of Gleason score ≥ 7 and cancer volumes ≥ 0.5 cm^3. With clinically insignificant cancers, percent free PSA and the Gleason score obtained at biopsy were the only significant predictors.

In men whose prostate cancers are detected at PSA-based screening, high total PSA levels in combination with low percent free PSA serum levels are suggestive of a potentially more aggressive type of cancer. This information may help both patients and clinicians in selecting the most appropriate therapeutic approach.

Correlation of Total PSA with Pathologic Stage and Tumor Volume in Patients Undergoing Radical Prostatectomy following PSA Screening with Low PSA Cut-Off Levels

Recent studies [19, 20] have shown that low cut-off values for total PSA in PSA-based screening may enhance the number of organ-confined prostate cancers detected at radical prostatectomy. In the following study the data of a subgroup of males from our screening program with PSA levels <3.99 ng/ml who underwent radical prostatectomy were evaluated.

Serial whole-mount sections from 95 patients with PSA levels 3.99 ng/ml who underwent radical prostatectomy were analyzed with regard to pathohistological stage, surgical margin status, Gleason grade and tumor volume. For statistical analysis the Mann-Whitney U-test was used.

Five men (group 1) had PSA levels <1.25 ng/ml, 27 (group 2) between 1.26 and 1.99 ng/ml, 30 (group 3) between 2.0 and 2.99 ng/ml and 33 (group 4) between 3.0 and 3.99 ng/ml. The mean tumor volume (g) in groups 1, 2, 3 and 4 was 0.80, 0.43, 0.92 and 0.79 g respectively. The results for percent free PSA, age, tumor volume, Gleason score as well as pathologic stage and surgical margin status are shown in table 17. With the exception of the tumor volume in group 2, none of the parameters in the different groups showed a statistically significant difference.

The results of this evaluation indicate that the radical prostatectomy specimens in patients with low total PSA values who were diagnosed with prostate cancer exhibit low tumor volumes and low Gleason grades; however, all of these cancers were clinically significant. Furthermore, all patients had organ-confined prostate cancers with negative surgical margins.

PSA-Based Screening with Very Low PSA Cut-Off Values: Correlation between Age and Clinical and Pathologic Features in the 40- to 59-Year Age Group

Recent data indicate that older men are more likely to have extensive disease compared to younger men with the same PSA levels [21]. To determine whether age has an impact on the extension of prostate cancer, the data of a subgroup of males aged between 40 and 59 years from our PSA screening program who presented with PSA levels <2.5 ng/ml were evaluated.

Sixty-four males undergoing radical retropubic prostatectomy for prostate cancer detected by PSA-based screening were evaluated in terms of pathohistologic stage, surgical margin status, Gleason grade, and tumor volume (g). The results obtained were subjected to statistical analysis to investigate whether there are statistically significant differences between the two groups. Of the 64 patients evaluated, 19 were between 40 and 49 (group 1) and 45 between 50 and 59 years of age (group 2). The mean values in group 1 for total PSA was 1.7 ng/ml, for percent free PSA 12.6, for Gleason score 5.5 and for the tumor volume 0.26 g. In group 2 the mean values for total PSA, percent free PSA, Gleason score and tumor volume was 1.9 ng/ml, 14.2, 5.3 and 0.78 g respectively. In both groups all patients had organ-confined prostate cancer and all had a negative surgical margin status (table 18).

Table 18. Mean values for total PSA, percent free PSA, Gleason score, tumor volume, pathohistological stage and surgical margin status in males aged 40–49 and 50–59 years

	Group 1 aged 40–49 (n = 19)	Group 2 aged 50–59 (n = 45)
Mean total PSA, ng/ml	1.7	1.9
Range, ng/ml	0.9–2.4	1.1–2.4
Mean free PSA, %	12.6	14.2
Range, %	6.2–19.1	4.3–21.9
Mean Gleason score	5.5	5.3
Range	4–7	4–7
Mean tumor volume, g	0.26	0.78
Range, g	0.13–0.49	0.17–0.59
Pathohistologic stage	Organ-confined	Organ-confined
Surgical margin status	Negative	Negative

The difference in tumor volumes between the two groups was statistically significant ($p \leq 0.001$). All other parameters (total PSA, percent free PSA and Gleason score) were statistically not significant. Two patients in each group had clinically insignificant prostate cancers according to the definition by Epstein et al. [14]. These data suggest that older men more likely have larger tumor volumes compared to younger men with the same PSA levels. Furthermore, the data suggest that in PSA-based screening low cut-off values may increase the detection rate of organ-confined tumors with negative surgical margins that are potentially curable.

References

1 Brawer MK, Chetner MP, Beattie J, et al: Screening for prostatic carcinoma with prostate-specific antigen. J Urol 1992;147:841–845.

2 Catalona WJ, Smith DS, Ratliff TL, et al: Measurement of prostate-specific antigen in serum as a screening test for prostate cancer. N Engl J Med 1991;324:1156–1161.

3 Labrie F, Dupont A, Suburu R, et al: Serum prostate-specific antigen as pre-screening test for prostate cancer. J Urol 1992;147:846–852.

4 Imai K, Ichinose Y, Kubota Y, et al: Diagnostic significance of prostate-specific antigen and the development of a mass screening system for prostate cancer. J Urol 1995;154:1085–1089.

5 Oesterling JE, Jacobsen SJ, Chute CG, et al: Serum prostate-specific antigen in a community-based population of healthy men: Establishment of age-specific reference ranges. JAMA 1993;270:860

6 Oesterling JE, Jacobsen SJ, Cooner WH: The use of age-specific reference ranges for serum prostate-specific antigen in men 60 years old or older. J Urol 1995;153:1160–1163.

7 McNeal JE, Redwine EA, Freiha FS, et al: Zonal distribution of prostatic adenocarcinoma: Correlation with histologic pattern and direction of spread. Am J Surg Pathol 1988;12:897–906.

8 Reissigl A, Pointner J, Horninger W, et al: Comparison of different prostate-specific antigen cutpoints for early detection of prostate cancer: Results of a large screening study. Urology 1995;46:662–665.

9 Hudson MA, Bahnson RR, Catalona WJ: Clinical use of prostate-specific antigen in patients with prostate cancer. J Urol 1989;142:1011–1017.

10 Lange P, Ercole C, Lightner D, Fraley E, Vessella R: The value of serum prostate-specific antigen determinations before and after radical prostatectomy. J Urol 1989;141:873–879.

11 Reissigl A, Klocker H, Pointner J, et al: Improvement of prostate cancer screening by determination of the ratio free/total PSA in addition to PSA levels. Prostate 1997;30:243.

12 Reissigl A, Klocker H, Pointner J, Fink K, Horninger W, Ennemoser O, et al: Usefulness of the ratio free/total prostate-specific antigen in addition to total PSA levels in prostate cancer screening. Urology 1996;48:62–66.

13 Jewett H: The present status of radical prostatectomy for stages A and B prostatic cancer. Urol Clin North Am 1975;2:105–124.

14 Epstein J, Pauli G, Eggleston J, Walsh P: Prognoses of untreated stage A1 prostatic carcinoma: A study of 94 cases with extended follow-up. J Urol 1986;136:837–839.

15 Gilliland FD, Hunt WC, Key CR: Improving survival for patients with prostate cancer diagnosed in the prostate-specific antigen era. Urology 1996;48:67–71.

16 Perrotti M, Rabbani F, Rosso P, Solomon MC, Fair WR: Early prostate cancer detection and potential for surgical cure in men with poorly differentiated tumors. Urology 1998;52:106–110.

17 Stamey TA, et al: Prostate-specific antigen in the diagnosis and treatment of adenocarcinoma of the prostate. Radical prostatectomy-treated patients. J Urol 1989;141:1067.

18 Rainwater LM, Morgan WR, Klee GG, Zincke H: Prostate-specific antigen testing in untreated and treated prostatic adenocarcinomas. Mayo Clin Proc 1990;65:1118.

19 Hoedemaeker RF, Rietbergen JB, Kranse R, van der Kwast TH, Schröder FH: Comparison of pathologic characteristics of T1c and non-T1c cancers detected in a population-based screening study, the European Randomized Study of Screening for Prostate Cancer. World J Urol 1997;15:339–345.

20 Littrup PJ: Future benefits and cost effectiveness of prostate carcinoma screening. American Cancer Society. Cancer 1997;80:1864–1870.

21 Carter BH, Epstein JI, Walsh PC, Partin AW: Age, PSA and the chance of curable prostate cancer among men with non-palpable disease. J Urol 1998;159:279.

European Urology

Eur Urol 1999;35:539–543

The European Randomized Study of Screening for Prostate Cancer (ERSPC): An Update

Fritz H. Schröder[a] Ries Kranse[a] John Rietbergen[a] Robert Hoedemaeker[b] Wim Kirkels[a] and members of the ERSPC, Section Rotterdam

Departments of [a]Urology and [b]Pathology, Erasmus University and Academic Hospital, Rotterdam, The Netherlands

Key Words

Prostate cancer · Screening · Randomized study · Screening tests · Preliminary results

Abstract

Screening for prostate cancer is controversial. While in some parts of the world screening is practised as a healthcare policy, it is strongly rejected in other areas, because solid evidence of effectiveness of screening combined with early treatment with respect to lowering the mortality of prostate cancer has not been shown. It is for this reason that a large European study is installed to establish or rule out the value of screening for this frequent disease. The present paper presents the goal of the study and elaborates on the value of presently available screening tests. Preliminary results with respect to the first round of screening in the Rotterdam area relating to 32,000 randomized men are presented. Evidence of effectiveness of screening through other studies and mechanisms is discussed.

The European Randomized Study of Screening for Prostate Cancer (ERSPC) was initiated in 1994 after pilot studies had been conducted in Antwerp and Rotterdam. The study is coordinated by the first author, with Prof. Louis Denis of Antwerp as co-coordinator. There are at present 7 study centers in the following countries: Belgium, Finland, Italy, The Netherlands, Portugal, Spain, and Sweden [1, 2].

The Goal of the Study

The goal of the study is to demonstrate or to rule out an effect of early detection and treatment on prostate cancer mortality. The study should result in information that is suitable to guide the governments of participating countries and of other countries to come to a rational decision with respect to the possible introduction of prostate cancer screening as a health care policy. Obviously, a negative study would be a strong argument against the introduction of prostate cancer screening, at least with the methodology applied in this protocol. Other endpoints are the evaluation of quality of life and the calculation of quality-adjusted life years (QUALYs). Additionally, this study group aims at producing information with regard to the optimization of screening procedures. Data in this respect were supposed to be used to streamline the screening procedure within the protocol, but also to serve for advice in opportunistic screening that may be requested by males who are at risk, and that cannot be refused by urologists and other medical professionals.

KARGER

Fax + 41 61 306 12 34
E-Mail karger@karger.ch
www.karger.com

0302–2838/99/0356–0539$17.50/0

Accessible online at:
http://BioMedNet.com/karger

Fritz H. Schröder, MD, Professor and Chairman
Department of Urology, Erasmus University and Academic Hospital
PO Box 1738, NL–3000 DR Rotterdam (The Netherlands)
Tel. +31 10 463 3607, Fax +31 10 463 5838
E-Mail vanalphen@urol.azr.nl

Sample Size and Power

The international study group is conducting a randomized study with randomization between screening and early intervention compared to a control population to which present health care policies in the individual countries are applied. The study group wishes to show or to exclude an advantage in prostate cancer mortality of 20% with a power of 90%. The original sample size was calculated to be 132,000 men, half of these randomized to each arm. Unfortunately, opportunistic screening within the study population cannot be avoided. Careful evaluation and monitoring is necessary since the opportunistic use of the screening procedures within the study population enters the formula used to calculate sample size as a square. Assuming a contamination rate of 10%, the sample size was recalculated to be 190,000.

Table 1 shows a recent summary of the contribution of the individual countries. It is evident that the group has a capacity of randomizing up to 230,000 men in the age group 50–75. This sample can be increased by addition of about 70,000 men randomized within the Prostate, Lung, Colon and Ovary Study of the National Cancer Institute of the United States. Altogether, a significant result can be expected from this very large enterprise. At this time, in July 1998, about 160,000 men have been included in Europe. The International Prostate Screening Trial Evaluation Group (IPSTEG), which included European and American centers, has agreed upon a prospective common plan for data collection and evaluation [3].

Screening produces lead-time and length time. Lead-time is the time that is added to the time until a clinical diagnosis would be made. Early estimates of lead-time vary between 3 and 10 years [4, 5]. On the basis of such information, the group has determined the re-screening interval to be 4 years. Adjustment may be necessary if necessitated by the interim evaluation of interval cancers and the distribution of prognostic factors in those men who have entered the pilot studies in the time between 1992 and 1994, and who are presently being re-screened. A recent review of the international effort combined within IPSTEG is given by de Koning et al. [6].

The Screening Tests

The study group in Rotterdam, The Netherlands, has taken on the task of evaluating the value of the individual screening tests, rectal examination (DRE), transrectal ultrasonography (TRUS), and prostate-specific antigen (PSA). Initially, within the population randomized to screening, all three screening tests were used. This resulted in a biopsy indication in 1 man of 4, and a positive again in 1 of 5 biopsies that were actually carried out.

Table 1. ERSPC, January 1998 – participation and recruitment

Center	Randomized	Capacity
Belgium	7,914	20,000
Finland	39,446	75,000[1]
Italy	3,338	40,000
Netherlands	28,075	40,000
Portugal	2,123	32,000
Spain	No participant in 1998	
Sweden	32,298	32,000[1]
Total	113,194	239,000

1 Randomization control/screening = 2/1.

Improving Specificity

This comes down to a false-positive rate of biopsy indications of ±80%, and a detection rate between 4 and 5%. Several options, including the use of age-specific reference ranges, the ratio of free to total PSA, the use of PSA density or the exclusion of men who had very low PSA values at the time of screening, all led to an improvement of the specificity of the procedure by 30–40% with a variable loss of cancers which would otherwise be diagnosed (loss of sensitivity). The possibilities of altering the screening procedure were subject to multiple published evaluations by the Rotterdam study group [7–10], and the study groups in other countries. Data on 4,800 screened men who underwent DRE, PSA and TRUS are summarized in table 2 [9]. Table 2 indicates the effect of changing the screening procedure in 4,800 men. It has to be taken into account that biopsies were only taken with PSA values >4. The table indicates the proportion of biopsies saved (improvement in specificity), and the proportion of cancers lost (loss of sensitivity) with the different treatment regimens. Where necessary, estimates based on logistic regression analysis are used. The first column and the lower three lines of this diagram indicate the effect of applying PSA as a prescreening test. In these algorithms, DRE and/or TRUS would still remain in action above the cut-off of the prescreening values of PSA 1.0, 2.0 or 3.0

Table 2. Simulation of case selection based on 4,800 men randomized to screening, 976 biopsies were done and 190 prostate cancers (PCs) were found

Prescreen (PSA, ng/ml)	Biopsy[1] indication	Number bx/PC	Reduction biopsies % (SE)	Loss PC % (SE)	bx/PC
	PSA, DRE, TRUS	976/190	–	–	5.1
	PSA age, DRE	583/149	40.3 (1.6)	21.6 (3.0)	3.9
–	PSA density (≥0.12), DRE	581/163	40.5 (1.6)	14.2 (2.5)	3.6
–	F/T ratio (<0.2), DRE	649/170	33.5 (1.5)	10.5 (2.2)	3.8
>1.0	PSA ≥4, DRE, TRUS	811/168	16.9 (1.2)	2.1 (1.0)	4.8
>3.0	PSA ≥4, DRE, TRUS	559/160	42.7 (1.6)	15.8 (2.6)	3.5

[1] Biopsies were indicated if PSA was ≥4.0 ng/ml or if DRE and/or TRUS were suspicious. It is assumed that *only* men with PSA values above the prescreen level undergo DRE and TRUS.

ng/ml. The diagram does not include the option of biopsying everybody above this prescreening range. Prescreening, however, means that no DRE and/or TRUS is carried out below the prescreening PSA values indicated. Obviously, any change of the screening procedure would bear the risk of eliminating cancer cases that would contribute in a major way to the outcome of the study. It was therefore essential, prior to applying changes, to not only know the effect of possible changes on sensitivity and specificity of the screening procedure, but also to know what kind of tumors would be excluded. Such an evaluation was carried out by comparing the results of the screening tests, and their modification to the results of the careful study of prognostic factors in more than 100 radical prostatectomy specimens coming from the study section of Rotterdam.

The Rotterdam group was encouraged by the experience of the Swedish section of ERSPC, which used PSA-based screening from the very beginning on. In this procedure, every man with a PSA >3.0 ng/ml would be biopsied. No other screening tests were applied. It was shown that the detection rate of cancers between PSA 3.0 and 3.9 was 12%. Furthermore, there was certainly no accumulation of nonaggressive cases. At this time the Rotterdam group was aware of Labrie's suggestion to use a PSA cut-off of 3 implemented by DRE and ultrasound where necessary. Labrie recommended a cut-off of 3.0 because sensitivity and specificity of the screening procedure were both highest at this point. In the meantime, it remains unknown what kind of cancers would be missed with PSA levels <3 and what the effect of applying such a procedure to a population-based study such as ERSPC would be [11, 12].

Table 3. Results of screening by DRE, PSA and TRUS (old regimen, n = 4,413 screened men aged 55–74) compared to PSA-based screening (PSA ≥3.0 is a biopsy indication, no screening <3.0, new regimen)

Parameters	Old regimen, %	New regimen, %
DRE + TRUS	100	20
Detection (cancers/screened)	4.8	4.7
Biopsied	23.7	19.8
False-positive biopsy indication	19.8	15.1
Clinically confined	78	76
Pathologically confined	60	56
Negative margins	72	68
Grade 3	12	15

Several methods of calculation, including logistic regression analysis, resulted in similar results: the use of a PSA value of 3.0 as a prescreening cut-off point would preserve sensitivity almost at an identical level, while specificity would be improved by almost 20% (table 3). This table shows a comparison of the previous regimen of using PSA, DRE and TRUS in all men as compared to the new regimen recommended subsequently to ERSPC in which men with a PSA <3.0 would receive an 'all-clear' message until re-screening, while those who have a PSA of 3.0 ng/ml or higher would all be biopsied. The data are based on three different evaluation techniques, extrapolation of predictive values for prostate cancer in the PSA range ≥4 ng/ml, where all men were biopsied, determined through extrapolation of predictive values for prostate cancer with or without positive DRE and/or TRUS, or determined through a logistic regression-based predictive index model. All three calculations yielded very similar results which are summarized in table 3. The reason why the detection rate remains almost unchanged obviously lies in the fact that all men between 3 and 4 undergo a biopsy. This is at variance with the data presented in table 2. The proportion of biopsied men is decreased by about 4%, the proportion of false biopsy indications by about 5%. The proportion of pathologically confined cases and those who have negative margins, drops slightly. However, the proportion of grade III disease (which may be curable if locally confined) increases. This is due to the fact that very few grade III cases are present in the population of men who have a PSA of 0–2.9 ng/ml which is omitted from the new regimen. Further pathological anatomical studies of 105 radical prostatectomy specimens from the Rotterdam screening study showed that those tumors that might be missed were usually well differentiated and had a volume of <0.5 cm^3. This analysis further confirmed that the proportion of cases that might be considered insignificant on the basis of presently available criteria, is strongly dependent and inversally correlates with PSA levels. Of 30 cancers in the PSA range 0–2.9, 15 were considered minimal. In the PSA range 3–10, minimal characteristics were seen in 13%. This was the same figure for PSA 3–3.9 ng/ml. Knowledge of characteristics of tumors missed give a more rational basis to changes of the screening procedure. It was recommended to the European study group to switch to the new regimen. This change was adopted by most of the European centers during the year of 1998.

Preliminary Results

As is evident from table 3, the study group has randomized far more than half of the necessary sample. In Antwerp, Belgium, Rotterdam, The Netherlands, and Göteborg, Sweden, the second round of screening has already started. A review of the present status of the study has recently been written and is at present submitted for publication [6].

In the Rotterdam area about 32,000 men have been randomized by now, 16,000 have been screened, and about 800 prostate cancers have been diagnosed. Obviously, an interim analysis with respect to the main endpoint, prostate cancer mortality, is not available, not even to the study group. However, a review of intermediate endpoints has recently been carried out. A significant reduction of stage and grade is seen with respect to the cancers found in the control group. While control populations in The Netherlands show up to 24% of men with metastatic disease, within the screening group this percentage has dropped to below 1%. These are encouraging signs but do not allow anticipation on the final result of the study. If a reduction of stage and grade were not visible at this time, probably the randomized screening study would no longer be justified and would be discontinued.

Other Evidence

Recently, data from the randomized study of screening for prostate cancer conducted in Quebec City since 1989 have been presented by Labrie et al. [13]. According to the authors the data presented suggest a strong effect of screening and early aggressive treatment on prostate cancer mortality with a 3.7 times higher risk of dying of prostate cancer in a not screened group of men. However, the study and its evaluation show very strong methodological flaws and has been severely criticized. The study is not considered as presenting a final answer at this time. In the USA in several areas where screening is prevalent, prostate cancer mortality has been decreasing. Also, recently a decrease of prostate cancer mortality overall in the USA of 6.3% has been described [14]. This decrease is more pronounced in the relevant age group of men who are 55–75 years old. The possibility that this is an effect of screening cannot be excluded. However, positive proof requires more than the available information. At present, unless data become more convincing over time, it seems that a randomized study remains necessary and is most likely to produce the definite answer on the issue of screening and early treatment of prostate cancer.

References

1 Schröder FH, Damhuis RAM, Kirkels WJ, de Koning HJ, Kranse R, Nijs GHT, Blijenberg BG: European randomized study of screening for prostate cancer – the Rotterdam pilot studies. Int J Cancer 1996;65:145–151.

2 Schröder FH, Bangma CH: The European Randomized Study of Screening for Prostate Cancer (ERSPC). Br J Urol 1997;79(suppl 2):68–71.

3 Auvinen A, Rietbergen JBW, Denis LJ, Schröder FH, Prorok PhC, for the International Prostate Cancer Screening Trial Evaluation Group: Prospective evaluation plan for randomised trials of prostate cancer screening. J Med Screen 1996;3:97–104.

4 Parkes CJ, Wald NJ, Murphy P, George L, Watt HC, Kirby R, Knekt P, Helzlsouer KJ, Tuomilehto J: Prospective observational study to assess value of prostate-specific antigen as screening test for prostate cancer. BMJ 1995; 311:1340–1343.

5 Stenman UH, Hakama M, Knekt P, Aromaa A, Teppo L, Leinonen J: Serum concentrations of prostate-specific antigen and its complex with α_1-antichymotrypsin before diagnosis of prostate cancer. Lancet 1994;334:1594–1598.

6 de Koning HJ, Auvinen A, Berenguer Sanchez A, Calais da Silva F, Ciatto S, Denis L, Gohagan J, Hakama M, Kranse R, Nelen V, Prorok PC, Schröder FH: Large-scale randomized prostate cancer screening trials: Program performances in the ERSPC and PLCO trials (European Randomized Screening for Prostate Cancer and Prostate, Lung, Colorectal and Ovary Cancer trials). 1999, in press.

7 Bangma ChrH, Kranse R, Blijenberg B, Schröder FH: The value of screening tests in the detection of prostate cancer. I. Results of a retrospective evaluation of 1,726 men. Urology 1995;46:773–778.

8 Bangma CH, Kranse R, Blijenberg BG, Schröder FH: The free-to-total serum prostate-specific antigen ratio for staging prostate carcinoma. J Urol 1997;157:544–547.

9 Rietbergen JBW, Hoedemaeker RF, Boeken Kruger AE, Kirkels WJ, Schröder FH: The changing pattern of prostate cancer at the time of diagnosis: Characteristics of prostate cancers detected in a population-based screening study (ERSPC data, Rotterdam region). J Urol 1999, in press.

10 Bangma CH, Rietbergen JBW, Schröder FH: Prostate-specific antigen as a screening test. Urol Clin North Am 1997;24:307–314.

11 Lodding P, Aus G, Bergdahl S, Frösing R, Lilja H, Pihl CG, Hugosson J: Characteristics of screening-detected prostate cancer in men 50 to 66 years old with 3 to 4 ng/ml prostate-specific antigen. J Urol 1998;159:899–903.

12 Labrie F, Dupont A, Suburu R, Cusan L, Tremblay M, Gomez JL, Emond J: Serum prostate-specific antigen as pre-screening test for prostate cancer. J Urol 1992;147:846–852.

13 Labrie F, Dupont A, Candas B, Cusan L, Gomez JL, Diamond P, Bélanger A, Brousseau J, Levesque J: Decrease of prostate cancer death by screening: First data from the Quebec Prospective Randomized Study. Proc ASCO, vol 17, 1998, abstr 4, p 2A.

14 National Cancer Institute: Cancer death rate declined for the first time ever in the 1990s. Press release, National Cancer Institute, Nov 1996.

European Urology

Eur Urol 1999;35:544–547

Prostate Cancer Prevention Trial (PCPT) Update

Charles A. Coltman, Jr.[a] Ian M. Thompson, Jr.[b] Polly Feigl[c]

[a]Southwest Oncology Group; [b]Brooke Army Medical Center, San Antonio, Tex., and
[c]Fred Hutchinson Cancer Research Center, Seattle, Wash., USA

Key Words
Prostate cancer · Prevention · Finasteride · Intergroup clinical trial

Abstract
The Prostate Cancer Prevention Trial is an intergroup effort in the USA managed by the Southwest Oncology Group (SWOG) in collaboration with the Eastern Cooperative Oncology Group (ECOG) and the Cancer and Leukemia Group B (CALGB). This 10-year study began approximately 5 years ago and will achieve its primary endpoint in October 2004. At the start of the study, 18,882 men, aged over 55 years, and with normal digital rectal examination (DRE) and serum prostate-specific antigen (PSA) levels of ≤3.0 ng/ml were randomized to take finasteride (5 mg/day) or placebo (1 tablet/day). DRE and PSA have been determined yearly (PSA in a central laboratory). When DRE is abnormal or PSA rises to >4.0 ng/ml, a biopsy is recommended. Because of the effect finasteride has on PSA, the PSA value has been indexed to equalize the number of biopsies in both arms. At 7 years all survivors will undergo a sextant biopsy to determine the period prevalence of prostate cancer. The critical assumptions are: (1) finasteride-induced PSA changes result in a simple downward shift; (2) the assessment of adherence is sensitive enough to detect nonadherence affecting PSA level interpretation: (3) factors affecting biopsy loss will be equal in both arms; (4) finasteride does not affect the sensitivity or specificity of DRE on transrectal ultrasound nor the sensitivity of biopsy; (5) bias resulting from transurethral resection of the prostate in benign prostate hyperplasia cases will be negligible.

Introduction

In 1998, it is anticipated that there will be 184,500 new cases of prostate cancer and 39,200 prostate cancer deaths [1]. The focus of the past decade has been on early detection and treatment. This approach results in a potential overtreatment, and resultant morbidity, and increased cost, with unknown efficacy [2]. An ideal alternative to the reduction of morbidity and mortality is through primary prevention of prostate cancer.

There is clear evidence that androgens have an influence on prostate cancer. Men with lower androgen levels have a lower incidence of carcinoma of the prostate [3]. Circulating testosterone is 10–15% higher in African-Americans than in US Caucasians. The risk of prostate cancer is higher in African-Americans for both incidence and mortality [4]. Testosterone and dihydrotestosterone are responsible for prostatic development and androgen

KARGER
Fax + 41 61 306 12 34
E-Mail karger@karger.ch
www.karger.com

0302–2838/99/0356–0544$17.50/0

Accessible online at:
http://BioMedNet.com/karger

Charles A. Coltman, Jr., MD, Chairman
Southwest Oncology Group, 14980 Omicron Drive
San Antonio, TX 78245-3217 (USA)
Tel. +1 210 677 8808, Fax +1 210 677 0006
E-Mail charles_coltman@msmtp.idde.saci.org

deprivation results in prostatic involution [5]. There is a small group of kindreds with inherited deficiency of 5α-reductase [6], the enzyme which catalyzes the conversion of testosterone to dihydrotestosterone, who develop a form of male pseudohermaphroditism with mild external genital abnormalities at birth. These males have normal serum testosterone levels, virilize at puberty, and have underdeveloped prostates [7]. The development of benign prostatic hyperplasia (BPH) or carcinoma of the prostate has not been reported in these individuals. Finasteride, a 4-aza-steroid competitive inhibitor of human 5α-reductase, has been synthesized. It produces a profound reduction in prostatic dihydrotestosterone similar to the inherited deficiency [8].

In view of the fact that the development of prostate cancer is influenced by the androgenic milieu, the choice of finasteride, which reduces the dihydrotestosterone levels in the prostate, has relatively low risks of side effects [9], and inhibits growth of prostate cancer cells in vitro [10], is a rational choice for a primary chemopreventive strategy.

Study Design

There are some problems associated with the choice of finasteride as a chemopreventive agent. Finasteride leads to a 20% reduction in prostate size over a 6-month period of time [9]. This could result in a digital rectal examination bias (DRE Bias) with either underdetection or overdetection of prostate cancer. If a smaller gland is homogeneous, it may result in a lower number of biopsies and thus underdetection. On the other hand, if gland shrinkage results in a nodular gland, more biopsies will occur with potential overdetection. In addition, a standard sextant biopsy of a smaller gland will result in sampling a larger fraction of the prostate gland, potentially resulting in overdetection.

In addition, finasteride reduces the serum prostate-specific antigen (PSA), a principal method of prostate cancer detection, by 50%. If the PSA is employed to identify participants with prostate cancer, more participants receiving the placebo will undergo biopsy. Because of the relationship of biopsy rate and cancer detection, the placebo detection rate would rise, resulting in PSA Bias. Because of these potential biases, steps were taken to index the PSA to assure an equal number of biopsies were performed in both the finasteride and the placebo arms.

At least five different study designs were considered. An initial design included, as the ideal endpoint, prostate cancer-specific mortality. This design was rejected because of sample size. Using a 26% relative risk reduction, a 5% two-sided α, and a 90% power, a sample size of 51,000 would be required in a 15-year study. This design was rejected because of the huge sample size and length of study. The final design selection was to recruit normal, healthy men, age 55 and older, with a 10-year life expectancy, to a randomized double-blind, placebo-controlled trial of 10 years in length, 3 years of accrual and 7 years of treatment. Each had a normal DRE, a PSA ≤ 3 ng/ml. A prostate biopsy during the trial would be prompted by an abnormal DRE or PSA >4 ng/ml. Blinded indexed PSAs assured that the biopsy rate would be the same percentage in the finasteride group as in the placebo group. A sample size of 18,000 men, following a 3-month placebo run-in, would be randomly assigned to placebo or finasteride. Each would be followed every 3 months by telephone, and would undergo an annual DRE and PSA, with a biopsy of the prostate if either or both were abnormal. All surviving participants would be biopsied at 7 years.

The objectives of the study are: (1) to test the difference in biopsy-proven period prevalence of carcinoma of the prostate; (2) to test the effect of finasteride on the stage and grade at diagnosis; (3) to assess the toxicity of long-term administration of finasteride; (4) to estimate the difference in prostate cancer-specific mortality; (5) to estimate the difference in incidence and severity of BPH and (6) to estimate sensitivity, specificity, and predictive values of the DRE and PSA as screening tests for prostate cancer.

The trial was designed to have a 92% power to detect a 25% reduction in the period prevalence of biopsy-proven disease using a two-sided test with an α equal to 0.05. The critical assumptions, which must be maintained in order to assure the integrity of the clinical trial design, are: (1) A total 7-year biopsy loss of 40%, with 20% due to mortality; 15% loss to follow-up, and a 5% biopsy refusal. Those factors affecting loss will be the same in both arms. (2) The original PSA rank on the finasteride arm is preserved. (3) Finasteride does not affect the sensitivity or specificity of the DRE or the transrectral ultrasound (TRUS), nor does finasteride affect the sensitivity of the prostate biopsy. (4) The finasteride nonadherence is less than 10% and placebo contamination less than 5%. (5) Any bias resulting from transurethral resection of the prostate in men with a BPH incident cases will be negligible. All critical elements are being monitored by an independent Data and Safety Monitoring Committee every 6 months throughout the trial.

Table 1. Cooperative groups

	Sites	Randomized	%
SWOG	107	11,571	61
ECOG	77	5,281	28
CALGB	35	2,030	11
Total	219	18,882	

Table 2. Age of the men randomized

	Randomized	%
Median age	63	
Age range	55–86	
Distribution		
55–59 years	5,626	30
60–64 years	5,816	31
65+ years	7,440	39
Total	18,882	

Table 3. Race of the men randomized

Race	Randomized	%
Caucasian	17,272	92
African-American	702	4
Other	782	4
Unknown	126	
Total	18,882	

Table 4. Highest education level

	Randomized	%	
Grade school	258	1	
Some high school	553	3	
High school graduate	2,739	15	
Voc./training school	846	5	
Some college	4,603	25	} 76
College graduate	3,092	16	} 76
Post-grad. education	6,649	35	} 76
Unknown	142		
Total	18,882		

Table 5. PSA level

	Randomized	%
Median	1.1	
Range	0.2–3	
Distribution		
≤1.0	9,121	48
1.1–2.0	6,715	36
2.1–3.0	3,045	18
Total	18,882	

Interim Results

This intergroup prevention trial included 219 sites. Table 1 shows the number of men randomized to PCPT from each of the three Cooperative Groups: Southwest Oncology Group (SWOG), Eastern Cooperative Oncology Group (ECOG), and Cancer and Leukemia Group B (CALGB). The clinical trial opened October 13, 1993, and 3 years to the day (October 13, 1996) from the initiation of the study, sufficient men were enrolled to randomize a total of 18,000. On December 6, 1996, the registrations were formally closed, and in the final analysis, 18,882 men were randomly assigned to finasteride or placebo.

Demographics

Tables 2 and 3 show the age and race of those 18,882 men randomized. The median age is 63, with 39% over the age of 65. Table 3 shows that only 4% of those randomized were African-American, which is substantially lower than the 8% estimate of African-American men ≥55 years of age in the US population. Aggressive recruitment of Black men did not influence that percentage. Table 4 demonstrates that the PCPT participants were highly educated, with 76% having at least some college experience. There was no difference in education level of African-American men when compared to the total sample. The percentage of African-American men, within the age range recruited, is likely to be less than the 8% in the US population. These data demonstrate that those men in the upper socioeconomic strata are those most concerned with prevention. The median PSA is 1.1, with 48% ≤1.0 ng/ml (table 5). These data are a reflection of the normal healthy men enrolled and the eligibility requirements of

Table 6. PCPT sexual dysfunction (placebo)

	Baseline, %		Two years, %	
	some	total	some	total
Impotence	13	5	25	13
Loss of libido	12	1	25	3
Ejaculatory volume	8	2	21	5

the protocol. Fifteen percent of those in the trial are of high risk as a result of having a first-degree relative with prostate cancer.

Adverse Effects

The most important adverse effects of the use of finasteride, as reported in a randomized double-blind, placebo-controlled clinical trial of finasteride in the management of BPH, are decreased libido (4.7 vs. 1.3%, $p < 0.05$), ejaculatory dysfunction (4.4 vs. 1.7%, $p < 0.05$) and impotence (3.4 vs. 1.7%, NS) [9]. With Data and Safety Monitoring Committee permission, the sexual function information among men on the placebo arm of PCPT was made available to share with the men on PCPT to put the impact of sexual dysfunction of men on this trial in proper perspective. Those data are shown in table 6. This initial level of sexual dysfunction among the men on the placebo arm of this study are substantially higher than those on the placebo arm of the trial of BPH (see above). This difference may be due to the fact that the PCPT sexual dysfunction data were documented by detailed personal interviews with each man rather than by self-reporting.

Discussion

This National Cancer Institute, Division of Cancer Prevention and Control Intergroup Cancer Prevention Trial is proceeding well some 5 years into the study. Critical assumptions would appear to be on target, as no indication to the contrary has been provided by the DSMC. With the period prevalence of prostate cancer as the primary endpoint, it will not be reached before May 2004, when all of the surviving men will have undergone a sextant biopsy. It is anticipated that the majority of those who have been taking a pill for 7 years will be anxious to know their prostate status. A prostate biopsy video is in production, which will be shown to men as they approach time for their biopsy, to encourage their commitment to that important endpoint.

References

1 Landis SH, Murray T, Bolden S, Wingo PA: Cancer Statistics, 1998. CA Cancer J Clin 1998;48:6–30.
2 Von Eschenbach A, Ho R, Murphy GF, Cunningham M, Lins N: American Cancer Society guidelines for the early detection of prostate cancer. Cancer 1997;80:1805–1807.
3 Huggins C, Hodges CV: Studies on prostate cancer. I. The effect of castration, of estrogen, and of androgen injection on serum phosphatases in metastatic carcinoma of the prostate. Cancer Res 1941;1:293.
4 Ross RK, Bernstein L, Lobo RA et al: Evidence for reduced 5-alpha-reductase activity in Japanese compared to US white and black males: Implications for prostate cancer risk. Lancet 1992;339:887–889.
5 Peters CA, Walsh PC: The effect of nafarelin acetate, a luteinizing hormone-releasing hormone agonist, on benign prostatic hyperplasia. N Engl J Med 1987;317:599–604.
6 Imperato-McGinley J, Guerreo L, Gautier T et al: Steroid 5-alpha-reductase deficiency in man: An inherited form of male pseudohermaphroditism. Science 1974;186:1213–1215.
7 Walsh PC, Madden JD, Harrod MJ et al: Familial incomplete male pseudohermaphroditism, type 2: Decreased dihydrotestosterone formation in pseudovaginal perineoscrotal hypospadias. N Engl J Med 1974;291:944–949.
8 Metcalf BW, Levy MA, Holt DA: Inhibitors of steroid 5-alpha-reductase in benign prostatic hyperplasia, male pattern baldness and acne. Trends Pharmacol Sci 1989;10:491–495.
9 Gormley GJ, Stoner E, Bruskewitz RC et al: The effect of finasteride in men with benign prostatic hyperplasia. N Engl J Med 1992;327:1185–1191.
10 Bologna M, Muzi P, Biordi L et al: Antiandrogens and 5-alpha-reductase inhibition of the proliferation rate in PC3 and DU145 human prostatic cancer cell lines. Curr Ther Res 1992;51:799–813.

Author Index Vol. 35, No. 5–6, 1999

European Urology

Algaba, F. 496
Altshuler, D. 355

Bairati, I. 388
Bartels, H.G. 484
Bartels, P.H. 468, 484
Bartsch, G. 413, 523
Bayne, C.W. 439
Boone, Ch.W. 342
Bosland, M.C. 459
Bostwick, D.G. 479, 492
Boyle, P. 370
Bretsky, P. 355
Bussemakers, M.J.G. 408

Cato, A.C.B. 413
Cheng, L. 492
Coetzee, G.A. 355
Collette, L. 519
Coltman, Ch.A., Jr. 544
Crawford, E.D. 511
Crowell, J.A. 342
Culig, Z. 413

Daley, G. 355
Denis, L. 377, 443
Duval da Silva, V. 484

Eder, I.E. 413
Ekman, P. 362
ERSPC, Section Rotterdam 539

Feigl, P. 544
Fradet, Y. 388

Ghosh, J. 395
Griffiths, K. 377, 443
Grizzle, W. 429

Habib, F.K. 439
Hamilton, P.W. 468, 484
Henderson, B.E. 355
Hobisch, A. 413
Hoedemaeker, R. 539
Horninger, W. 523

Jenkins, R.B. 479

Kelloff, G.J. 341, 342, 429
Kirkels, W. 539
Klocker, H. 413, 523
Kolonel, L.N. 355
Kopelovitch, L. 342
Kranse, R. 539
Kwast, Th.H. van der 508

Labrie, F. 508
Lander, E. 355
Lieberman, R. 342, 429
Lubet, R.A. 342

McCormick, D.L. 464
Malone, W.A. 342
Manne, U. 429
Markiewicz, M. 429
Marshall, M. 429
Meijden, A.P.M. van der 515
Meyer, F. 388
Mohler, J. 429
Montironi, R. 468, 484
Moore, L. 388
Morton, M.S. 377, 443
Moul, J.W. 399
Myers, Ch.E. 395
Myers, R. 429

Nessler-Menardi, C. 413
Neumann, R. 492
Newling, D. 504
Nupponen, N. 351

Pearce, C.L. 355
Peehl, D.M. 392
Perkins, D. 429
Peterziel, H. 413
Putz, Th. 413

Qian, J. 479, 492

Rao, K.V.N. 464
Reichardt, J.K.V. 355
Reissigl, A. 523
Rietbergen, J. 539
Rogatsch, H. 523
Ross, M. 439
Ross, R.K. 355

Sakr, W.A. 474
Scarpelli, M. 468
Schröder, F.H. 539
Schulman, C.C. 341, 498
Severi, G. 370
Shadmani, R. 388
Sigman, C.C. 342
Sporn, M.B. 420
Steele, V.E. 342
Studen, M. 523
Sylvester, R. 519

Têtu, B. 508
Thompson, D. 468, 484
Thompson, I.M., Jr. 544

Urban, D. 429

Vaught, L. 484
Visakorpi, T. 351
Volgger, H. 523

Waters, D.J. 456
Weiss, H. 429
Whelan, P. 424

Zlotta, A.R. 498

KARGER

Fax + 41 61 306 12 34
E-Mail karger@karger.ch
www.karger.com

Accessible online at:
http://BioMedNet.com/karger

European
Urology

Subject Index Vol. 35, No. 5–6, 1999

Ageing 370
Amplification 351
Androgen(s) 355
 deprivation therapy 492
 receptor 351, 413
 withdrawal 413
Animal models 456, 459
Apoptosis 395
Arachidonic acid 395

bcl-2 399
BPH 439
Breast cancer 424

Cancer 392, 399, 456
CaP 439
Carcinogenesis 456
Cervical cancer 424
Chemoprevention 342, 370, 377, 392, 420, 424, 429, 443, 456, 459, 464, 474, 492, 508, 511, 515, 519
Chromosomal anomaly 479
Comparative genomic hybridization 351

Dehydroepiandrosterone 464
Deletion 351
Deltanoids 420
Diet 362, 377, 388
Dietary fat 395
α-Difluoromethylornithine 464
DNA adducts 468
Drug development 342
Du-145 413

Efficacy testing 459
Endocrine therapy 508
Endpoints 519
Environment 362
Enzyme-altered foci 468
Epidemiology 370, 474
Epidermal growth factor 395

Fat 388
Fenretinide 429
Finasteride 544
Fluorescence in situ hybridization 351, 479
Free prostate-specific antigen 523

Gene expression 408
Genetic alterations 351, 479
Genetics 355, 362
Glutathione S-transferase 468

Head and neck cancer 424
Histometry 484
Histopathology 508
Hormonal therapy 492
Hormone-refractory disease 351
(4-Hydroxyphenyl)retinamide 429
N-(4-Hydroxyphenyl)retinamide (fenretinide) 464

Image analysis 468
Intergroup clinical trial 544
Intracellular signalling 443
Invasive adenocarcinoma 468
Isoflavonoids 443

Karyometry 484
Ki-67 399

Liarozole fumarate 464
Ligand-independent activation 413
Lignans 443
5-Lipoxygenase 395
LNCaP 413
Lung cancer 424

Malignancy-associated changes 468
Marker 408
Metastasis 479
mRNA expression 439

Oltipraz 464
Organ-confined tumors 523

p53 399
Paracrine control 439
Phyto-oestrogens 377
PIN I/III 504
Practical aspects 515
Predictive value 459
Preliminary results 539
Premalignant nature 456
Prevention 544
Probability of prostate cancer 523
Prognosis 399

Progression index 484
Proliferative activity 508
Prostate 342, 392, 399, 456, 468
 biopsy 496
 cancer 362, 370, 377, 388, 408, 424, 429, 459, 464, 474, 504, 515, 519, 539, 544
 neoplasms 492
Prostate-specific antigen 523
 transition zone density 523
Prostatic cancer 496
 carcinoma 479, 492
 intraepithelial neoplasia 468, 474, 479, 484, 492, 496, 498, 508
 neoplasms 355, 498
PSA 413
 as surrogate marker 511
 screening 523

Radiation therapy 492
Radical prostatectomy 399
Randomized study 539
Receptors 362
5α-Reductase isoenzymes 439
Reporter gene 413
9-*cis*-Retinoic acid 464
Retinoids 420, 424

Screening 539
 tests 539
L-Selenomethionine 464
Stage migration 523
Statistical considerations 519
Surrogate endpoint biomarker 429

Tamoxifen 420
Telomerase 468
Therapy 408
Timing treatment 504
DL-α-Tocopherol (vitamin E) 464
Transcriptional activity 413
Transitional zone cancer 523

Vitamin D 392
 E 388

KARGER

Fax + 41 61 306 12 34
E-Mail karger@karger.ch
www.karger.com

Accessible online at:
http://BioMedNet.com/karger

European Urology

Forthcoming Papers

Reviews

Ballanger P et al: An Overview of Female Urinary Incontinence
Bemelmans B et al: Neuromodulation by Implant for Treating Lower Urinary Tract Symptoms and Dysfunction
de Sèze M et al: Intravesical Instillation of Capsaicin in Urology. A Review of the Literature
Djavan B et al: A Meta Analysis on the Efficacy and Tolerability of Alpha 1-Adrenoceptor Antagonists in Patients with Lower Urinary Tract Symptoms Suggestive of Benign Prostatic Obstruction
Tiselius H: Factors Influencing the Course of Calcium Oxalate Stone Disease

Clinical Papers

Ahlgren G et al: Evaluation of DNA-Ploidy Combined with a Cytometric Proliferation Index of Imprints from Core Needle Biopsies in Prostate Cancer
Aragona F et al: No Evidence of Fluid Absorption during Continuous Low Pressure TURP. Assessment by Measuring the Expiratory Breath Ethanol Concentrations
Barré C et al: Improving Bladder Neck Division in Radical Retropubic Prostatectomy by Prior Dissection of the Seminal Vesicles and Vasa deferentia
Carter A et al: Quality of Life Changes following KTP/ND:YAG Laser Treatment of the Prostate and TURP
Carter P et al: The Role of Atrial Natriuretic Peptide in Nocturnal Polyuria in Elderly Males
Chautard D et al: Values for the Free to Total PSA Ratio as a Function of Age. Necessity of Reference Range Validation
Chung W et al: Is Obesity an Underlying Factor in Erectile Dysfunction?
Dawkins G et al: Sorbitol-Mannitol Solution for Urological Electrosurgical Resection – A Safer Fluid than Glycine 1.5%
Droupy S et al: Cavernospongious Shunts: Anatomical Study of Intrapenile Vascular Pathways
Fujii Y et al: Late Recurrence and Progression after a Long Tumor-Free Period in Primary TA and T1 Bladder Cancer
Gatti R et al: Histological Adaptation of the Orthotopic Ileal Neobladders Mucosa: 4 Year's Follow-Up of 30 Patients
Graefen M et al: Early PSA Relapse after Radical Retropubic Prostatectomy: Prediction on the Bases of Preoperative and Postoperative Tumor Characteristics
Guillonneau B et al: Laparoscopic Radical Prostatectomy: Technical and Early Oncological Assessment of 40 Operations
Gumus E et al: The Effect of Long-Term Sitting on Serum Prostate-Specific Antigen Levels
Harada Y et al: Clinical Study of Brain Metastasis of Renal Cell Carcinoma
Hatzichristou D et al: Hemodynamic Characterization of a Functional Erection: Arterial and Corporeal Veno-Occlusive Function in Patients with a Positive Intracavernosal Injection Test
Herranz Amo F et al: The Need for Intravenous Urography in Patients with Primary Transitional Carcinoma of the Bladder
Hess B et al: Effects of a 'Common Sense Diet' on Urinary Composition and Supersaturation in Patients with Idiopathic Calcium Urolithiasis
Hilz H et al: Molecular Heterogeneity of Free PSA in Sera of Patients with Benign and Malignant Prostate Tumors
Hofer C et al: Fluorine-18 Fluorodeoxyglucose (F-18 FDG) Positron Emission Tomography Is Useless for the Detection of Local Recurrence after Radical Prostatectomy
Ichiyanagi O et al: Relationship between Urodynamic Type of Obstruction and Histological Component of the Prostate in Patients with Benign Prostatic Hyperplasia
Keeley Jr et al: Clearance of Lower Pole Stones following SWL: Effect of Infundibulopelvic Angle
Klingler C et al: The Value of the Power Doppler - Sonography in the Investigation of Erectile Dysfunction
Knopf H et al: Nosocomial Infections after Transurethral Prostatectomy
Küpeli S et al: Penile Implants in Erectile Impotence: The Importance of Clinical Experience on Outcome
Leibovici D et al: Ureteral Catheterization and Patient Mobilization: Is Bed Restriction Mandatory?
Liukkonen T et al: The Prognostic Value of MIB-1 Score, p53, EGFr, Mitotic Index and Papillary Status in Primary Superficial (Stage pTA/T1) Bladder Cancer: A Prospective Comparative Study
Martin X et al: The Use of Long-Term Defunctionalized Bladder in Renal Transplantation. Is It Save?
Masuda M et al: The Worst Histologic Elements Predict Prognosis in Moderately-Differentiated Prostate Cancer Patients with Androgen-Withdrawal Endocrine Therapy
Matuszewski M et al: Laparoscopic Treatment of Parapubic Post-Prostatectomy Hernia
Mejean A et al: Mortality and Morbidity after Nephrectomy for Renal Cell Carcinoma Using a Transperitoneal Anterior Subcostal Incision
Millon R et al: Detection of Prostate-Specific-Antigen- or Prostate-Specific-Membrane-Antigen-Positive Circulating Cells in Prostatic Cancer Patients: Clinical Implications
Mirone V et al: Our Experience about Association of a New Physical and Medical Therapy in Patients Suffering for Induratio Penis Plastica
Morote Robles J et al: Intraindividual Variations of Total and Percent-Free Serum Prostatic-Specific Antigen Levels in Patients with Normal Digital Rectal Examination
Ogreid P et al: Tissue PSA and Androgen Receptor Immunoreactivity in Prostate Cancer Biopsies before, during and after Neo-Adjuvant Androgen Deprivation Followed by Radiotherapy
Ou J et al: Transitional Cell Carcinoma in Dialysis Patients
Palmberg C et al: PSA Decline Is an Independent Prognostic Marker in Hormonally Treated Prostate Cancer
Patrick D et al: Cultural Adaptation of a Quality-of-Life Measure for Urinary Incontinence
Pesce C et al: Ureterovascular Hydronephrosis in Children: Is the Pyeloplasty Always Necessary?
Post P et al: Trend and Variation in Treatment of Localised Prostate Cancer in the Southern Part of the Netherlands, 1988–1996
Pu Y et al: Antiandrogen Hepatotoxicity in Patients with Chronic Viral Hepatitis
Puppo P et al: Primary Endoscopic Treatment of Ureteric Calculi: A Review of 378 Cases
Radosevi-Jelic L et al: Concomitant Radiotherapy and Carboplatin in Locally Advanced Bladder Cancer
Riedl C et al: Bacterial Colonization of Ureteral Stents
Sasagawa I et al: Influence of Carbon Dioxide on Respiratory Function during Posterior Retroperitoneoscopic Adrenalectomy in Prone Position
Schatzl G et al: The Impact of Urinary Extravasation after Radical Retropubic Prostatectomy on Urinary Incontinence and Anastomotic Strictures
Sözen S et al: Comparison of the Nuclear Matrix Protein 222 with Voided Urine Cytology and BTA stat Test in the Diagnosis of Transitional Cell Carcinoma of the Bladder

Pediatric Urology

Abd-El-Gawad G et al: Kock Urinary Reservoir Maturation in Children and Adolescents: Consequences for Kidney and Upper Urinary Tract
Angwafo III F et al: Pediatric Urolithiasis in Sub-Saharan Africa: A Comparative Study in Two Regions of Cameroon
Heidenreich A et al: Nephrogenic Adenoma – A Rare Bladder Tumor in Children
Nonomura K et al: Impact of Congenital Narrowing of the Bulbar Urethra (Cobb's Collar) and Its Transurethral Incision in Children
Pesce C et al: Ureterovascular Hydronephrosis in Children: Is the Pyeloplasty Always Necessary?
Radmayr C et al: Importance of Renal Resistive Index in Children Suffering from Vesicoureteral Reflux
Vereecken R et al: A Review of 92 Obstructive Megaureters in Children
Vögeli T et al: Urological Treatment and Clinical Course of BK-Polyomavirus Associated Hemorrhagic Cystitis in Children after Bone Marrow Transplantation

Basic Science

Höfner K et al: Tamsulosin 0.4 mg Once Daily: Effect on Sexual Function in Patients with Lower Urinary Tract Symptoms Suggestive of Benign Prostatic Obstruction
Hughes A et al: A Community Study of Uncomplicated Lower Urinary Tract Symptoms among Male Italian Immigrants in Sydney, Australia

KARGER

Fax+ 41 61 306 12 34
E-Mail karger@karger.ch
www.karger.com

Access to full text and tables of contents, including tentative ones for forthcoming issues:
www.karger.com/journals/eur/eurcont.htm

European
Urology

Acknowledgement to the Reviewers

The Editor-in-Chief and the Board of Editors greatly appreciate the support of the numerous reviewers who contributed by their collaboration to help them in the scientific evaluation and reviewing process of manuscripts submitted for publication from September 1998 to February 1999.

Abbou, C.-C., Créteil
Aigrain, Y., Paris
Albers, P., Bonn
Algaba, F., Barcelona
Alken, P., Mannheim
Andersson, K.E., Lund
Anidjar, M., Paris
Atala, A., Boston, Mass.
Austoni, E.A., Milan
Baert, L., Leuven
Bassi, P., Padua
Bloom, D.A., Ann Arbor, Mich.
Boccon-Gibod, L.M., Paris
Boccon-Gibod, L.A., Paris
Bussemakers, M.J.G., Nijmegen
Camby, I., Brussels
Chapple, C.R., Sheffield
Colombel, M., Lyon
D'Hallewin, M., Leuven
Danguy, A., Brussels
de la Rosette, J.J.M.C.H., Nijmegen
De Ridder, D., Leuven
De Sy, W.A., Ghent
Denis, L.J., Antwerpen
Desgrandchamps, F., Paris
Dieckmann, K.P., Hamburg
Djavan, B., Vienna
Dodat, H., Lyon
Englert, Y., Brussels
Eschwege, P., Le Krémlin-Bicêtre
Feitz, W.F.J., Nijmegen
Fisch, M., Mainz
Fitzpatrick, J.M., Dublin
Frey, P., Lausanne
Frick, J., Innsbruck
Habib, F.K., Edinburgh
Hamdy, F.C., Sheffield
Hammerer, P.G., Hamburg
Hargreave, T.B., Edinburgh
Hatzichristou, D.G., Thessaloniki
Heidenreich, A., Marburg
Hendry, W.F., London
Hjälmas, K., Göteborg
Hohenfellner, M., Mainz
Jacqmin, D., Strasbourg
Jünemann, K.-P., Mannheim
Kirby, R.S., London
Klocker, H., Innsbruck
Krautschick, A., Gotha
Lacombe, L., Québec
Leyh, H., Munich
Lobel, B., Rennes
Loch, T., Kiel
Madersbacher, S., Vienna
Mansson, W., Lund
Manzoni, G.M., Varese
Marberger, M., Vienna
Martin, X., Lyon
Merckx, L., Ghent
Meuleman, E.J.M., Nijmegen
Michel, M.C., Essen
Mickisch, G.H.J., Rotterdam
Montironi, R., Ancona
Montorsi, F., Milan
Mouriquand, P.D.E., Lyon
Mundy, A.R., London
Naber, K.G., Straubing
Nativ, O., Haifa
Noldus, J., Hamburg
Oosterlinck, W., Ghent
Oosterwijk, E., Nijmegen
Pagano, F., Padua
Petein, M.L., Brussels
Pizzocaro, G., Milan
Pomerol, J.M., Barcelona
Prayer-Galetti, T., Padua
Pummer, K., Graz
Puppo, P., Genoa
Rassweiler, J.J., Heilbronn
Ravery, V., Paris
Riedmiller, H., Würzburg
Robson, C.N., Newcastle upon Tyne
Sarramon, J.P., Toulouse
Schmitz-Dräger, B.J., Fürth
Schulman, C.C., Brussels
Stenzl, A., Innsbruck
Stief, C.G., Hannover
Struelens, M.J., Brussels
Studer, U.E., Bern
Thalmann, G.N., Bern
Thomas, D.F.M., Leeds
Thompson, I.M., San Antonio, Tex.
Tiselius, H.-G., Hudding
Turek, P.J., San Francisco, Calif.
Van Cangh, P.J., Brussels
van der Meijden, A.P.M., Den Bosch
Van Kerrebroeck, P.E.V., Maastricht
Van Poppel, H., Leuven
Virag, R., Paris
Weil, E.H.J., Maastricht
Whelan, P., Leeds
Wirth, M.P., Dresden
Witjes, J.A., Nijmegen
Woodhouse, C.R.J., London
Wullich, B., Homburg/Saar
Wyndaele, J.J., Antwerpen
Zlotta, A., Brussels

KARGER
Fax + 41 61 306 12 34
E-Mail karger@karger.ch
www.karger.com

0302–2838/99/0356–0551$17.50/0
Accessible online at:
http://BioMedNet.com/karger

Author Index Vol. 35, 1999

European Urology

Supplement Issues No. 1 and 2 have their own Author Index

Aarnink, R.G. 9
Abbou, C.-C. 289
Abu-Arafeh, W. 285
Algaba, F. 496
Allen, F.J. 223
Allhoff, E.P. 204
Altshuler, D. 355
Altwein, J.E. 9, 177
Amar, E. 312
Amorosi, A. 32
Anderl, H. 304
Aragona, F. 98
Aubert, J. 89

Bairati, I. 388
Balincourt, C. de 267
Banerjee, M. 210
Bartels, H.G. 484
Bartels, P.H. 468, 484
Bartsch, G. 413, 523
Bassi, P. 52
Bastús, R. 323
Bayne, C.W. 439
Beerlage, H.P. 9
Behringer, D. 70
Bellot, J. 289
Berenguer, A. 26, 228
Berresheim, U. 304
Biasoni, D. 93
Bichler, K.H. 21
Billebaud, T. 298
Birch, B.R. 327
Blanc, E. 298
Boccon-Gibod, L. 52, 239, 298, 312
Bolla, M. 23
Bon, D. 89
Boone, C.W. 342
Borrat, P. 323
Bortuzzo, G. 98
Bosland, M.C. 459
Bostwick, D.G. 479, 492
Bouvet, E. 239
Boyle, P. 370
Brausi, M. 267
Bretsky, P. 355
Bruwer, G. 223
Burger, B. 177
Bussemakers, M.J.G. 408

Caballero, J.M. 323
Casalots, J. 323
Cato, A.C.B. 413
Chapple, C.R. 119
Cheng, L. 492
Chertin, B. 285
Chopin, D. 289
Cirera, L. 323
Coba, J.M. 228
Coetzee, G.A. 355
Collette, L. 519
Colombel, M. 289
Coltman, C.A., Jr. 544
Conort, P. 52
Cooper, A.J. 327
Costello, A.J. 138
Crawford, E.D. 511
Crew, J.P. 2
Crowell, J.A. 342
Culig, Z. 413
Currò, A. 93

Daley, G. 355
Debruyne, F.M.J. 9, 197
De Caro, R. 98
De Lisa, A. 233
Delmas, V. 239, 298, 312
Del Nero, A. 93
Denis, L. 377, 443
Desgrandchamps, F. 89, 257
Di Loro, F. 32
Duval da Silva, V. 484

Eder, I.E. 413
Ekman, P. 362
Encabo, G. 294
EORTC-GU Group Superficial Bladder Committee 267
ERSPC, Section Rotterdam 539
Esposito, N. 93
Everaert, K. 57

Famiglietti, G. 210
Fanfani, A. 32
Farkas, A. 285
Feigl, P. 544
Fernández, P. 228
Fidas, A. 102
Fisch, P. 70
Fitzpatrick, J.M. 117
Fradet, Y. 388
Fujimoto, K. 185
Gerharz, E. 217
Gheiler, E.L. 210
Ghosh, J. 395
Gilling, P.J. 155
Girman, C.J. 277
Gomez de Segura, G. 323
González, G. 323
Grayson, T. 210
Griffith, D.P. 257
Griffiths, K. 377, 443
Grizzle, W. 429
Gruss, A. 204
Guess, H.A. 277

Habib, F.K. 439
Hadas-Halperin, I. 285
Hajivassiliou, C.A. 36
Hamilton, P.W. 468, 484
Hayashi, Y. 185
Hayes, M.C. 327
Heicappell, R. 81, 249
Henderson, B.E. 355
Hentrich, I. 70
Hermieu, J.-F. 239, 298
Herrero, A. 26
Heyns, C.F. 223
Hirao, Y. 185
Hobisch, A. 413
Hoebeke, P. 57
Hoedemaeker, R. 539
Höfner, K. 129
Homma, Y. 45
Horenblas, S. 197
Horninger, W. 523

Iklé, D.N. 70
Irani, J. 89
Ishak, L. 52
Issa, M.M. 119

Jacobsen, S.J. 277
Janitzky, V. 272
Jenkins, R.B. 479
Jennings, A.M. 327
Jesuiter, H. 70
Johnston, R.S. 192

Kabalin, J.N. 138
Kälble, T. 217
Kaplan, S.A. 166
Kawabe, K. 45
Keane, P.F. 192
Keller, T. 21
Kelloff, G.J. 341, 342, 429
Kienle, E. 27
Kırkalı, Z. 109
Kirkels, W. 539
Kishino, T. 185
Kleinhans, B. 217
Klocker, H. 413, 523
Köhler, G. 70
Kolonel, L.N. 355
Kopelovitch, L. 342
Kosmehl, H. 272
Kranse, R. 539
Krause, H. 249
Kulmburg, P. 70
Kunzmann, R. 70
Kurek, R. 27
Kurth, K.-H. 267
Kwast, Th.H. van der 508

Labrie, F. 508
Lahn, M. 70
Lander, E. 355
Le Duc, A. 89, 155
Lefrère-Belda, M.-A. 289
Leyh, H. 52
Liberopoulos, K. 102
Lieber, M.M. 277
Lieberman, R. 342, 429
Lindemann, A. 70
López, M. 294
Lotti, T. 17
Louca, G. 102
Lovisolo, J.A.J. 210
Lübben, G. 27
Lubet, R.A. 342
Luján, M. 26, 228
Lupa, S. 285
Lykourinas, M. 102
Lynch, J.H. 129

McCormick, D.L. 464
Malone, W.A. 342
Mangiarotti, B. 93
Manne, U. 429
Marberger, M. 52
Markiewicz, M. 429
Marshall, M. 429
Martí, Ll. 323
Martín, E. 26
Meijden, A.P.M. van der 267, 515

KARGER
Fax + 41 61 306 12 34
E-Mail karger@karger.ch
www.karger.com

Accessible online at:
http://BioMedNet.com/karger

Melekos, M. 217
Meyer, F. 388
Millán-Rodríguez, F. 318
Miller, K. 81, 249
Millet, C. 89
Miyagawa, I. 242
Mohler, J. 429
Montanari, E. 93
Montironi, R. 17, 468, 484
Moore, L. 388
Moriel, E.Z. 285
Morita, T. 45
Morote, J. 294
Morton, M.S. 377, 443
Moul, J.W. 399
Moulinier, F. 239, 298
Müller, M. 81, 249
Mungan, U. 109
Murillo, N. 228
Muschel, B. 70
Muschter, R. 147
Myers, C.E. 395
Myers, R. 429

Nessler-Menardi, C. 413
Neumann, R. 492
Nikolakopoulou, Z. 102
Ninković, M.M. 304
Nupponen, N. 351

Okajima, E. 185
Oldford, G. 210
Oosterlinck, W. 267
Otani, T. 185
Özkara, E. 109
Ozono, S. 185

Páez, A. 26, 228
Pagano, F. 52, 98
Palou, J. 318
Parenti, A. 98
Pasandoro, V. 52
Patard, J.-J. 289
Pearce, C.L. 355
Peehl, D.M. 392
Perkins, D. 429
Perlmutter, A.P. 161
Peterziel, H. 413
Pisani, E. 93
Polito, M. 17
Ponchietti, R. 32
Pontes, J.E. 210
Porru, D. 233
Porsche, C. 249
Powell, I.J. 210
Prévot, M.-H. 239
Prezioso, D. 17
Putz, T. 413

Qian, J. 479, 492

Rainer, C. 304
Rambeaud, J.-J. 32
Rao, K.V.N. 464
Ravery, V. 52, 239, 298
Reichardt, J.K.V. 355
Reichelt, O. 272
Reiher, F. 204
Reissigl, A. 523
Renneberg, H. 27
Rhodes, T. 277
Riedmiller, H. 217
Rietbergen, J. 539
Ristol, J. 323
Roberts, R.O. 277
Rogatsch, H. 523
Rosette, J.J.M.C.H. de la 9, 173
Ross, M. 439
Ross, R.K. 355
Roukema, J.A. 197

Sachsinger, J. 249
Sağol, Ö. 109
Sakr, W.A. 474
Salomon, L. 289
Samland, D. 204
Sánchez, E. 26
Sauter, Th. 81
Sauty, L. 239
Scarpa, R.M. 233
Scarpelli, M. 468
Schlichter, A. 272
Schmidt, U. 204
Schostak, M. 81
Schröder, F.H. 539
Schubert, J. 272
Schulman, C.C. 1, 341, 498
Schwabegger, A.H. 304
Sejima, T. 242
Serrago, M.P. 93
Settesoldi, D. 2
Severi, G. 370
Shadmani, R. 388
Sharpe, P. 327
Sica, G. 2
Sigman, C.C. 342
Solomon, L.Z. 327
Sporn, M.B. 420
Steele, V.E. 342
Steinbach, F. 204
Steiner, U. 81
Stenzl, A. 304
Sternberg, C. 52
Strigaris, K. 102
Strohmaier, W.L. 21
Studen, M. 523
Sylvester, R. 267, 519

Taille, A. de la 312
Takeda NHT Italian Group 17
Tefilli, M.V. 210
Têtu, B. 508
Thompson, D. 468, 484
Thompson, I.M., Jr. 544
Tiguert, R. 210
Torre-Holguera, P. de la 318
Torres, I. de 294
Toubert, M.-E. 89
Toublanc, M. 298
Treiber, U. 52
Trinchieri, A. 93
Tunn, U.W. 27
Urban, D. 429
Usai, E. 233

Vallancien, G. 161
Vande Walle, J. 57
Van Gool, J.D. 57
Van Laecke, E. 57
Vaught, L. 484
Vayreda-Martija, J.M. 318
Veelken, H. 70
Vicente-Rodríguez, J. 318
Villavicencio-Mavrich, H. 318
Visakorpi, T. 351
Volgger, H. 523

Walsh, I.K. 192
Waters, D.J. 456
Weidner, W. 177
Weiner, D.M. 166
Weingärtner, K. 217
Weiss, H. 429
Wettig, I.C. 81
Whelan, P. 424
Whitfield, H. 147
Wijkstra, H. 9
Woo, H. 119
Wood, D.P., Jr. 210
Wunderlich, H. 272

Yamanishi, T. 45
Yasuda, K. 45
Yörükoğlu, K. 109

Zanetti, G. 93
Zelano, G. 2
Zerbib, M. 1, 37
Zermann, D.-H. 272
Zilberman, M. 285
Zlotta, A.R. 173, 498

Subject Index Vol. 35, 1999

European Urology

Supplement issue No. 1 has its own Subject Index
Supplement issue No. 2 does not have a Subject Index

Adenocarcinoma 223
Adjuvant hormonal treatment 23
Adrenalectomy, indications 272
Ageing 370
AIDS 239
Alkaline phosphatase 21
Amplification 351
AMS 800 36
Androgen(s) 355
  deprivation therapy 492
  receptor 351, 413
  suppression 32
  withdrawal 413
Angiogenesis 2
Angiomyolipoma 249
Animal models 456, 459
Antigens 26
Apoptosis 395
Arachidonic acid 395
Artificial implants 36
  organs 257
  sphincter 36
bcl-2 242, 399
Benign prostatic hyperplasia 119, 129, 138, 147, 155, 161, 177, 185
Biopsy 289, 298
Bladder 257, 323
  cancer 2, 52, 89, 93
  disease 257
  neoplasms 52, 228
  tumor antigen 93
α-Blocker 45
Bone 197
  scan 21, 223
BPH 439
Breast cancer 424
BTA 89
  stat™ test 52

Cancer 392, 399, 456
CaP 439
Carcinogenesis 456
Carcinoma, transitional cell: diagnosis, pathology, urine 81
Cell line 70
Cervical cancer 424
Chemoprevention 342, 370, 377, 392, 420, 424, 429, 443, 456, 459, 464, 474, 492, 508, 511, 515, 519
Chemotherapy 323
Chromosomal anomaly 479
Coagulation 166
Community study 277
Comparative genomic hybridization 351
Complications 36, 210
Computer interpretation 9
Computed tomography 318
Confocal microscopy 327
Contrast agents 9
Cost 210
CT scan 21
Cytokines 70
Cytology 52, 93

Dehydroepiandrosterone 464
Deletion 351
Deltanoids 420
Desiccation 166
Diagnosis 26, 298
Diet 362, 377, 388
Dietary fat 395
α-Difluoromethylornithine 464
DNA adducts 468
Double-blind study 45
Drug development 342
Du-145 413
Dysfunctional voiding 57

Efficacy testing 459
Electrovaporization 166
Endocrine therapy 508
Endpoints 519
Endorectal coil magnetic resonance imaging 32
Enhanced Doppler imaging 9
Enucleation 155
Environment 362
Enzyme-altered foci 468
Epidemiology 277, 370, 474
Epidermal growth factor 395
Epirubicin 327
Estramustine 327

Fat 388
Fenretinide 429
Finasteride 544
Flow cytometry 327
Fluorescence in situ hybridization 351, 479

KARGER

Fax + 41 61 306 12 34
E-Mail karger@karger.ch
www.karger.com

Accessible online at:
http://BioMedNet.com/karger

Gene expression 408
Genetic alterations 351, 479
Genetics 355, 362
Glutathione S-transferase 468
GM-CSF 70

Head and neck cancer 424
Histology 17
Histometry 484
Histopathology 508
Holmium 155
Holmium:YAG laser 233
Hormonal therapy 492
Hormone dependence 32
Hormone-refractory disease 351
Hydronephrosis 102
(4-Hydroxyphenyl)retinamide 429
N-(4-Hydroxyphenyl)retinamide (fehretinide) 464

IL-2 204
IL-6 70
IL-8 70
IL-10 70
Image analysis 468
Impotence 312
Incontinence 217
Indicator-dilution curves 9
Indinavir 239
Inguinal defect 304
Ischaemia 36
Interferon-α 204
Intergroup clinical trial 544
Intermittent hormone therapy 32
Interstitial laser therapy 147
Intestinal mucosa 98
Intracavernous injection 312
Intracellular signalling 443
Intravesical therapy 2
Invasive adenocarcinoma 468
Isoflavonoids 443

Karyometry 484
Ki-67 399
Kidney cancer 249
  neoplasms 204

Laser 138, 155
  prostatectomy 147
  surgery 285
Liarozole fumarate 464
Ligand-independent activation 413
Lignans 443
5-Lipoxygenase 395
LNCaP 413
Long-term follow-up, impotence 312
Lower urinary tract symptoms 277

Lung 197
  cancer 424

Magnetic resonance urography 102
Malignancy-associated changes 468
Marker 408
Metastases 197, 223, 479
Microvascularization 109
Morbidity 36
Morcellation 155
mRNA expression 439
Mucins 98
Multidrug resistance 327

Needle biopsy 109
Neoadjuvant hormonal treatment 17
Neodymium:YAG 138
Neurogenic bladder 45
Neuromodulation 192
NMP22 93
Noninvasive diagnosis 102

Oltipraz 464
Oncocytoma 249
Organ-confined tumors 523
Orthotopic neobladder 98

p53 242, 399
Palliation 304
Paracrine control 439
Phyto-oestrogens 377
PIN I/III 504
Power 166
Practical aspects of clinical trials 515
Predictive value 459
Preliminary results 539
Premalignant nature 456
Pressure/flow study 45
Prevention 544
Primary tumor cell culture 70
Probability of prostate cancer 523
Prognosis 399
Progression index 484
Proliferating cell nuclear antigen 242
Proliferative activity 508
Prostate 119, 138, 223, 285, 342, 392, 399, 456, 468
  biopsy 496
  cancer 9, 17, 23, 32, 210, 289, 294, 298, 362, 370, 377, 388, 408, 424, 429, 459, 464, 474, 504, 515, 519, 539, 544
  carcinoma 109
  neoplasms 492
  size 277
  vaporization 161
Prostatectomy 138, 155, 285, 289
Prostate-specific antigen 21, 223, 523

intraepithelial neoplasia 468, 474, 479, 484, 492, 496, 498, 508
neoplasms 26, 355, 498
Prostatitis 177
Prostatodynia 177
Prosthesis 36
PSA 413
as surrogate marker 511
screening 523

Quality of life 177, 277

Radiation therapy 492
Radical prostatectomy 17, 210, 217, 399
Radiofrequency 119
Radiotherapy 23, 323
Random biopsies 267
Randomized study 539
Receptors 362
Reconstruction 304
Recurrence, bladder cancer 2
5α-Reductase isoenzymes 439
Renal cell carcinoma 70, 197, 204, 242, 249, 272
dilatation 102
obstruction 102
pelvis neoplasm 318
Reporter gene 413
Resection 155
Resistance 166
9-*cis*-Retinoic acid 464
Retinoids 420, 424
Reversal 327

Screening 539
tests 539
L-Selenomethionine 464
Sexuality 177
Silicone 36
Small cell bladder carcinoma 323
intestine 98
Soft tissue defect 304
Sonography 21
Stage migration 523
Staging 289
Statistical considerations 519
Superficial bladder cancer 327
Suprapubic region 304
Surgery 197
Surrogate endpoint biomarker 429
Survival 197
Systematic biopsies 294

Tamoxifen 420
Ta,T1 bladder cancer 267
Telomerase 468
activity 249
TGF-β_1 70
Therapeutic options 9
Therapy 197, 408
Thermal therapy 119
Thermotherapy 129
Timing treatment 504
TNF-α 70
DL-α-Tocopherol (vitamin E) 464
Transcriptional activity 413
Transcutaneous electrical neurostimulation 192
Transition zone biopsies 294
index 185
volume 185
Transitional cell 228
carcinoma 318
zone cancer 523
Transurethral microwave thermotherapy 129
needle ablation 119
resection, prostate 161, 185
vaporization, prostate 161
Tumor markers 89
biological: urine 81
surgery 304
volume 32
Tumor-associated antigen 52
Ultrasonography 26
Ultrasound 9
Urapidil 45

Ureter neoplasm 318
Ureteral dilatation 102
stones 233
Ureterolithotripsy 233
Ureteroscopy 233
Urethra 36
Urge syndrome 57
Urinary cytology 228
diversion 98, 257
Urine marker 93
Urodynamic study 57
Urodynamics 57, 217
Urolithiasis 239
Urologic neoplasms: pathology, urine 81

Vaporizing loop 161
Vascular endothelial growth factor 2
Vitamin D 392
E 388
Voiding dysfunction 192

Vol. 35, 1999

Official Journal of the

European Association of Urology

EORTC — European Organization for Research and Treatment of Cancer – Genito-Urinary Group

ESUOE — European Society for Urological Oncology and Endocrinology

European Urology

KARGER

Basel · Freiburg · Paris · London · New York · New Delhi · Bangkok · Singapore · Tokyo · Sydney

S. Karger
Medical and Scientific Publishers
Basel · Freiburg · Paris · London
New York · New Delhi · Bangkok
Singapore · Tokyo · Sydney

Drug Dosage
The authors and the publisher have exerted every effort to ensure that drug selection and dosage set forth in this text are in accord with current recommendations and practice at the time of publication. However, in view of ongoing research, changes in government regulations, and the constant flow of information relating to drug therapy and drug reactions, the reader is urged to check the package insert for each drug for any change in indications and dosage and for added warnings and precautions. This is particularly important when the recommended agent is a new and/or infrequently employed drug.

P.O. Box, CH–4009 Basel (Switzerland)
Printed in Switzerland on acid-free paper by
Druckerei Schüler AG, Biel

KARGER

Fax + 41 61 306 12 34
E-Mail karger@karger.ch
www.karger.com

Contents Vol. 35, 1999

European Urology

No. 1

1 **Editorial**

Review

2 **Vascular Endothelial Growth Factor: An Important Angiogenic Mediator in Bladder Cancer**
Crew, J.P. (Oxford)

Clinical Papers

9 **Contrast Angiosonography: A Technology to Improve Doppler Ultrasound Examinations of the Prostate**
Aarnink, R.G.; Beerlage, H.P.; de la Rosette, J.J.M.C.H.; Debruyne, F.M.J.; Wijkstra, H. (Nijmegen)

21 **Follow-Up in Prostate Cancer Patients: Which Parameters Are Necessary?**
Strohmaier, W.L. (Coburg); Keller, T.; Bichler, K.H. (Tübingen)

26 **Final Results of a Screening Campaign for Prostate Cancer**
Martín, E.; Luján, M.; Sánchez, E.; Herrero, A.; Páez, A.; Berenguer, A. (Madrid)

32 **Estimation of Prostate Cancer Volume by Endorectal Coil Magnetic Resonance Imagings vs. Pathologic Volume**
Ponchietti, R.; Di Loro, F.; Fanfani, A.; Amorosi, A. (Florence)

36 **A Review of the Complications and Results of Implantation of the AMS Artificial Urinary Sphincter**
Hajivassiliou, C.A. (Glasgow)

45 **A Multicenter Placebo-Controlled, Double-Blind Trial of Urapidil, an α-Blocker, on Neurogenic Bladder Dysfunction**
Yamanishi, T. (Chiba); Yasuda, K.; Homma, Y.; Kawabe, K.; Morita, T. (Tokyo)

52 **Comparison of the BTA *stat*™ Test with Voided Urine Cytology and Bladder Wash Cytology in the Diagnosis and Monitoring of Bladder Cancer**
Leyh, H. (Munich); Marberger, M. (Vienna); Conort, P. (Paris); Sternberg, C.; Pansadoro, V. (Rome); Pagano, F.; Bassi, P. (Padua); Boccon-Gibod, L.; Ravery, V. (Paris); Treiber, U. (Munich); Ishak, L. (Redmond, Wash.)

Pediatric Urology

57 **Assessment of Lower Urinary Tract Dysfunction in Children with Non-Neuropathic Bladder Sphincter Dysfunction**
Hoebeke, P.; Vande Walle, J.; Everaert, K.; Van Laecke, E. (Ghent); Van Gool, J.D. (Utrecht)

Basic Science

70 **Pro-Inflammatory and T Cell Inhibitory Cytokines Are Secreted at High Levels in Tumor Cell Cultures of Human Renal Cell Carcinoma**
Lahn, M.; Fisch, P.; Köhler, G.; Kunzmann, R.; Hentrich, I.; Jesuiter, H.; Behringer, D.; Muschal, B.; Veelken, H.; Kulmburg, P. (Freiburg); Iklé, D.N. (Denver, Colo.); Lindemann, A. (Freiburg)

81 **Quantitative Detection of Human Complement Factor H-Related Protein in Transitional Cell Carcinoma of the Urinary Bladder**
Heicappell, R.; Wettig, I.C.; Schostak, M.; Müller, M.; Steiner, U.; Sauter, T.; Miller, K. (Berlin)

8, 44, 87 **Congress Calendar**

88 **Forthcoming Papers**

Curriculum in Urology 1.1

Pediatrics
Phimosis and Circumcision in Children
Büyükalpelli, R.; Sarıkaya, Ş.; Ascı, R. (Samsun)

No. 2

Clinical Papers

89 **BTA *stat* and BTA TRAK: A Comparative Evaluation of Urine Testing for the Diagnosis of Transitional Cell Carcinoma of the Bladder**
Irani, J. (Poitiers); Desgrandchamps, F. (Paris); Millet, C. (Poitiers); Toubert, M.-E. (Paris); Bon, D.; Aubert, J. (Poitiers); Le Duc, A. (Paris)

93 **Evaluation of Urinary Level of NMP22 as a Diagnostic Marker for Stage pTa-pT1 Bladder Cancer: Comparison with Urinary Cytology and BTA Test**
Del Nero, A.; Esposito, N.; Currò, A.; Biasoni, D.; Montanari, E.; Mangiarotti, B.; Trinchieri, A.; Zanetti, G.; Serrago, M.P.; Pisani, E. (Milan)

98 **Abnormal Patterns of Mucin Secretion in Ileal Neobladder Mucosa: Evidence of Preneoplastic Lesion?**
Parenti, A.; Aragona, F.; Bortuzzo, G.; De Caro, R.; Pagano, F. (Padua)

102 **MR Urography in the Diagnosis of Urinary Tract Obstruction**
Louca, G.; Liberopoulos, K.; Fidas, A.; Nikolakopoulou, Z.; Lykourinas, M.; Strigaris, K. (Athens)

109 **Comparison of Microvascularization in Diagnostic Needle Biopsies and Radical Prostatectomies in Prostate Carcinoma**
Yörükoğlu, K.; Sağol, Ö.; Özkara, E.; Mungan, U.; Kırkalı, Z. (Izmir)

113 **Congress Calendar**

114 **Forthcoming Papers**

KARGER

Fax +41 61 306 12 34
E-Mail karger@karger.ch
www.karger.com

Access to full text and tables of contents, including tentative ones for forthcoming issues:
www.karger.com/journals/eur/eur_bk.htm

Alternative Instrumental Treatments in BPH
Guest Editors: J. de la Rosette, Nijmegen; A.R. Zlotta, Brussels

117 **Introduction**
Fitzpatrick, J.M. (Dublin)

119 **Transurethral Needle Ablation (TUNA™)**
A Critical Review of Radiofrequency Thermal Therapy in the Management of Benign Prostatic Hyperplasia
Chapple, C.R. (Sheffield); Issa, M.M. (Atlanta, Ga.); Woo, H. (Sydney)

129 **Transurethral Microwave Thermotherapy**
Lynch, J.H. (Washington, D.C.); Höfner, K. (Hannover)

138 **Side-Firing Neodymium:YAG Laser Prostatectomy**
Costello, A.J. (Melbourne); Kabalin, J.N. (Scottsbluff, Nebr.)

147 **Interstitial Laser Therapy of Benign Prostatic Hyperplasia**
Muschter, R.; Whitfield, H. (Munich)

155 **Holmium Laser Resection of the Prostate**
Le Duc, A. (Paris); Gilling, P.J. (Tauranga)

161 **Thick Loop Transurethral Resection of the Prostate**
Perlmutter, A.P. (New York, N.Y.); Vallancien, G. (Paris)

166 **Electrosurgery: VaporTrode**
Weiner, D.M.; Kaplan, S.A. (New York, N.Y.)

173 **Future Perspectives**
de la Rosette, J.J.M.C.H.; Zlotta, A.R. (Brussels)

Curriculum in Urology 2.3

Infections and Stones
Septicaemia and Shock
Ryan, D.W. (Newcastle upon Tyne)

No. 3

Review

177 **Prostate and Sexuality: An Overview**
Burger, B. (Munich); Weidner, W. (Giessen); Altwein, J.E. (Munich)

Clinical Papers

185 **A New Parameter in Decision Making for Transurethral Electroresection of Benign Prostate Hyperplasia**
Otani, T.; Hayashi, Y.; Kishino, T.; Fujimoto, K.; Hirao, Y.; Ozono, S.; Okajima, E. (Nara)

192 **Transcutaneous Sacral Neurostimulation for Irritative Voiding Dysfunction**
Walsh, I.K.; Johnston, R.S.; Keane, P.F. (Belfast)

197 **Metastasectomy in Renal Cell Carcinoma: A Multicenter Retrospective Analysis**
van der Poel, H.G. (Nijmegen); Roukema, J.A. (Tilburg); Horenblas, S. (Amsterdam); van Geel, A.N. (Rotterdam); Debruyne, F.M.J. (Nijmegen)

204 **Results of Immunochemotherapy with Interleukin-2, Interferon-α2 and 5-Fluorouracil in the Treatment of Metastatic Renal Cell Cancer**
Samland, D.; Steinbach, F.; Reiher, F.; Schmidt, U.; Gruss, A.; Allhoff, E.P. (Magdeburg)

210 **Results of a Clinical Care Pathway for Radical Prostatectomy Patients in an Open Hospital – Multiphysician System**
Gheiler, E.L.; Lovisolo, J.A.J.; Tiguert, R.; Tefilli, M.V.; Grayson, T.; Oldford, G.; Powell, I.J.; Famiglietti, G.; Banerjee, M.; Pontes, J.E.; Wood, D.P., Jr. (Detroit, Mich.)

217 **Changes of Urodynamic Findings after Radical Retropubic Prostatectomy**
Kleinhans, B.; Gerharz, E.; Melekos, M.; Weingärtner, K.; Kälble, T.; Riedmiller, H. (Marburg)
[Editorial Comment by K.-P. Jünemann, Mannheim]

223 **Influence of Local Tumour Stage and Grade on Reliability of Serum Prostate-Specific Antigen in Predicting Skeletal Metastases in Patients with Adenocarcinoma of the Prostate**
Bruwer, G.; Heyns, C.F.; Allen, F.J. (Tygerberg)

228 **Reliability of the Routine Cytological Diagnosis in Bladder Cancer**
Páez, A.; Coba, J.M.; Murillo, N.; Fernández, P.; de la Cal, M.A.; Luján, M.; Berenguer, A. (Madrid)

233 **Holmium:YAG Laser Ureterolithotripsy**
Scarpa, R.M.; De Lisa, A.; Porru, D.; Usai, E. (Cagliari)

239 **Urolithiasis and the Protease Inhibitor Indinavir**
Hermieu, J.-F.; Prévot, M.-H.; Ravery, V.; Sauty, L.; Moulinier, F.; Delmas, V.; Bouvet, E.; Boccon-Gibod, L. (Paris)

Basic Science

242 **Expression of Bcl-2, p53 Oncoprotein, and Proliferating Cell Nuclear Antigen in Renal Cell Carcinoma**
Sejima, T.; Miyagawa, I. (Yonago)

249 **Telomerase Activity in Malignant and Benign Renal Tumors**
Müller, M.; Heicappell, R.; Krause, H.; Sachsinger, J.; Porsche, C.; Miller, K. (Berlin)

238, 248 **Congress Calendar**
256 **Forthcoming Papers**

Curriculum in Urology 6.3

Oncology
Primary Carcinoma in situ of the Urinary Bladder: Diagnosis and Management
Boccon-Gibod, L. (Paris)

No. 4

Review

257 **The Artificial Bladder**
Desgrandchamps, F. (Paris); Griffith, D.P. (Huston, Tex.)

Clinical Papers

267 **Significance of Bladder Biopsies in Ta,T1 Bladder Tumors: A Report from the EORTC Genito-Urinary Tract Cancer Cooperative Group**
van der Meijden, A. ('s-Hertogenbosch); Oosterlinck, W. (Gent); Brausi, M. (Capri); Kurth, K.-H. (Amsterdam); Sylvester, R.; de Balincourt, C.; Members of the EORTC-GU Group Superficial Bladder Committee (Brussels)

272 **Real Indications for Adrenalectomy in Renal Cell Carcinoma**
Wunderlich, H.; Schlichter, A.; Reichelt, O.; Zermann, D.-H.; Janitzky, V.; Kosmehl, H.; Schubert, J. (Jena)

277 **Association of Health-Related Quality of Life and Benign Prostatic Enlargement**
Girman, C.J. (West Point, Pa./Rochester, Minn.); Jacobsen, S.J. (Rochester, Minn.); Rhodes, T. (West Point, Pa.); Guess, H.A. (West Point, Pa./Rochester, Minn./Chapel Hill, N.C.); Roberts, R.O.; Lieber, M.M. (Rochester, Minn.)

285 **Laser Prostatectomy.** Long-Term Follow-Up of 303 Patients
Chertin, B.; Moriel, E.Z.; Hadas-Halperin, I.; Abu-Arafeh, W.; Lupa, S.; Zilberman, M.; Farkas, A. (Jerusalem)

289 **Value of Ultrasound-Guided Systematic Sextant Biopsies in Prostate Tumor Mapping**
Salomon, L.; Colombel, M.; Patard, J.-J.; Lefrère-Belda, M.-A.; Bellot, J.; Chopin, D.; Abbou, C.-C. (Créteil)

294 **Value of Routine Transition Zone Biopsies in Patients Undergoing Ultrasound-Guided Sextant Biopsies for the First Time**
Morote, J.; López, M.; Encabo, G.; deTorres, I. (Barcelona)

Prostatitis and Urethritis

M. Ludwig, W. Weidner
Urologische Klinik, Justus-Liebig-Universität Giessen, Deutschland

The prostatitis syndrome is of great significance for urologists as has been demonstrated in recent studies dealing with epidemiologic data. A new classification has been suggested. A detailed standardized diagnostic procedure remains mandatory to differentiate the various forms of prostatitis. Though new insights into pathogenic factors have been achieved, the genesis of chronic prostatitis often remains uncertain. Treatment options must be considered according to the diagnostic results; however, they are often limited and aimed at improving symptoms. Logically, the therapy of infectious urethritis should follow a standardized diagnostic procedure, so as to administer antimicrobials effective against the underlying etiologic cause.

Definitions

Epidemiologic research during the last decade has indicated 'prostatitis' to be one of the major medical healthcare problems in urology. Recent data revealed that, in 1985, there were more office visits for prostatitis than for BPH or prostate cancer resulting in 2 million office visits per year in the early 1990s and representing the most common urologic diagnosis in men less than 50 years of age [overview in 1].

Traditionally, prostatitis has been classified into four clinical entities: acute bacterial (ABP) and prostatic abscess as sequelae of ABP, chronic bacterial (CBP), non- or abacterial prostatitis (NBP) and prostatodynia (Pd) [2, 3]. Whereas the first three types had widely been accepted as being of inflammatory origin, Pd described a condition when, despite clinical symptoms, neither signs of inflammation nor of infection have been detectable. Though being rarely questioned, this classification system did not address adequately several important problems concerning the diagnostic work-up. The major questions still to be answered have recently been summarized by Nickel [1]:

M. Ludwig, MD
Urologische Klinik, Justus-Liebig-Universität Giessen
Klinikstrasse 29, D-35385 Giessen (Germany)
Tel. +49 641 9944501, Fax +49 641 9944509
E-Mail: w.weidner@chiru.med.uni-giessen.de

Eur Urol 1999;35/5–6 (Curric Urol 2.4:1–10)
Published in cooperation with European Urology and Karger

Table 1. The new National Institutes of Health classification of the prostatitis syndrome

Category	Name	Description
I	Acute bacterial prostatitis	Acute infection of the prostate gland
II	Chronic bacterial prostatitis	Recurrent infection of the prostate
III	Chronic abacterial prostatitis/ chronic pelvic pain syndrome (CPPS)	No demonstrable infection
IIIA	Inflammatory chronic pelvic pain syndrome	White cells in semen, expressed prostatic secretions or post-prostatic massage urine
IIIB	Non-inflammatory chronic pelvic pain syndrome	No white cells in semen, expressed prostatic secretions or post-prostatic massage urine
IV	Asymptomatic inflammatory prostatitis	No subjective symptoms, detected either by prostate biopsy or the presence of white cells in expressed prostatic secretions or semen during evaluation for other disorders

- In 'bacterial prostatitis', the etiologic relevance of enterococci, coagulase-negative staphylococci, chlamydia, and anaerobes has remained unsolved. In patients with an initial diagnosis of bacterial prostatitis and lack of positive cultures in case of symptom recurrence, it is not known whether the pathogen was eradicated ('nonbacterial prostatitis'). It might well be that due to antimicrobial and immunologic threat, bacteria have formed small microcolonies surrounded by a protective coat of extrapolymeric slime (still: bacterial prostatitis), thus sustaining symptoms by plugging prostatic ducts.
- The origin of 'nonbacterial prostatitis' has remained even more mysterious. Immunological and autoimmunological factors have been discussed. On the other hand, there has been evidence that in some cases 'nonbacterial prostatitis' may be secondary to nonuropathogenic or cryptic microorganisms. In these cases, the term 'nonbacterial' is not fully correct.
- The term 'prostatodynia' has always provoked the most confusion. Though being defined by the absence of leukocytes in expressed prostatic secretions (EPS) it has never been validated. It has been suggested that this entitiy may not be related to the prostate but rather to a neuromuscular disorder of the pelvic floor/perineal neuromuscular unit.
- Finally, the occurrence of asymptomatic inflammation of the prostate noted histologically in BPH specimens, prostate biopsies or detected in EPS during evaluation for other disorders has not been addressed in the traditional nomenclature. This implies on the other hand that 'symptomatic' disease should best be defined by a standardized questionnaire.

Therefore, in order to acquire a better definition and understanding of the prostatitis syndrome, a new classification system has recently been proposed by a meeting of the National Institue of Diabetes, Digestive, and Kidney Diseases (NIDDK) [1] (table 1). This new classification system focuses on the clinical and diagnostic problems concerning chronic prostatitis and has become the reference standard for research studies on these diseases and disorders.

Microbiology

ABP, CBP, and, even more, prostatic abscess are important but uncommon diseases. The most common etiologic causes of bacterial

prostatitis are gram-negative pathogens, predominantly strains of *Escherichia coli* which have been identified in 65–80% of infections [4–6]. *Pseudomonas aeruginosa, Serratia, Klebsiella,* and *Enterobacter aerogenes* have been isolated in 10–15% [4].

Controversies exist regarding the role of gram-positive bacteria as pathogens in bacterial prostatitis. Whereas enterococci may cause bacterial prostatitis and associated recurrent urinary tract infections (UTI), the significance of other gram-positive bacteria is doubtful. Though they are believed to represent commensals of the anterior urethra, these bacteria may become pathogenic under certain circumstances [7]. Sporadical incidences of *Staphylococcus saprophyticus,* hemolytic streptococci [4], *Staphylococcus aureus* and coagulase-negative staphylococci [8] as well as *Neisseria gonorrhoeae, Mycobacterium tuberculosis, Salmonella, Clostridia,* and parasitic or mycotic organisms have been reported. Moreover, immunocompromised states, particularly HIV infection and AIDS, may well lead to an increase of bacterial forms of prostatitis and to an increasing significance of uncommon pathogens.

The role of *Chlamydia trachomatis* and mycoplasma, particularly *Ureaplasma (U.) urealyticum,* in some cases of chronic prostatitis remains highly equivocal. Some authors were able to associate the finding of *C. trachomatis* and high numbers of *U. urealyticum* in prostatic secretions with symptomatic disease whereas, in contrast, others did not confirm these results [overviews in 4, 9]. In patients with NBP, some authors tried to demonstrate chlamydial infection of the prostate by transrectal biopsy, open surgery and transurethral resection [overview in 4]. However, results have remained contradictory. Culture for *C. trachomatis* or demonstration of the antigen by immunofluorescence test was typically negative after transperineal puncture of the prostate. In contrast, after transrectal or transurethral procedures, positive results were obtained, which, unfortunately, did not exclude contamination via the prostatic urethra or the rectum. Recently, new techniques (immunofluorescence, in situ hybridization, and transmission electron microscopy) have shown evidence of a true infection of the prostate epithelium with *C. trachomatis* [10, 11].

The prostate gland is known to be capable of both a systemic and local immune response to invading pathogens. In acute bacterial prostatitis, serum *and* prostatic fluid antigen-specific IgG and IgA antibodies against gram-negative pathogens have been found, whereas, in CBP, serum antibodies were not detectable [overview in 12]. On the other hand, antigen-specific antibodies were not increased in chronic prostatitis patients with mycoplasmal or chlamydial infection compared to those without evidence of these pathogens [13]. In contrast, in chronic prostatitis, a Japanese study group has found a correlation with IgA antibodies specific for *C. trachomatis* and anti-heat shock protein IgA in EPS by immunoblotting (Western blot) [14].

The role of *U. urealyticum* is still being discussed. It has been agreed that pathogen counts of $<10^3$ cfu/ml should be judged as normal urethral contamination [overview in 4]. Although several studies investigating prostatitis identified this pathogen with chronic idiopathic prostatitis, increased titers of antiureaplasmal IgA in EPS were not present [13]. In summary, these pathogens may be capable of ascending to the prostate gland, but definite evidence for prostatic infection in chronic idiopathic prostatitis has yet to be confirmed by further immunohistological, immunocytological or molecular biological studies.

Antibody-coated bacteria (ACB) have been described in the ejaculate of patients with CBP in contrast to patients with inflammatory and noninflammatory chronic pelvic pain syndrome (CPPS) or normal controls. A hypothesis of bacteria serving as an antigen stimulus and thereby initiating an immunological process that results in (bacterial) prostatitis has been proposed. The known and unknown immunological aspects of chronic prostatitis have recently been re-evaluated [15] (table 2).

Recent data indicate that bacteria may have an etiological role in patients with chronic idiopathic prostatitis after exclusion of CBP. Krieger et al. [16] integrated molecular meth-

Table 2. Immunological aspects of prostatitis [15]

Antibody-coated bacteria
Serum and prostatic fluid antigen-specific IgG and IgA antibodies
Altered phagocytotic activity
Mast cell degranulation
Cytokine production (particularly interleukin-6)
Autoantibodies
T-lymphocyte-mediated autoimmunity

ods in the bacteriological examination of men experiencing chronic pelvic pain and found procaryotic 16s RNA significantly more often in patients with increased leukocyte numbers in their prostatic secretions than in those without. These findings suggest that the prostate may harbor microorganisms not detectable by traditional approaches. Even when analyzing transperineal prostate biopsies by traditional culture, Berger et al. [17] demonstrated a significantly higher bacterial isolation, more positive cultures for anaerobic bacteria, higher bacterial counts, and more bacterial species isolated in men with inflammatory cells in their EPS. In patients with Pd, positive cultures of bacteria, mostly coagulase-negative staphylococci, were found in prostatic secretions [18]. However, the significance of these findings remains uncertain for implicating a bacterial etiology in some cases of CPPS and needs further evaluation.

Diagnosis

Only in ABP is it possible to establish the diagnosis on clinical grounds: Dysuria, pollakisuria and perineal pain as well as pain during defecation, and even acute urinary retention have been described. Systemic symptoms include fever and shivering rigors. Urosepsis may develop. Digital rectal examination (DRE) is extremely painful due to a markedly tender prostate. The clinical diagnosis of prostatic abscess is based on fluctuation during DRE and imaging procedures, especially transrectal ultrasonography (TRUS) (see following section).

The remaining forms of the prostatitis syndrome cannot be differentiated on the basis of their clinical symptoms. They include typical local signs of inflammation, diffuse anogenital symptoms, bladder voiding disturbances, and sexual dysfunction. Chronic pelvic pain has been suggested to be a leading symptom [19]. As there are multidimensional associations to physical and mental health status, a comprehensive symptomatic evaluation appears necessary using appropriate questionnaires with the aim of providing the possibility to ask for typical 'true' prostatitis symptoms and to quantify symptom severity. First experience with different scoring systems are available: these include the University of Washington Symptom Score, the Prostatitis Symptom Severity Index and the Giessen Prostatitis Symptom Score [overview in 20].

As clinical symptomatology does not allow a differentiation, the only way to discriminate inflammatory CPPS or CBP from noninflammatory CPPS is the demonstration of leukocytes and lipid-laden macrophages in the case of inflammatory CPPS and CBP. Controversies exist on the criterion number of white blood cells indicative for inflammation. The cutoff point for inflammatory disease has been suggested at ≥ 10 and ≥ 15 white blood cells per high-power field, respectively [overview in 20]. When insufficient or no EPS is obtained for analysis, the presence of ≥ 10 granulocytes/high-power field in urine after prostatic massage has been proposed to be indicative of inflammation [overview in 20]. In some cases, this technique appears to simplify the rationale of diagnostic procedures, provided that first and midstream urine are free of leukocytes. Staining procedures simplify identification and quantification of leukocytes. Recent data indicate an increased sensitivity to detect inflammation when using a counting chamber [21].

Laboratory diagnosis of CBP is based on the four-specimen test for bacterial localization [3]. Its principle is to perform sequential quantitative bacteriologic cultures of the urethra, bladder urine and prostatic secretions both in EPS and urine after prostatic massage (VB 3). The diagnosis is confirmed when quantifiable path-

ogenic bacteria can clearly be ascribed to the prostate gland. The growth of only small numbers of bacteria of prostatic fluid is pathognomonic in CBP. There exists no absolute count in cfu/ml to diagnose CBP; instead, the counts of bacteria in the above-mentioned specimens must be compared. Demonstration of bacteria in EPS or VB 3, when the urethra and midstream urine specimens show no growth, is highly suggestive of CBP. Alternatively, a significant increase of a log or more in the bacterial count in the prostatic specimens when compared to urethral and bladder specimens is considered diagnostic.

The hallmark of CBP is relapsing bacteriuria. If UTI is present, the diagnosis of CBP is hampered by a high bacterial count in the midstream urine. In these cases, 3 days' administration of nitrofurantoin prior to the performance of the 'four-specimens test' has been recommended. Nitrofurantoin is able to clear the midstream urine of pathogens, whereas the number of bacteria in prostatic secretions is untouched due to the inability of nitrofurantoin to penetrate prostatic tissue.

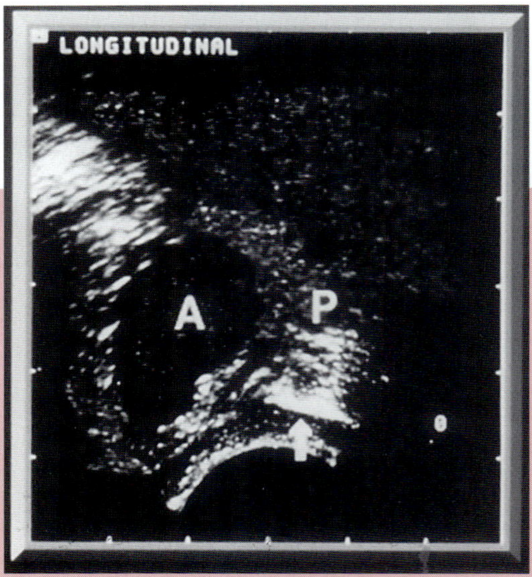

Fig. 1. Transrectal drainage of prostatic abscess (image digitally remastered). A = Abscess; P = prostate gland; arrow = needle.

Ejaculate Analysis

An ejaculate analysis is done to obtain further information about whether the prostate is part of a generalized infection of the male accessory sex glands. After exclusion of urethritis and bladder infection, the presence of $\geq 10^6$ peroxidase-positive white blood cells/ml ejaculate indicates an inflammatory process [22]. In these cases a culture should be performed. A concentration of $\geq 10^3$ cfu/ml of urinary tract pathogens in the ejaculate is regarded as a significant finding. It must be kept in mind that the ejaculate analysis does not allow a definitive localization of the inflammatory process, because the ejaculate represents a mixture of different genital secretions and is usually contaminated by pathogens from the anterior urethra.

In patients with inflammatory CPPS, increased peroxidase-positive leukocytes and PMN-elastase levels seem to be present as compared to noninflammatory CPPS and controls. Recently an increase in the concentration of interleukin-6 in seminal plasma has been desribed as indicator of accessory gland inflammation. In CBP, a significant bacteriospermia with the same pathogen as isolated by the four-specimens technique is demonstrable in about 50% of cases [overview in 20].

Some authors have reported on poor sperm quality (reduced sperm count, abnormal motility, morphologic defects), but these results remain controversial due to a possibly inprecise definition of the inflammatory patient groups [overview in 20].

Screening of Bladder Voiding

The evaluation of the bladderemptying process is accepted to be a mandatory diagnostic step in patients with prostatitis-like symptoms. However, discrepancies exist about the prevalence of urodynamic abnormalities in these patients. Whereas the Giessen prostatitis study group found urodynamic changes in approximately 33–45 % of patients following the analysis of urinary flow patterns, other

a

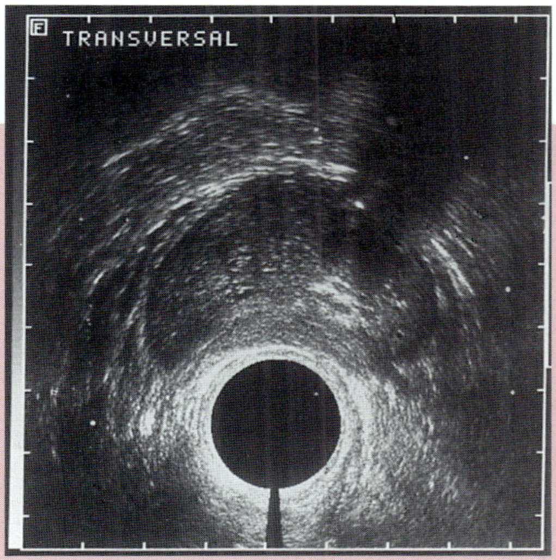

b

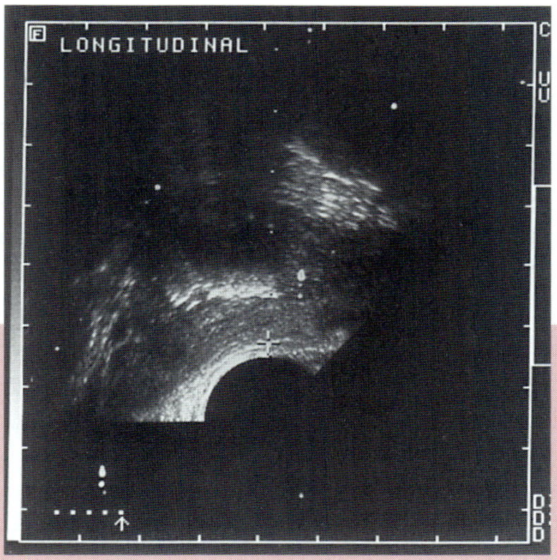

Fig. 2. TRUS image of diffuse prostatic calcification with acoustic shadow. **a** Transverse diameter; **b** Longitudinal diameter with upper prostatic pole on the left-hand side.

authors demonstrated a significant bladder outlet obstruction in only a few patients as assessed by a complete urodynamic evaluation [overview in 20].

Ultrasound Appearances

TRUS has proven the best sonographic approach to visualize the prostate gland in case of acute or chronic inflammation [overview in 23]. Today, 7.5- to 10-MHz transducers are used as standard.

Prostatic abscess

TRUS has led to an increased sensitivity in detecting prostatic abscess and has turned out to be the preferable imaging procedure as it is the most cost-effective, has a better contrast resolution than CT/MRI, and is easily accessible. Typical signs of prostatic abscess are particularly a hypo- or anechoic area with thick walls or perifocal edema [overview in 24] (fig. 1). Repeated examinations allow an exact observation of the success of therapeutical strategies. In case of drainage procedures, TRUS should be performed for correct placement of the needle (fig. 1).

Table 3. TRUS signs that indicate prostatic inflammation [overview in 25]

Solitary and diffuse prostatic calculi
Echo-poor periurethral zone
Heterogeneous internal echo pattern
Irregularities of the prostatic capsule and the periprostatic venous plexus
Uni- and bilateral seminal gland abnormalities

Chronic Bacterial Prostatitis/CPPS

A number of sonographic abnormalities have been used to identify patients with chronic prostatitis in contrast to normal controls [overview in 25] (table 3). Some authors tried to compare sonographic irregularities to histological findings obtained by biopsy [26]. However, most of these studies have been performed with old 3.5- to 4-MHz scanners which cannot match the images of today's high-resolution transducers. Thus, these results remain questionable. The Giessen Prostatitis Study Group demonstrated a significantly higher prevalence of prostatic calculi, particularly diffuse calcifications, in patients with inflammatory vs. noninflammatory CPPS [25] (fig. 2a, b). These results gain clinical importance, because infected prostatic stones, similar to kidney

Table 4. Antimicrobial therapy for CBP

	Substance	Duration	Dosis	Remarks
First line therapy	Trimethoprim or trimethoprim/ sulfamethoxazole	3 months	2 × 200 mg 2 × 160/800 mg	Cure rate 50 % Hampered diffusion into alkaline inflammatory prostate secretions
	Fluoroquinolones	4 weeks	For example: Ciprofloxacin 2 × 500 mg or Ofloxacin 2 × 200 mg	Cure rate about 70% Therapy failure due to infected prostatic calculi Therapy failure due to glycocalix protected bacterial microcolonies
Long-term therapy	Trimethoprim Nitrofurantoin	3–6 months	50–100 mg/day 50–100 mg/day	Suppression of recurrent urinary tract infections

stones, may be impregnated with pathogens that are shielded from antibacterial agents and thereby lead to recurrent prostatitis as well as to relapsing UTI [12]. Seminal vesicle asymmetry in case of inflammation is also a frequent finding. Asymmetry may be due to enlargement of one vesicle as a consequence of ductal obstruction or due to shrinking on the part of one infected vesicle.

Management

Prostatic Abscess

In the treatment of prostatic abscess, both conservative and surgical strategies have been described [overview in 24]. Under TRUS control, the administration of high-dosage antimicrobials together with the placement of a suprapubic catheter may lead to cure of the abscess in some patients. However, most patients will require drainage procedures. Surgical options in the case of prostatic abscess must always be accompanied by antibiotic treatment. Transurethral incision, transurethral resection, and transperineal and transrectal prostatic puncture under TRUS guidance have become standard procedures [24].

Acute and Chronic Bacterial Prostatitis

In ABP, after taking a midstream urine for pathogen culture, antibiotic therapy must be given. As drug of first choice, we prefer the initial administration of a parenteral fluoroquinolone, followed by oral administration. The symptomatic application of analgetics and antipyretics may be useful. A suprapubic catheter is recommended whereas a transurethral catheter is said to block prostatic drainage and therefore should not be used. In spite of the correct treatment, chronic prostatitis may develop. It is not known how often this occurs.

Antimicrobial therapy is the most important part of the treatment strategy for CBP. Antimicrobials must fulfill the following prerequisites to be effective in the treatment of bacterial prostatitis: lipid solubility, low protein binding, dissociation constant close to plasma pH and a pH gradient between plasma and prostatic secretions between 7.4 and 6.4 [overview in 27]. According to these criteria, trimethoprim and the fluoroquinolones are available as the drugs of first choice. Cure rates range from 50 to 70 %. In case of treatment failure, a long-term antimicrobial prophylaxis is started, aimed at controlling symptoms and at preventing recurrent bacteriuria. It is not capable of eliminating the pathogen in the prostate gland (table 4). In patients with associated infection with *C. trachomatis* or *U. urealyticum*, oral treatment with tetracyclin (e.g. doxycyclin 100–200 mg/day) or erythromycin (3–4 × 500 mg/day) should be initiated.

Two alternative treatment modalities have been discussed [overview in 28]: (1) the transperineal injection of antibiotics, usually with amikacin; long-term results with regard to bacteriological cure are disappointing, and (2) in an immunological approach a cell vaccine

Table 5. Suggested management for patients with inflammatory CPPS after failed antimicrobial therapy
α-Blocker therapy (particularly in concomitant subvesical obstruction)*
α-Blocker plus antimicrobial*
Allopurinol*
Transurethral microwave therapy*
Phytotherapy
Anti-inflammatory agents
Finasteride
Repetitive prostate massage

* Proven effect in prospective randomized single-blind/double-blind trials.

Table 6. Suggestions for the treatment of noninflammatory CPPS [overviews in 1, 28]
α-Blocker therapy
Muscle relaxant therapy
Analgesics
Reduction of stress
Biofeedback

made from several inactivated uropathogenic bacteria has been used without convincing results.

Depending on the patient's age, patients over 50 years with refractory symptoms in spite of repeated antibiotic therapy may be considered for a radical transurethral resection. The inflammation most severe in CBP is known to be located in the peripheral zone of the prostate, not in the periurethral or central zone. Furthermore, prostatic calculi as possible foci of infection often develop in ducts of the true prostate and accumulate in the interface between adenomatous tissue and the peripheral (or true) prostate. Thus, to enable successful surgery, the resection must remove all areas of infected tissue and prostatic calculi and, therefore, all intracapsular tissue, especially laterally, along the floor, and at the apices. By this way, prostatic calculi causing recurrent inflammations are to be eliminated. In the current literature, 27 patients have been reported to be treated by this method. In 19 patients, symptoms ceased after operation [overview in 28].

Inflammatory CPPS

As obstruction of prostatic ducts or failure to demonstrate fastidious pathogens may lead to the incorrect diagnosis of inflammatory CPPS instead of CBP, it is justifiable to perform one course of antimicrobials. After failure of antimicrobial therapy, further therapeutical approaches remain symptomatic and are aimed at improving drainage of the prostatic secretions and suppressing the inflammatory situation. Table 5 summarizes treatment suggestions that have been described in the current literature [overviews in 1, 28, 29]. Supportive strategies include lifestyle changes and psychotherapeutical approaches.

Noninflammatory CPPS

The unknown etiology of noninflammatory CPPS makes a therapeutical algorithm problematic. Antimicrobial therapy should not be given as it is ineffective and leads to patients' fixation on a nonexistent infectious cause for his problems. The delimitation of psychosomatic problems is one of the greatest challenges for urologists concerned with prostatitis. Psychosexual therapy should be initiated particularly when sexual problems were preexisting for a long time, fear of failure is present, partner problems are serious and sexual advice has hitherto not been possible [overview in 28]. Treatment options are summarized in table 6. However, prospective randomized blinded studies do not exist.

Asymptomatic Inflammatory Prostatitis

Asymptomatic inflammation of the prostate does not require therapy.

Acute Urethritis in the Male

Infectious, sexually acquired urethritis may be caused by varying pathogens such as *C. trachomatis*, *U. urealyticum* and *N. gonorrhoeae* being the most frequent (table 7) [overview in 30]. Noninfectious causes of urethritis include mechanical irritation or trauma.

Table 7. Frequent and infrequent causes of infectious urethritis

	Frequency 5%	Frequency 95%
Sexually transmitted	*Candida* spp. *Trichomonas vaginalis* Herpes simplex virus II	*Chlamydia trachomatis* *Ureaplasma urealyticum* *Neisseria gonorrhoeae*
Normally not sexually transmitted	Enterobacteriaceae spp. *Streptococcus* spp. *Staphylococcus* spp.	

Urethral discharge and bladder voiding difficulties are the predominant symptoms of acute urethritis. Asymptomatic infections are estimated to occur in 5–10 % and constitute an important epidemiologic problem because they remain untreated.

Cytological diagnosis is based on the analysis of a urethral smear and first-catch urine (VB 1). According to the Giessen urethritis protocol, evidence of ≥4 granulocytes per microscopic field (1,000×) in a urethral smear, or ≥15 granulocytes/microscopic field (400×) in the smear of the sediment of 3 ml VB 1 have been considered pathognomonic [overview in 30]. Etiologic classification is based on the following criteria: (1) evidence of *C. trachomatis, N. gonorrhoeae, Trichomonas vaginalis,* and (2) evidence of significantly high numbers of conventional bacteria, *Candida* spp., *Mycoplasma* spp., i.e. $\geq 10^4$ cfu/ml of urethral discharge, and $\geq 10^3$ cfu/ml VB 1.

Sexually transmitted diseases treatment guidelines according to the Centers of Disease Control have recently been reviewed [31]. As in most cases of acute urethritis, the etiology is unknown at the time of diagnosis, the Giessen urethritis study group prefers an empiric treatment of one single dose of a fluoroquinolone followed by a 2 weeks' regimen with doxycycline. Thus, treatment is effective against both gonococcal and (coexisting) chlamydial/ureaplasmal infection.

References

1 Nickel JC: Prostatitis: Myths and realities. Urology 1998; 51:362–366.
2 Drach GW, Meares EM, Fair WR, Stamey TA: Classification of benign diseases associated with prostatic pain: Prostatitis or prostatodynia. J Urol 1978;120:266.
3 Meares EM, Stamey TA: Bacteriologic localization patterns in bacterial prostatitis and urethritis. Invest Urol 1968;5: 492–518.
4 Weidner W, Schiefer HG, Krauss H, Jantos C, Friedrich HJ, Altmannsberger M: Chronic prostatitis: A thorough search for etiologically involved microorganisms in 1,461 patients. Infection 1991;19(suppl 3):119–125.
5 Lopez-Plaza I, Bostwick DG: Prostatitis; in Bostwick DG (ed): Pathology of the Prostate. New York, Churchill Livingstone, 1990, pp 15–30.
6 Stamey TA: Pathogenesis and Treatment of Urinary Tract Infections. Baltimore, Williams & Wilkins, 1980, pp 343–429.
7 Bergman B: On the relevance of gram-positive bacteria in prostatitis. Infection 1994;22(suppl 1):22.
8 Nickel JC, Costerton JW: Coagulase-negative *Staphylococcus* in chronic prostatitis. J Urol 1992;147:398–401.
9 Krieger JN: Chronic urogenital infections in the man. Urologe A 1994;33:196–202.
10 Bruce AW, Reid G: Prostatitis associated with *C. trachomatis* in six patients. J Urol 1989;142:1006–1007.
11 Corradi G, Bucsek M, Pánovics J, Verebélyi A, Kardos M, Kádár M, Frang D: Detection of *Chlamydia trachomatis* in the prostate by in-situ hybridization and by transmission electron microscopy. Int J Androl 1996;19:109–112.
12 Meares EM: Acute and chronic prostatitis and prostatodynia; in Fitzpatrick JM, Krane RJ (eds): The Prostate. Edinburgh, Churchill Livingstone, 1989, pp 62–75.
13 Shortliffe LMD, Sellers RG, Schachter J: The characterization of nonbacterial prostatitis: Search for an etiology. J Urol 1992;148:1461–1466.
14 Koroku M, Kumamoto Y, Hirose T: A study of the role of *Chlamydia trachomatis* in chronic prostatitis – Analysis of anti-*Chlamydia trachomatis* specific IgA in expressed prostate secretion by Western-blotting method. Kansenshogaku Zasshi 1995;69:426–437.
15 Moon TD: Immunology of chronic prostatitis: Etiological and therapeutic considerations. Curr Opin Urol 1998;8: 39–43.
16 Krieger JN, Riley DE, Roberts MC, Berger RE: Procaryotic DNA sequences in patients with chronic idiopathic prostatitis. J Clin Microbiol 1996;34:3120–3128.
17 Berger RE, Krieger JN, Rothman I, Muller CH, Hillier SL: Bacteria in the prostate tissue of men with idiopathic prostate inflammation. J Urol 1997;157:863–865.

18 Lowentritt JE, Kawahara K, Hunan LG, Hellstrom WJG, Dominque GJ: Bacterial infection in prostatodynia. J Urol 1995;154:1378–1381.
19 Krieger JN, Egan KJ, Ross SO, Jacobs R, Berger RE: Chronic pelvic pains represent the most prominent urogenital symptoms of 'chronic prostatitis'. Urology 1996; 48:715–722.
20 Weidner W, Ludwig M: Patient assessment in chronic prostatitis. Curr Opin Urol 1998;8:51–54.
21 Muller H, Mohr L, Berger RE, Krieger JN: Evaluation of microscopic methods for detection of inflamed expressed prostatic secretion. J Urol 1997;157(suppl):247, abstr 943.
22 World Health Organization: WHO Laboratory Manual for the Examination of Human Semen and Semen-Cervical Mucus Interaction. New York, Cambridge University Press, 1992.
23 Clements R, Griffiths GJ, Peeling WB: Ultrasonographic features of prostatitis; in Weidner W, Madsen PO, Schiefer HG (eds): Prostatitis. Berlin, Springer, 1994, pp 66–90.
24 Ludwig M, Schroeder-Printzen I, Schiefer HG, Weidner W: Diagnosis and therapeutic management in 18 patients with prostatic abscess. Urology 1999;53:340–345.
25 Ludwig M, Weidner W, Schroeder-Printzen I, Zimmermann O, Ringert RH: Transrectal prostatic sonography as a useful diagnostic means in patients with chronic prostatitis or prostatodynia. Br J Urol 1994;73:664–668.
26 Doble A, Thomas BJ, Walker MM, Harris JRW, Witherow R, Taylor-Robinson C: The role of *Chlamydia trachomatis* in chronic abacterial prostatitis: A study using ultrasound-guided biopsy. J Urol 1991;141:332–333.
27 Madsen PO, Drescher P, Gasser TC: Basis for antibacterial treatment of prostatitis: Experimental and clinical pharmacokinetic studies and models; in Weidner W, Madsen PO, Schiefer HG (eds): Prostatitis. Berlin, Springer, 1994, pp 110–122.
28 Ludwig M, Weidner W: Prostato-Urethritis; in Hofstetter A (ed): Urogenitale Infektionen. Berlin, Springer, 1998, pp 297–319.
29 Neal DE Jr: Treatment of chronic prostatitis: An etiologically based approach. Curr Opin Urol 1998,8:55–58.
30 Schiefer HG: Microbiology of male urethroadnexitis: Diagnostic procedures and criteria for aetiologic classification. Andrologia 1998;30(suppl 1);30:7–13.
31 Krieger JN: New sexually transmitted diseases treatment guidelines. J Urol 1995;154:209–213.

European Association of Urology

MEMBERSHIP APPLICATION

Name: . . . .
(last) (first & middle) (title)

Date of birth: ... - ... -19..

Mailing address: . . . .

. . . .

Zip code/City: . . . .

Country: . . . .

Phone number: . . . . FAX number: . . . .

❑ Active membership ❑ Affiliated membership

❑ Corresponding membership

❑ Junior membership

Please mark with x the membership you are applying for.

Certification as Urologist

- Country: . . . .
- Date of certification: . . . .
- Authority which had delivered the certification: . . . .
  (please enclose copy)

Sponsor (Name of a *Active Member* of the EAU who supports your application)

. . . .

Certification as Urologist-in-Training **(only necessary when you apply for Junior membership)**

- Country: . . . .
- Date of starting the education as urologist in training: . . . .
- Statement of Chief of your department indicating that you are a urologist-in-training
  (please enclose copy)

Sponsor (Name of a Active Member of the EAU who supports your application)

. . . .

MEMBERSHIP CATEGORIES

Admission Regulations

Active membership
Active membership is open to all registered urologists in Europe.
The application has to be endorsed by one Active Member of the EAU. Active Members have the right to vote at the General Assembly.
Application is made directly to the EAU Central Office, accompanied by a certificate of registration as a urologist in the applicant's European country.

Junior membership
Junior membership is open to European urologists-in-training. The application has to be endorsed by one Active Member of the EAU. Junior Members have no right to vote at the General Assembly.
Application is made directly to the EAU Central Office accompanied by a letter from the Chief of his/her department indicating that he/she is a urologist-in-training.
Upon registration as a urologist, Junior members may apply to become Active Members

Senior membership
Senior membership is open to Active Members officially retired (at their own request)
Senior members have no right to vote at the General Assembly.
Senior members are exempted from any fees payable to the Association.

Corresponding membership
Corresponding membership is open to all registered non-European urologists. The application has to be endorsed by two Active Members of the EAU.
Corresponding Members have no right to vote at the General Assembly.
Application is made directly to the EAU Central Office, accompanied by a certificate of registration as a urologist in the applicant's own country or an endorsement by their national society.

Affiliate membership
Affiliate membership is open to all scientists or others who have contributed significantly to the specialty of urology. The application has to be endorsed by two Active members.
Application is made directly to the EAU Central Office accompanied with a curriculum vitae and other pertinent information as well as a signed document that they are not connected with any commercial or pharmaceutical company.

Honorary membership
Honorary membership may be awarded to scientists and others who have had an important influence on European urology. Their election will be recommended by the Board and must be approved by the General Assembly.

MEMBERSHIP FEES

Active members will have to pay NLG 250 per year (including subscription to European Urology).
Corresponding members will have to pay NLG 315 per year (including subscription to European Urology).
Junior members will have to pay NLG 150 per year (including subscription to European Urology).
Affiliated members will have to pay NLG 200 per year (including subscription to European Urology).

Please enclose payment with your membership application.

Methods of payments

Please make your bank transfer or cheque, in Dutch guilders only, payable to:

European Urological Foundation (EAU), account number: 22.59.17.726.
Bank relation: F. van Lanschot, bankers, Nijmegen, the Netherlands.

Credit cards: ❑ **American Express** ❑ **Visa** ❑ **Euro/Mastercard**

card number: .... **expiry date:** ....

signature: .... **name creditcard holder:** ....

PLEASE RETURN THIS APPLICATION TO:

The EAU Office
P.O. Box 204
6600 AE Wijchen
the Netherlands

phone: +31-24-6452510
fax: +31-24-6450769

492 **Reversibility of Prostatic Intraepithelial Neoplasia: Implications for Chemoprevention**
Bostwick, D.G.; Neumann, R.; Qian, J.; Cheng, L. (Rochester, Minn.)

496 **Evolution of Isolated High-Grade Prostate Intraepithelial Neoplasia in a Mediterranean Patient Population**
Algaba, F. (Barcelona)

498 **Clinical Evolution of Prostatic Intraepithelial Neoplasia**
Zlotta, A.R.; Schulman, C.C. (Brussels)

504 **PIN I–III: When Should We Interfere?**
Newling, D. (Amsterdam)

508 **Prostatic Intraepithelial Neoplasia and Endocrine Manipulation**
van der Kwast, Th.H.; Labrie, F.; Têtu, B. (Rotterdam/Québec)

511 **The Utility of Prostate-Specific Antigen as a Surrogate Marker for Identification of High-Risk Cohorts and Assessing Response in Chemoprevention Trials**
Crawford, E.D. (Denver, Colo.)

Clinical Trial Designs for Chemoprevention of Prostate Cancer

515 **Practical Aspects of Clinical Trials on Chemoprevention of Prostate Cancer**
van der Meijden, A.P.M. ('s-Hertogenbosch)

519 **Statistical Considerations of Chemoprevention Clinical Trials in Prostate Cancer**
Sylvester, R.; Collette, L. (Brussels)

523 **Prostate Cancer Screening in Tyrol, Austria: Experience and Results**
Horninger, W.; Reissigl, A.; Rogatsch, H.; Volgger, H.; Studen, M.; Klocker, H.; Bartsch, G. (Innsbruck)

539 **The European Randomized Study of Screening for Prostate Cancer (ERSPC): An Update**
Schröder, F.H.; Kranse, R.; Rietbergen, J.; Hoedemaeker, R.; Kirkels, W. (Rotterdam); and members of the ERSPC

544 **Prostate Cancer Prevention Trial (PCPT) Update**
Coltman, C.A., Jr.; Thompson, I.M., Jr. (San Antonio, Tex.); Feigl, P. (Seattle, Wash.)

354, 423 **Congress Calendar**
548 **Author Index Vol. 35, No. 5–6, 1999**
549 **Subject Index Vol. 35, No. 5–6, 1999**
550 **Forthcoming Papers**
551 **Acknowledgement to the Reviewers**

552 **Author Index Vol. 35, 1999**
554 **Subject Index Vol. 35, 1999**

Curriculum in Urology 2.4

Infections and Stones
Prostatitis and Urethritis
Ludwig, M.; Weidner, W. (Giessen)

Suppl. 1

Hormonal Effects on Prostate Cancer Growth: Recent Scientific Progress and Clinical Outcome
Edited by M. Zerbib (Paris)

Suppl. 2

XIVth Congress of the European Association of Urology
April 1999, Stockholm
Edited by the Members of the Scientific Committee of the XIVth EAU Congress

298 **Diagnostic Value of Ten Systematic TRUS-Guided Prostate Biopsies**
Ravery, V.; Billebaud, T.; Toublanc, M.; Boccon-Gibod, L.; Hermieu, J.-F.; Moulinier, F.; Blanc, E.; Delmas, V.; Boccon-Gibod, L. (Paris)

304 **Reconstruction of Large Soft Tissue Defects in the Inguinal and Suprapubic Region Using a Variety of Flaps**
Schwabegger, A.H.; Rainer, C.; Berresheim, U.; Stenzl, A.; Anderl, H.; Ninković, M.M. (Innsbruck)

312 **Reasons of Dropout from Short- and Long-Term Self-Injection Therapy for Impotence**
de la Taille, A.; Delmas, V.; Amar, E.; Boccon-Gibod, L. (Paris)

318 **Conventional CT Signs in Staging Transitional Cell Tumors of the Upper Urinary Tract**
Millán-Rodríguez, F.; Palou, J.; de la Torre-Holguera, P.; Vayreda-Martija, J.M.; Villavicencio-Mavrich, H.; Vicente-Rodríguez, J. (Barcelona)

323 **Small Cell Carcinoma of the Urinary Bladder Treated with Chemotherapy and Radiotherapy: Results in Five Cases**
Bastús, R.; Caballero, J.M.; González, G.; Borrat, P.; Casalots, J.; Gomez de Segura, G.; Martí, Ll.; Ristol, J.; Cirera, L. (Barcelona)

Basic Science

327 **Estramustine Reversal of Resistance to Intravesical Epirubicin Chemotherapy**
Jennings, A.M.; Solomon, L.Z.; Sharpe, P.; Hayes, M.C.; Cooper, A.J.; Birch, B.R. (Southampton)

297, 303, 317 **Congress Calendar**
336 **Forthcoming Papers**

Curriculum in Urology 1.2

Pediatrics
Congenital Urine Flow Impairments of the Upper Urinary Tract
Wilcox, D.T.; Mouriquand, D.E. (London)

No. 5–6

341 **Introduction**
Schulman, C.C. (Brussels); Kelloff, G.J. (Bethesda, Calif.)

342 **Chemoprevention of Prostate Cancer: Concepts and Strategies**
Kelloff, G.J.; Lieberman, R.; Steele, V.E.; Boone, C.W.; Lubet, R.A.; Kopelovitch, L.; Malone, W.A.; Crowell, J.A. (Bethesda, Md.); Sigman, C.C. (Mountain View, Calif.)

Genetic and Environmental Factors in Prostate Cancer Genesis

351 **Molecular Biology of Progression of Prostate Cancer**
Nupponen, N.; Visakorpi, T. (Tampere)

355 **Androgen Metabolism and Prostate Cancer: Establishing a Model of Genetic Susceptibility**
Ross, R.K.; Coetzee, G.A.; Pearce, C.L.; Reichardt, J.K.V.; Bretsky, P. (Los Angeles, Calif.); Kolonel, L.N. (Honolulu, Hawaii); Henderson, B.E. (Los Angeles, Calif.); Lander, E.; Altshuler, D.; Daley, G. (Boston, Mass.)

362 **Genetic and Environmental Factors in Prostate Cancer Genesis: Identifying High-Risk Cohorts**
Ekman, P. (Stockholm)

370 **Epidemiology of Prostate Cancer Chemoprevention**
Boyle, P.; Severi, G. (Milan)

377 **Diet and Its Preventive Role in Prostatic Disease**
Denis, L. (Antwerp); Morton, M.S.; Griffiths, K. (Cardiff)

388 **Dietary Fat and Prostate Cancer Progression and Survival**
Fradet, Y.; Meyer, F.; Bairati, I.; Shadmani, R.; Moore, L. (Québec)

Molecular Targets for Chemoprevention of Prostate Cancer

392 **Vitamin D and Prostate Cancer Risk**
Peehl, D.M. (Stanford, Calif.)

395 **Lipoxygenase Inhibition in Prostate Cancer**
Myers, C.E.; Ghosh, J. (Charlottesville, Va.)

399 **Angiogenesis, p53, *bcl-2* and Ki-67 in the Progression of Prostate Cancer after Radical Prostatectomy**
Moul, J.W. (Washington, D.C./Bethesda, Md.)

408 **Changes in Gene Expression and Targets for Therapy**
Bussemakers, M.J.G. (Nijmegen)

413 **Mechanism of Androgen Receptor Activation and Possible Implications for Chemoprevention Trials**
Klocker, H.; Culig, Z.; Eder, I.E.; Nessler-Menardi, C.; Hobisch, A.; Putz, T.; Bartsch, G. (Innsbruck); Peterziel, H.; Cato, A.C.B. (Karlsruhe)

420 **New Agents for Chemoprevention of Prostate Cancer**
Sporn, M.B. (Hanover, N.H.)

424 **Retinoids in Chemoprevention**
Whelan, P. (Leeds)

429 **Evaluation of Biomarker Modulation by Fenretinide in Prostate Cancer Patients**
Urban, D.; Myers, R.; Manne, U.; Weiss, H. (Birmingham, Ala.); Mohler, J. (Chapel Hill, N.C.); Perkins, D.; Markiewicz, M. (Birmingham, Ala.); Lieberman, R.; Kelloff, G. (Bethesda, Md.); Marshall, M.; Grizzle, W. (Birmingham, Ala.)

439 **Factors Controlling the Expression of 5α-Reductase in Human Prostate: A Possible New Approach for the Treatment of Prostate Cancer**
Habib, F.K.; Ross, M.; Bayne, C.W. (Edinburgh)

443 **Certain Aspects of Molecular Endocrinology That Relate to the Influence of Dietary Factors on the Pathogenesis of Prostate Cancer**
Griffiths, K.; Morton, M.S. (Cardiff); Denis, L. (Antwerp)

Preclinical Models for Drug Discovery

456 **High-Grade Prostatic Intraepithelial Neoplasia in Dogs**
Waters, D.J. (West Lafayette, Ind.)

459 **Use of Animal Models in Defining Efficacy of Chemoprevention Agents against Prostate Cancer**
Bosland, M.C. (New York, N.Y.)

464 **Chemoprevention of Hormone-Dependent Prostate Cancer in the Wistar-Unilever Rat**
McCormick, D.L.; Rao, K.V.N. (Chicago, Ill.)

Surrogate Endpoint Biomarkers for Clinical Trials of Prostate Cancer Chemoprevention

468 **Subtle Morphological and Molecular Changes in Normal-Looking Epithelium in Prostates with Prostatic Intraepithelial Neoplasia or Cancer**
Montironi, R. (Ancona); Hamilton, P.W. (Belfast); Scarpelli, M. (Ancona); Thompson, D.; Bartels, P.H. (Tucson, Ariz.)

474 **Prostatic Intraepithelial Neoplasia: A Marker for High-Risk Groups and a Potential Target for Chemoprevention**
Sakr, W.A. (Detroit, Mich.)

479 **Genetic and Chromosomal Alterations in Prostatic Intraepithelial Neoplasia and Carcinoma Detected by Fluorescence in situ Hybridization**
Qian, J.; Jenkins, R.B.; Bostwick, D.G. (Rochester, Minn.)

484 **Tissue Architecture Analysis in Prostate Cancer and Its Precursors: An Innovative Approach to Computerized Histometry**
Bartels, P.H. (Tucson, Ariz.); Montironi, R. (Ancona); Duval da Silva, V. (Brasília/Porto Alegre); Hamilton, P.W. (Belfast); Thompson, D.; Vaught, L.; Bartels, H.G. (Tucson, Ariz.)